LECTURE NOTES ON PHARMACOLOGY

RUTH E. GRAHAM.

CW00369989

Lecture Notes on Pharmacology

H. F. GRUNDY
MD, BChir, MA, BSc
Emeritus Fellow
Trinity Hall
Cambridge

SECOND EDITION

OXFORD

BLACKWELL SCIENTIFIC PUBLICATIONS

LONDON EDINBURGH BOSTON
MELBOURNE PARIS BERLIN VIENNA

© 1985, 1990 by
Blackwell Scientific Publications
Editorial offices:
Osney Mead, Oxford, OX2 0EL
25 John Street, London WCIN 2BL
23 Ainslie Place, Edinburgh EH3 6AJ
3 Cambridge Center, Cambridge,
  Massachusetts 02142, USA
54 University Street, Carlton
  Victoria 3053, Australia

Other Editorial Offices:
Arnette SA
2, rue Casimir-Delavigne
75006 Paris
France

Blackwell Wissenschaft
Meinekestrasse 4
D-1000 Berlin 15
Germany

Blackwell MZV
Feldgasse 13
A-1238 Wien
Austria

First published 1985
Second edition 1990
Reprinted with corrections 1991

Set by Times Graphics, Singapore;
printed and bound in Great Britain
by Hartnolls Ltd, Bodmin, Cornwall

DISTRIBUTORS

Marston Book Services Ltd
PO Box 87
Oxford OX2 0DT
(*Orders*: Tel: 0865 791155
          Fax: 0865 791927
          Telex: 837515)

USA
Mosby-Year Book, Inc.
11830 Westline Industrial Drive
St Louis, Missouri 63146
(*Orders*: Tel: (800) 633–6699)

Canada
Mosby-Year Book, Inc.
5240 Finch Avenue East
Scarborough, Ontario
(*Orders*: Tel: (416) 298-1588)

Australia
Blackwell Scientific Publications
(Australia) Pty Ltd
54 University Street
Carlton, Victoria 3053
(*Orders*: Tel: (03) 347–0300)

British Library
Cataloguing in Publication Data

Grundy, H.F.
  Lecture notes on pharmacology,
    —2nd ed.
  1. Medicine. Drug therapy
  I. Title
  615.5'8

ISBN 0-632-02558-1

Contents

Preface

This second edition has been extensively updated to present as modern a view as possible of current pharmacological knowledge.

During the twentieth century, pharmacology has progressed from being a predominantly descriptive subject towards a deductive discipline based on established principles. Here, an attempt is made to enunciate fundamental propositions on which the student can gradually build a corpus of knowledge and thus be spared much of the drudgery of learning isolated, unrelated facts. A further simplification is achieved by a full description of the pharmacology of 'type substances' within many sections, stressing their respective advantages and disadvantages so that sensible criteria can be established against which newer compounds may be evaluated.

Without personal contact, it is impossible to convey the exact nuances essential to a full appreciation of the subject. Nevertheless this is the primary aim of this book—to give the reader a true feeling for pharmacology, both in its own right and in relation to associated scientific (including clinically applied) disciplines. This involves the realisation that facts can be derived or approached from differing angles. For this reason the book contains many cross-references. These insertions should not be allowed to fragment straightforward reading of the text but they are available for immediate confirmation of previously unknown or unappreciated connections. This text does not include general references for two main reasons: first, the student's own teacher can best recommend the appropriate reading, which often changes rapidly as new discoveries are made; secondly, it would be invidious to select extended texts from the many excellent ones available.

Drugs are prescribed preferably under their non-proprietary names: these are either pharmacopoeial, i.e. published in the current pharmacopoeia of a particular country, or the approved name (US: adopted name), i.e. the designation of a drug which has not yet attained pharmacopoeial status. Proprietary names indicate trademarks which are copyright to particular manufacturers; these are included in the text *only* when they are helpful to the recognition of a particular substance and are indicated by the superscript ®.

The author is the sole writer of this textbook to whom any errors and misjudgements are attributable. However, he wishes gratefully to acknowledge the criticism and advice of a few friends. In particular, Figures 19.9 and 19.11 are the handiwork, respectively, of Doctors Kareen Thorne and Clive Grundy.

Warmest thanks are due to typists and secretaries, Clare Grundy and Thelma Jeffs. Stuart Taylor of Blackwell Scientific Publications has been most helpful in the production of this textbook and special thanks to Rowena Millar for seeing the work through to bound book.

Part 1

Pharmacokinetics

1   Pharmacokinetics

A drug (Gk:* *pharmakon*) may be defined as a substance which modifies some function of a biological system. Pharmacology—the study of drugs—is divisible into:

• *pharmacodynamics* (Gk: *dynamis*, power): the actions upon cells (or subcellular fragments), tissues or organs and

• *pharmacokinetics* (Gk: *kinesis*, movement): the processes whereby drug concentrations at effector sites are achieved, maintained and diminished.

This chapter will be concerned with some fundamental pharmacokinetic concepts. As shown in Fig. 1.1 the following, often sequential, categories may be involved:

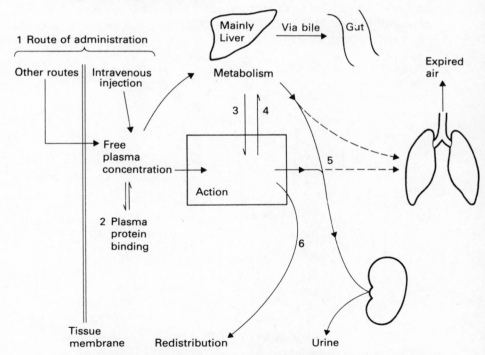

Fig. 1.1 Factors involved in pharmacokinetics (*see* text for numbers). Interrupted lines indicate uncommon routes.

*Gk, Greek.

3

1 Route of administration.
2 Plasma protein binding.
3 Activation, i.e. conversion to a more effective compound.
4 Inactivation, i.e. conversion to a less active agent.
5 Excretion—either as the unchanged drug or in the form of its metabolites.
6 Redistribution, i.e. passage to inactive sites.

An understanding of some of these processes involves an appreciation of the mechanisms by which drugs cross membranes.

1.1 Passage of drugs across biological membranes

The plasma membranes of mammalian cells have three main organic chemical structural components (usually arranged as in Fig. 1.2).

Lipids
A bilayer of phospholipids and cholesterol forms the main framework. The hydrophilic ends—glyceryl phosphate attached to an amine (choline, ethanolamine or serine) or the cyclic polyhydric alcohol (inositol—*see* Fig. 4.7a) in the case of the phospholipids or the terminal hydroxyl group of cholesterol—orientate themselves at both the inner and outer surfaces, while the hydrophobic portions—hydrocarbon chains of phospholipids or the main bulk of the cholesterol molecule—occupy the centre of the membrane.

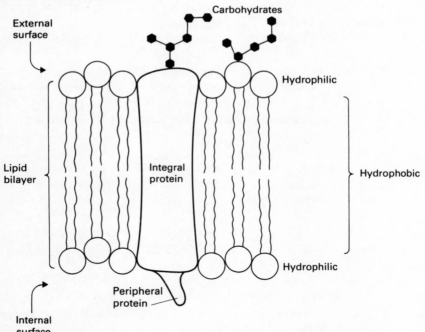

Fig. 1.2 Structure of the mammalian membrane (diagrammatic).

Proteins
Integral proteins extend the full width of the membrane and show a predominance of either hydrophilic or hydrophobic groups at their surfaces contiguous to the corresponding lipids according to their depth within the membrane. *Peripheral* proteins are attached *either* to integral proteins at the inner side of the membrane and are predominantly hydrophilic (like cytoplasmic proteins) *or* to the hydrophilic ends of lipids at either surface.

Carbohydrates
Glycoproteins or glycolipids are formed on the *outer* surface of the membrane by the attachment of different polymeric arrangements of monosaccharides (galactose, mannose, fucose, i.e. 6-desoxygalactose), amino-sugar derivatives (*N*-acetyl glucosamine, *N*-acetyl galactosamine), or one of these condensed with pyruvate: the sialic acids (e.g. *N*-acetyl neuraminic acid, NANA).

All these elements can manifest mobility over periods of minutes to days mainly in a lateral direction.

Inorganic components of significance include: *membrane-bound water* which coats polar, ionised groups and thus tends to restrict the transverse mobility of proteins, producing a barrier to hydrophilic diffusion across the membrane; *ions* (particularly Ca^{2+}) which can separate negatively charged phospholipid heads and thereby alter the charge distribution within the membrane.

It is important to realise that the typical membrane (as depicted in Fig 1.2)
• is not only asymmetrical morphologically but also electrically, so that excitation or inhibition can occur by an appropriate alteration of the ionic disposition inside or outside
• contains pores or intracellular (through cells) or paracellular (between cells) spaces along which small molecules (molecular weight up to about 100) can diffuse
• is dynamic insofar as ionic channels can be formed by integral proteins (e.g. Fig. 7.2), and phase transitions from (rigid) gel to liquid states can occur widely or locally, e.g. in the presence of general anaesthetics (p. 224)
• often has carrier substances which, by protecting polar molecules with a hydrophobic coating, facilitate membrane passage, e.g. Na^+, K^+-activated ATPase (p. 108)
• links extra- to intracellular events via receptors, which can modify ion-conductances and/or enzyme activities (*see* Receptor–response linking, p. 106 *et seq.*).
Atypical membranes (e.g. capillary wall, blood–brain barrier) are dealt with later in this chapter.

The three fundamental mechanisms by which physiological, pharmacological and pathological agents traverse biological membranes are

1 *Diffusion*, either through water-filled pores (ultrafiltration), paracellular spaces or directly via the lipoprotein structure (simple diffusion). The latter is the most common method by which drugs gain access to, are distributed within and are, finally, eliminated from the body.

2 *Facilitated diffusion*. This process proceeds more rapidly than simple diffusion* due to the intervention of a specific, saturable carrier (protein) system but cannot occur against a gradient (*see* below).

3 *Active movements*. These can proceed against concentration, electrical, hydrostatic or osmotic gradients and have the ability to produce a selective concentration of a particular substance at one side of a biological membrane. They require an energy supply and, often in addition, a carrier substance, e.g. Na^+, K^+–activated ATPase. For example, L-dopa (p. 173) and a-methyldopa (p. 257) are both actively absorbed from the gut via the usual transport mechanism for aromatic amino acids.

Simple (transcellular) diffusion requires not only a favourable concentration gradient of the drug but also sufficient lipid solubility to pass through the membrane. Strongly ionised molecules (irrespective of whether the charge is positive-cation or negative-anion) attract a considerable shell of water molecules around themselves, which effectively precludes significant passage through the hydrophobic centre of the membrane. Less-ionised substances pass slowly whereas unionised drugs, with their much greater lipid solubility, cross readily.

Each ionisable group in a drug has a pK_a value, i.e. a pH at which equal numbers of the ionised and of the non-ionised forms are present. At other pH values, the relative preponderance of one or the other form is dependent on the following equations.

For an acid (proton donor):

$$R.COOH \underset{\text{(add OH}^-)}{\overset{\text{add H}^+}{\rightleftharpoons}} R.COO^-(+H_2O), \text{ e.g. aspirin}$$

$$R.OH \rightleftharpoons R.O^- (+H_2O), \text{ e.g. a barbiturate (enol form, *see* Table 1.3)}$$

(i.e. more of the drug is present in the ionised form as the pH is *in*creased).

For a base (proton acceptor):

$$R.NH_3^+ \underset{\text{(add OH}^-)}{\overset{\text{add H}^+}{\rightleftharpoons}} R.NH_2 (+H_2O), \text{e.g. amphetamine, Table 3.2}$$

*An exception occurs when integral proteins function as specific channels for small ions, e.g. Na^+, K^+, Ca^{2+}, Cl^- (*see* p. 106 *et seq.*) which cross the membrane *faster* then facilitated (carrier protein-mediated) diffusion.

(i.e. more of the drug is present in the ionised form as the pH is *de*creased).

Quantitatively the ratio of ionised to unionised forms can be calculated using the *general* Henderson–Hasselbalch equation:

$$pH = pK_a + \log\frac{[\text{'base'}]}{[\text{'acid'}]}$$

where the 'base' forms (of either an acid or a base) are those on the right-hand sides of the previous equations and the 'acid' forms are those on the left-hand sides. Simply, for each pH unit of displacement from the pK_a value the favoured form is increased tenfold. Thus, for aspirin with a pK_a of 3.4, at pH 7.4, the ionised concentration is 10^4 times that of the unionised amount.

These principles can be exemplified by following the absorption of an aspirin tablet from the alimentary canal (Fig. 1.3). Immediately

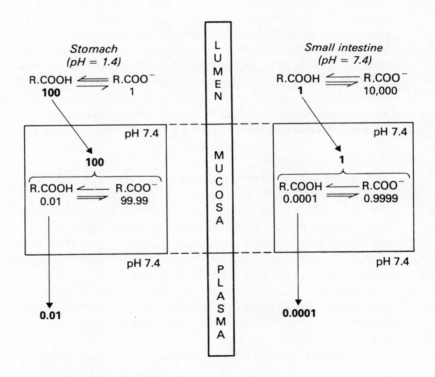

Fig. 1.3 Absorption of acetylsalicylic acid (aspirin, R.COOH, pK_a 3.4) through the mucosal cells of the stomach and the small intestine. Numbers indicate the relative proportions of unionised and ionised forms of the drug present in solution at relevant sites.

following ingestion, the low pH of the *stomach* contents results in most of the drug being present in the unionised form which allows ready passage into the mucosal cells. However, this entry is limited because aspirin is relatively insoluble at such a low pH and therefore not very concentrated in the intragastric fluid. But the aspirin which *is* absorbed, mainly (at the intracellular pH of 7.4, Fig. 1.3) reverts to the ionised form which can only slowly cross from the cells into the extracellular fluid (blood plasma). This process, whereby an ion passes a membrane and encounters a milieu of different pH from which it has difficulty in escaping, is known as 'ion-trapping'. In this specific example, the concentration of aspirin within the cells may contribute to the gastric irritation which can occur with this drug (*see* 7.9).

In the alkaline chyme of the *small intestine* (Fig. 1.3), the aqueous solubility of aspirin increases. Now, although the unionised form of the drug is present in much lower proportion, most of the passage into the bloodstream occurs due to the larger absorptive surface and the greater time spent in this part of the alimentary tract. Further, note that aspirin is much less concentrated in the mucosal cells of the small intestine compared with those of the stomach. So, solubility in the alimentary tract fluids (to achieve an adequate available concentration at the luminal surface of the absorptive membrane) and lipid solubility (to cross the cell membranes) are necessary prerequisites for drug absorption following oral (including sublingual) administration. Unless carrier molecules or active transport processes are involved, charged molecules are not adequately absorbed by these routes but this may be turned to advantage if a local effect upon the gut is desired.

Capillary wall passage

Most drugs at some stage have to traverse a capillary wall. The means by which they may do so are shown in Fig. 1.4. Lipid-soluble drugs pass almost instantaneously across the whole surface area of the capillary endothelium. Poorly lipid-soluble agents can negotiate 'pores' in the membrane (size variable but usually in the range 3–10 nm diameter: average 4–5 nm, corresponding to molecular weights—depending on shape of molecule—*c*. 15 000–30 000*) between the endothelial cells and then transit, in a matter of minutes, the enclosing basement membrane. Thus, for practically all drugs, the only factor which significantly delays absorption from the bloodstream is plasma protein binding.

An example of this is illustrated in b, Fig. 1.4. Diazepam—at the usual therapeutic dose—is 98% protein bound, so that initially only 2%

See Table 1.2. Heparin, molecular weight (mol. wt.) 15 000–20 000, is usually confined to the blood plasma but is also highly protein bound; dextrans, mol. wts, 40 000–110 000, are given as plasma expanders to maintain blood volume by remaining within the circulation.

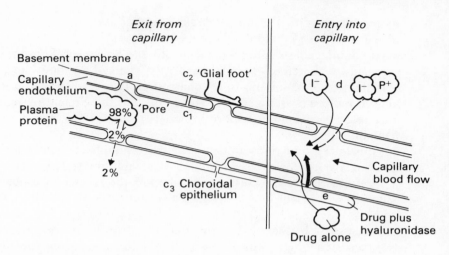

Fig. 1.4 Passage across capillary membranes (diagrammatic).
Exit from capillary: a, a 'pore' (schematic) in capillary wall; b, plasma protein binding (98%, e.g. for diazepam) delays passage into tissue fluid; c, anatomical blood–brain barrier: c_1 tight junction of capillary endothelial cell, c_2 pore covered by neuroglial process ('glial foot'), c_3 tight junction of choroidal epithelial cell. *Entry into capillary*: d, subcutaneous and intramuscular injections—more rapidly acting soluble Insulin (I^-, mol. wt. *c.* 6000) and a depot preparation with protamine (P^+); e, addition of hyaluronidase to increase the area of contact of the drug solution with the absorptive surface. Arrowed lines indicate relative rates of passage as follows: interrupted, slow; continuous, moderate; thick, fast.

passes into the tissues; this results in further dissociation from the protein so that eventually all the drug will be absorbed but in a delayed fashion. This principle can be exploited by the use of a heavily protein-bound agent to achieve a 'circulating depot preparation' which is satisfactory if only a low concentration of the drug is required over a prolonged period, e.g. hydroxocobalamin in pernicious anaemia (p. 378), e.g. sulphadimethoxine (a long-acting sulphonamide).

Conversely, as the capillary wall does not present a significant barrier to the passage of any drug, following intramuscular (i.m.) or subcutaneous (s.c.) injection, the relevant factors limiting intravascular absorption are
• local tissue binding. This slows absorption, e.g. following i.m. administration of chlorpromazine (*see also* footnote to Table 1.2)
• aqueous solubility, so that it can cross the tissue fluid and reach the capillary endothelium
• capillary blood flow.

Slowing of absorption
Since water-soluble compounds tend to be preferentially absorbed from i.m. and s.c. sites, slow-release ('depot') preparations can be produced

by the incorporation of lipid-soluble factors. Examples of this type of pharmacokinetic manipulation are

• protamine zinc insulin. Soluble insulin has an isoelectric point of c. 5.5 and is therefore overall negatively charged at body pH. Its combination with the positively charged protamine results in a more neutral molecule with a slower absorption into the circulation (d, Fig. 1.4) and, consequently, a more prolonged action. Similarly, procaine penicillin (p. 403)

• fluphenazine (a phenothiazine major tranquilliser, *see* Table 7.7) can be given i.m. as its decanoate in sesame oil, to last 2–4 weeks.

Also, the larger the particle size, the less the surface area per unit volume and the slower the absorption (insulin zinc suspensions, Table 14.8).

Drugs may be localised to subcutaneous sites by the addition of a vasoconstrictor, e.g. adrenaline with local anaesthetics (*see* Table 8.2). Conversely, in severe pain associated with peripheral circulatory failure (e.g. a road traffic accident), there is vascular stasis which necessitates an *i.v.* injection of morphine. A similar situation arises when insulin has to be infused i.v. in hyperglycaemic ketoacidosis (pp. 347–8).

Acceleration of absorption
To encourage absorption, hyaluronidase is sometimes added to s.c. or i.m. injections e.g. of ergometrine, p. 361. As shown in e, Fig. 1.4, the rationale behind this is that the enzyme breaks down intercellular ground substance and thus allows a greater area of contact between the drug and the absorptive surfaces.

Blood–brain barrier

The central nervous system capillaries are unusual in possessing either close ('tight') junctions between their endothelial cells (c_1, Fig. 1.4), an investment of neuroglial tissue ('glial foot', c_2, Fig. 1.4) or, in the case of the (intraventricular) choroid plexuses, an overlying modified ependymal layer—the choroidal epithelium—which has close ('tight') junctions (c_3, Fig. 1.4). These collectively constitute the *anatomical* blood–brain barrier which allows the passage (by simple diffusion) of the non-protein bound fractions of lipid-soluble drugs into the neuraxis and cerebrospinal fluid. Conversely, access by highly charged molecules is negligible unless specific transport mechanisms are involved, e.g. for physiologically important small ions, sugars, amino acids, or the protective membranes have been disrupted by pathological conditions, e.g. meningitis. There is also an *enzymatic* blood–brain barrier. The capillary endothelial cells contain aromatic L-amino acid decarboxylase (dopa decarboxylase) so that some of the precursors, L-dopa and L-5-hydroxytryptophan (*see* Table 6.3), are converted into dopamine and 5-

hydroxytryptamine, respectively. Dopamine, noradrenaline, adrenaline and 5-hydroxytryptamine—in addition to being highly ionised—are inactivated by monoamine oxidase (also present within the endothelial cells) and effectively excluded from entering the brain tissue. Some L-dopa does manage to gain access to produce beneficial effects in parkinsonism (7.2). α-Methyl dopa which exerts CNS actions in hypertension is not broken down by monoamine oxidase (Table 3.2, rule 6). The cells lining the brain capillaries also contain acetyl- and butyrylcholinesterases, thus precluding circulating substances inactivated by either of these enzymes from entering the cerebrospinal tissue in significant concentrations.

The ependyma lining the ventricles appears not to be limited either by tight junctions or by glial feet, so that drugs given experimentally into the cerebrospinal fluid will circumvent the blood–brain barrier. Nor does the latter seem to limit access to either the chemoreceptor trigger zone of the vomiting centre (13.4) or the anterior hypothalamic centres associated with heat regulation (p. 188).

The kidney

This organ shows a number of membrane-crossing mechanisms (Fig. 1.5). The glomerular membrane (capillary endothelium, basement membrane and Bowman's capsule epithelium) functionally has a larger than average pore size (approaching that of albumin, *average* mol. wt. *c.* 70 000 so that—apart from huge macromolecules, such as dextrans

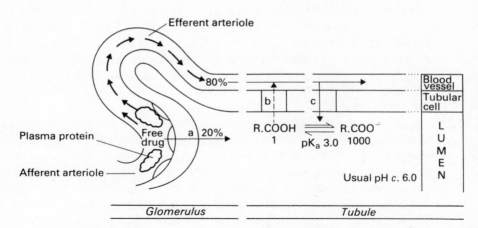

Fig. 1.5 Passage across membranes in the kidney illustrated diagrammatically for the major metabolite of aspirin in cases of poisoning (p. 195) viz. salicylic acid (R.COOH; pK_a 3.0): a, glomerular ultrafiltration (about 20% of free plasma concentration); b, passive reabsorption by simple diffusion of unionised form of the drug; c, active secretion of organic acids ('anion pump'—blocked by *probenecid*) into the *proximal* tubular fluid.

70 and 110 (average mol. wts 70 000 and 110 000 respectively)—the only drugs excluded from the ultrafiltrate are the plasma protein-bound fractions. From the tubular fluid, lipid-soluble substances can be absorbed by simple diffusion (because their concentration relative to that in plasma increases as water is progressively absorbed at many sites along the tubules, *see* Fig. 12.1). This is why substances such as DDT tend to concentrate in the body and, conversely, as catabolism usually makes drugs more water-soluble why their metabolites are more readily excreted via the kidney. Furthermore, pH changes in the tubular fluid as the glomerular filtrate is converted to urine (Fig. 1.5) alter the unionised to ionised ratios of drugs. In poisoning this can be exploited by deliberately altering the pH of the urine so that more of the ionised form is present. Thus, in the case of aspirin (Fig. 1.5), the normal urinary pH favours salicylate excretion which is intensified by alkalinisation up to pH 8.4 (with potassium citrate or sodium bicarbonate, p. 313) and is further helped by the active secretion of the organic acid (c, Fig. 1.5), — free and as conjugates, p. 195—into the tubular fluid by an active carrier-mediated process (anion pump); thus overall a life-saving, increased excretion of the drug can be achieved. With barbiturates, the differential effect is less significant. Phenobarbitone is the best: with a pK_a of 7.4, it gains a tenfold advantage of ionised to unionised at a pH of 8.4. This is useful and superior to those of the other barbiturates which have pK_as in the range 7.7–8.1. If the intention is to eliminate a *base* via the kidney, the opposite considerations apply. For drugs of this type which are excreted unchanged in any significant quantity (such as amphetamine, pK_a 9.8, *see also* p. 31; pethidine, (US: meperidine), pK_a 8.7, *see* p. 205) make the urine more acid with, e.g. ammonium chloride. Additionally there is an active, carrier-mediated process ('cation pump') which secretes organic *bases* into the *proximal* tubular fluid; this process is inhibited by cimetidine or ranitidine (p. 319), or trimethoprim (p. 408).

1.2   Routes of administration

The selection of a suitable route is dictated by considerations which may be grouped under the following headings: convenience, the patient's condition, action required, and achievement and maintenance of an adequate drug concentration at the requisite site. Illustrative examples are given—add others as you meet them.

Convenience and the patient's condition

Topical application, if the site is easily accessible, is both convenient and encouraging to the patient. The sublingual route is rapidly effective (e.g. glyceryl trinitrite in angina pectoris, p. 268). Otherwise, oral administration—for a local or systemic effect—is the most acceptable method, although it obviously depends upon the patient's compliance and is not feasible in severely myasthenic, unconscious or vomiting patients. Rectal administration is an alternative in such cases. Medical auxiliaries can give s.c. or i.m. injections but these may be ineffective, e.g. in shock or when rapid results are required. Under such conditions, registered general nurses or doctors are authorised to administer drugs intravenously; this is also useful if large volumes of fluid need to be given. Inhalational anaesthesia or intrathecal (including sacral) injections must only be performed by medically qualified personnel.

Action required

Speed
Intravenous injection or inhalation is essential if a rapid systemic effect is desired but both have obvious dangers (*see* Toxicity, below). In general, due to the greater blood supply to skeletal muscle than to subcutaneous tissues, the i.m. route usually produces a faster onset than s.c. injection. Drugs administered sublingually can act within a few minutes but, if swallowed, their systemic effects usually begin after about 20 minutes if the stomach is empty and longer if a meal has recently been taken.

Accuracy of dosage
Again, inhalational and i.v. routes allow (as in the production of general anaesthesia) 'fine tuning' of the administered drug. In fact, i.v. infusions may enable the therapeutic agent to be 'titrated' exactly to a desired end-point, e.g. oxytocin to induce labour (p. 360); sodium nitroprusside to lower blood pressure immediately (p. 258). Slightly 'less fine' examples are insulin in hyperglycaemia ketoacidosis (p. 348), and heparin in pulmonary embolism.

Duration
Because almost all penicillins only act during the division stages of susceptible bacteria (p. 400), i.v. injections which predispose to rapid excretion by the renal organic acid mechanism are much less sustained than i.m. administrations of benzylpenicillin. If lower concentrations of drugs are adequate, they can be maintained over longer periods by the use of depot preparations, *see* earlier, (including 'circulating depot preparations' and subcutaneous pellet implants).

Activation by metabolism
Hepatic conversion of prednisone to the active compound prednisolone is essential; so in ulcerative colitis, if an enema is given, it must contain prednisolone (p. 325). Other examples of necessary activations carried out by the liver are:

azathioprine→6-mercaptopurine (Fig. 19.7, Table 19.9)
cyclophosphamide→a nitrogen mustard (p. 411)

Toxicity
This may be local or general.

Local. Irritant substances should not be given either orally (otherwise vomiting, colic or diarrhoea can occur) or s.c./i.m. (to avoid tissue necrosis consequent upon a prolonged contact between the offending drug and susceptible tissues). Direct i.v. injection is usually satisfactory for an irritant drug because it is rapidly diluted in the circulating blood volume. However, even this route is contraindicated if the substance is extremely irritant locally, e.g. the nitrogen mustard, mustine (p. 411), must be given by injection into a *running* saline drip.

General. The main danger with the rapidly acting routes of administration (i.v. and inhalational) is that some vital area (e.g. respiratory or cardiovascular centres, myocardium) may suddenly be exposed to a lethal concentration of the drug. Avoid this by a slower rate of administration. Treatment of bronchial asthma with beclomethasone by inhalation minimises systemic side-effects but can cause hoarseness and/or super-infection locally (p. 285).

**Attainment and maintenance of an adequate
drug concentration at the active site**

Form
Gases or vapours can only be inhaled but particulate matter, especially between 2 and 5 μm in diameter, will reach the bronchioles without passing through into the alveoli and is thus useful in the treatment of bronchial asthma (e.g. salbutamol, sodium cromoglycate, 11.5). The formulation of drug preparations is a branch of pharmacy termed pharmaceutics which can make a great deal of difference to the onset, effectiveness, and duration of drug action, e.g. enteric-coated capsules or tablets (which do not release their contents until they reach the small or large intestine), e.g. slow-release preparations given i.m. or s.c.

Site of action
Topical application is obviously preferable if circumscribed local effects are to be produced (e.g. in a dermatological condition). In subacute bacterial endocarditis the poor vascularity of the vegetations results in a weak, inflammatory response—which demands that all bacteria must be killed—and difficulty of penetration of the site by the drug; therefore use *high* concentrations of bacteri*cidal* drugs (benzyl-penicillin plus gentamicin) given intravenously.

Absorption

The general principles involved have been discussed earlier. In the case of absorption from the alimentary tract (*see* 13.1, 13.2 and drug interactions, 20.5). Further examples of the latter involve calcium salts which are absorbed chiefly in the upper small intestine by a carrier mechanism initiated by activated vitamin D (Fig. 16.1). Osteomalacia can result either from antagonism of this action by adrenal glucocorticoids or by a decrease in the content of activated vitamin D caused by the long-term use of anticonvulsants such as phenytoin or phenobarbitone (p. 170).

The alveolar membrane is sufficiently permeable to allow all inhalational anaesthetics (which are of relatively low molecular size) to pass this and the underlying pulmonary capillary wall readily.

Inactivation by catabolism

This will be detailed later (1.9) but it is obviously inappropriate to give orally either insulin (a polypeptide) or adrenaline (destroyed by monoamine oxidase in the cells of the intestinal epithelium and the liver).

Inactivation by binding

Diazoxide when given i.v. over a few minutes is rendered less effective by massive plasma protein binding (*see* section 1.3): a rapid 'bolus' (Gk: *bolos*, lump) injection is therefore preferred.

Removal by excretion

See section 1.10.

1.3   Plasma protein binding

Drugs attach themselves (usually by electrostatic bonds—Table 4.1: less commonly by hydrophobic interactions) to plasma proteins. Acidic substances, e.g. warfarin, frusemide, tolbutamide, combine largely with albumins; basic and amphoteric agents, e.g. diazepam, chlorpromazine, propranolol, also bind to globulins—particularly α_1-acid glycoproteins. Light or moderate binding modifies drug pharmacokinetics and pharmacodynamics relatively little. Heavy protein binding (90–100% *as is the case with all the above examples*) results in a low free plasma concentration of the drug (Fig. 1.4) but this may be significantly raised under the three conditions specified in Table 1.1. In the first two cases the free plasma concentration increases induced are acute—levelling out because any increased free drug is rapidly more widely distributed and/or excreted in the urine or metabolised—as is any further drug given. Clearly, the immediate effects of a displaced drug are greater, the smaller its volume of distribution (1.4), its metabolism or its excretion unchanged.

Table 1.1 Situations which can result in a rise in the free plasma concentration of a heavily plasma protein bound drug, X

Plasma protein concentration	Situation	Free plasma concentration of drug X
Normal	Increased dosage of the same drug, X	Increased*
Normal	Additional dose of a displacing drug	Increased*
Low	Initial dose of drug X	Increased*†

* If the available plasma protein binding sites become saturated.
† Compared to free plasma concentration of drug X in patient with normal plasma protein concentration.

When the concentration of plasma proteins is low (as in hepatic disease or in malnutrition), heavily bound drugs should be administered in less than normal doses. In nephrotic syndrome the situation is complicated by the additional loss of plasma protein-bound drug in the urine, so that normal dosage may be appropriate (e.g. with phenytoin, 7.1). A high degree of binding may also necessitate *bolus* injection (p. 15) so that the drug is able to exert its effect before massive combination with the plasma proteins occurs (e.g. diazoxide in acute hypertensive episodes, p. 258).

In general, heavily plasma protein-bound substances tend to have prolonged actions due to slow passage into the tissues (b, Fig. 1.4) and delayed glomerular filtration, although secretion into the renal tubules is not affected, probably due to an increased rate of dissociation (from the proteins) induced by the active mechanism (c, Fig. 1.5). Finally, plasma protein binding will enhance alimentary absorption of drugs, by lowering the free plasma concentration and thus increasing the concentration gradient for diffusion from the gut lumen.

1.4   Volumes of distribution of drugs

To be effective, a drug must attain and maintain an adequate therapeutic concentration at its site of action. A knowledge of its volume of distribution (V_d) enables one to calculate the doses to be administered initially and subsequently to achieve these ends (*see* 1.7–1.8). The volume of distribution can be measured by injecting a known amount of a substance, e.g. D_2O i.v. and then determining its total (i.e. free plus combined) concentration in the plasma after a period of time adequate to allow its passage into that part of the total body water to which it can gain access. Ideally, in this connection, substances are divisible into three categories as shown in Table 1.2. In practice, however, for most drugs such an equilibrium is not attained because, before distribution is complete, the opposing processes of metabolism, excretion or concentration in specific sites have come into play.

Table 1.2 Ideal volumes of distribution

Fluid compartment	Mean volume V_d (1 kg^{-1})	Average value for 70 kg adult (1)	Approximate time for equilibration (t) of, for example, D_2O*	Type of substance with example(s)
Blood plasma	0.05	3.5	10 minutes	Highly plasma protein bound (e.g. warfarin) and/or molecular weight >15 000 (e.g. heparin, dextrans, p. 8)
Extracellular fluid	0.2	14	30 minutes	Highly ionised (e.g. D-tubocurarine, gentamicin)
Total body water	0.60	42	1 hour	Lipid-soluble (e.g. ethanol)

$$V_d = \frac{\text{dose of drug injected i.v. } (D)}{\text{total plasma concentration at time } t}$$

(*see also* definition of V_d obtained from Fig. 1.7)

Intermediate values for V_d indicate either insufficient time allowed for equilibration or the intervention of metabolic, excretory or redistributive factors during the equilibration period. (These factors also account for impossibly high values obtained for V_d ; e.g. chlorpromazine due to extensive tissue binding has a V_d of about 20 l kg^{-1}, i.e. *c.* 33 times the total body water.) As these factors commonly intervene, the calculated V_d is usually termed the *apparent* volume of distribution.

* D_2O is not greatly affected by metabolism, excretion or redistribution during its equilibration periods.

Conversely, in the simplified calculations shown in 1.7 and 1.8, it is assumed that the drug (given i.v.) is *immediately* distributed throughout its V_d; this is termed a single (one)-compartment model.

1.5 Redistribution: multiple-compartment models

The secondary dispersion of drugs into (usually) inactive sites is particularly associated with highly lipid-soluble substances. As such drugs readily cross cell membranes, the limiting factor in their access to particular tissues is the blood flow. Thus, organs with a rapid blood flow (e.g. brain, heart, liver, kidney) initially receive a high concentration of the drug but, with time, this is depleted as the agent redistributes into moderately and slowly perfused tissues (skeletal muscle and fat, respectively, Fig. 1.6). In particular, barbiturates have their duration of effect minimised to a varying extent by redistribution into, initially, skeletal muscle and, later, adipose tissue. The greater the lipid solubility of the drug, the more rapid its redistribution (A′ in Fig. 1.6 is about 3–10 minutes for methohexitone or thiopentone, Table 1.4). However, charged drugs *can* be redistributed; this mainly accounts for the short duration of action of edrophonium (p. 50). Redistribution also means that *repeated* doses of the drug can exert *prolonged* effects due to gradual

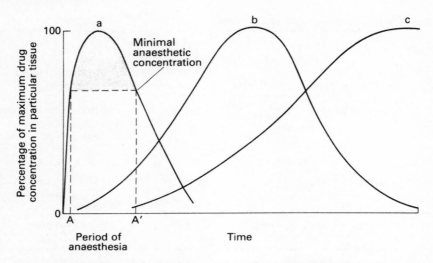

Fig. 1.6 Redistribution of lipid-soluble anaesthetic given i.v. in single dose. Relative drug concentrations plotted against time for: a, a rapidly perfused tissue, e.g. brain (shaded area AA′ indicates period of anaesthesia); b, a moderately perfused tissue, e.g. skeletal muscle; c, a slowly perfused tissue, e.g. fat.

passage from the saturated inactive sites back into the plasma over an extended period. This applies both to lipid-soluble agents, e.g. thiopentone, and to ionised agents, e.g. D-tubocurarine. Plasma and the 'rapid blood-flow organs' can be taken as one compartment; moderately and slowly perfused tissues represent second (and third) compartments.

1.6   Modification of drug duration of action, exemplified by the barbiturates

A high degree of lipid solubility will result in: increased absorption from the gastrointestinal tract, increased redistribution, and increased metabolism (producing compounds which are more water-soluble, p. 26 and thus more readily excreted via the kidney).

The general formula of the barbiturate molecule and the structural modifications which produce *increased* lipid solubility (as italicised in Table 1.3) are

R_4 S>O
R_3 methyl>hydrogen
R_1 allyl>ethyl
R_2 aliphatic (optimal 5–6 carbon atoms, chain branched, unsaturated) >aromatic.

So the range of lipid solubilities shown in Table 1.4 is obtained and from it the relative degrees of redistribution, metabolism and excretory products. The major factor determining the effective duration of a

Table 1.3 The formulae and main uses of some representative barbiturates

$$
\begin{array}{c}
\text{HN} \overline{}_6\ \text{CO} \\[2pt]
R_4{=}C\ _2 \qquad\qquad _5\ C{\raise2pt\hbox{$\diagdown$}}^{R_1}_{R_2} \\[2pt]
R_3{-}N\ \underline{}^{34}\ \text{CO}
\end{array}
$$

Barbiturate	R_4	R_3	R_1	R_2	Use	*See* page
Methohexitone*	O	*methyl*	*allyl*	*l-methyl-2-pentynyl*	i.v. anaesthetic†	220
Thiopentone*	*S*	H	ethyl	*l-methylbutyl*	i.v. anaesthetic†	220
Pentobarbitone*	O	H	ethyl	*l-methylbutyl*	Oral hypnotic‡	
Phenobarbitone*	O	H	ethyl	phenyl	Oral anticonvulsant	169

Italicised groups result in increased lipid solubility.
* In US terminology '-al' replaces the ending '-one'.
† Can cause some involuntary movements.
‡ Obsolete.

particular barbiturate is shown in *italics*. Thus, for the two i.v. anaesthetics the action is primarily terminated by *redistribution* into skeletal muscle (A′ in Fig. 1.6) and, to a lesser extent, into adipose tissue. Medium-acting barbiturates (e.g. pentobarbitone) are not now used as oral hypnotics, since they have been replaced by benzodiazepines (for the reasons stated on p. 177); but their duration of action was mainly determined by *metabolism*. Phenobarbitone, still occasionally used in the treatment of epilepsy (7.1) is wholly removed unchanged via *renal excretion* in the dog, which is *the* factor controlling its long duration of action in that species. In man (Table 1.4) metabolism is also important.

Table 1.4 Factors affecting the duration of action of some representative barbiturates when used as indicated in Table 1.3

Barbiturate	Mean duration of action	Lipid solubility	Redistribution	Metabolism	Renal excretion Unchanged (%)	As metabolites (%)
Methohexitone	3 minutes	++++	++++	++++*	0	100
Thiopentone	10 minutes	+++	+++	+++	0	100
Pentobarbitone	5 hours	++	++	++	10	90
Phenobarbitone	10 hours	+	+	+ (man)	25	75
				0 (dog)	*100*	0

++++ most, +++ much, ++ moderate, + less, 0 none.
* Probably accounts for less 'hangover' effect (compared with thiopentone).

1.7   Kinetics of drug absorption and elimination

Examples of absorption and elimination processes which obey zero-order or first-order kinetics are shown in Table 1.5.

A zero-order process is one which occurs a a constant *rate* and is, therefore, independent of the amount of drug present at the particular site(s) of drug absorption or elimination. Such a process requires a large excess of the drug available on the entry side (e.g. inhalational anaesthesia or intravenous infusion; roughly satisfied by slow-release preparations), or, on the exit side, a system whose capacity is limited. For example, the rate-limiting step in the metabolism of ethanol is the initial change to acetaldehyde (9.2). This has a low capacity so that the reaction is almost always zero-order at a rate of 10–15 ml per hour (*see* p. 231). Conversely, in the renal tubules, the active processes involved either in absorption or in secretion generally have high capacities so that only rarely (e.g. in the excretion of glucose by the diabetic) are zero-order kinetics involved. Some processes have moderate capacities and thus may switch from first- to zero-order kinetics (termed 'non-linear' kinetics) as the mechanism becomes saturated (e.g. hepatic metabolism of phenytoin as the therapeutically effective concentration is approached in some patients: if so, adjust the dosage in *small* increments to avoid adverse effects, Table 7.1).

First-order kinetics usually apply to processes involving diffusion or filtration and are the most common for both drug absorption and drug elimination (Table 1.5). Here the rate of the reaction is exponentially related to the amount of drug available which means that a constant *fraction* of the agent is absorbed or eliminated in unit time. The rate constants (k_{ab} and k_{el}) are quantitative measurements of these fractions (i.e. k_{ab} is the fraction of the drug present which is absorbed in unit time—minute, hour or day; k_{el} is a similar fraction for elimination).

To illustrate the points already stated, a simplified example is shown in Fig. 1.7. The drug is given intravenously and undergoes first-order

Table 1.5 Processes of drug entry and drug elimination exemplifying zero- and first-order kinetics

	Zero-order processes	First-order processes
Drug entry	Inhalation Continuous i.v. infusion (approximately). Slow-release, depot, preparations	Oral (also buccal, rectal) i.m. and s.c. injections (except depot preparations)
Drug elimination	Metabolism, e.g. of ethanol Renal excretion (above T_{max} absorption or T_{max} secretion)	Metabolism (of most drugs) Renal excretion (of most on drugs) Exhalation

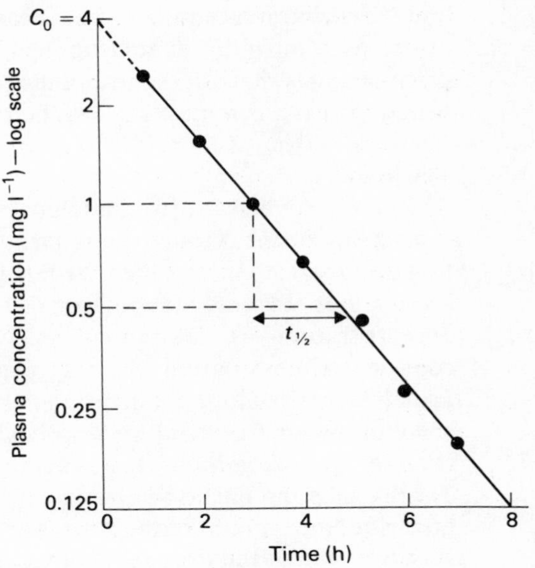

Fig. 1.7 Drug is given by i.v. injection in dose, D. One-compartment model. Dots indicate measured plasma concentrations at given time intervals after injection. Obtain C_0 and $t_{1/2}$ from the graph as shown. Then,

$$V_d = \frac{D}{C_0} \quad k_{el} = \frac{\log_e 2}{t_{1/2}} = \frac{0.693}{t_{1/2}}$$

CL_p (clearance from plasma)

$$= V_d \times k_{el}$$

elimination from the plasma; under these conditions, a plot of *log* plasma concentration against time is linear.

1 Measure $t_{1/2}$, i.e. the time taken for the concentration to halve, plasma half-life: calculate k_{el}.

2 Measure C_0, i.e. concentration at zero time: calculate V_d. This assumes the attainment of the latter to be immediate (in practice, this is never so, *see* 1.4).

3 Calculate the clearance from the plasma. This assumes that the V_d is constant over the whole time period (again this is never so, *see* 1.4).

A more accurate method assumes that clearance from the plasma is constant (even this is an approximation), in which case:

CL_p (clearance from the plasma)

$$= \frac{D \text{ (original dose)}}{AUC_{0 \to \infty} \text{ (area under the curve from time zero to complete elimination of the drug)}}$$

The required area is obtained from a graph of concentration (*not* log concentration) against time. (See extended texts dealing with pharmacokinetics for methods of determination of $AUC_{0 \to \infty}$ and for two compartment models which take cognisance of significant passage of a drug into moderately and slowly perfused tissues, p. 17.)

Note that the k_{el} from the plasma is the sum of the individual rate constants of elimination via metabolism, the various routes of excretion and redistribution. Similarly, the clearance from the plasma is the sum of the relevant individual clearances. Thus, if the clearance from the plasma equals that via the urine, the latter represents the only route by which the drug is removed from the plasma.

1.8   The plateau principle

This applies when a drug undergoes zero-order absorption and first-order elimination. Under these particular conditions, because absorption is at a constant rate, the time taken to reach a steady-state (plateau) level—after starting, stopping or changing the concentration of drug administration—is determined solely by the reciprocal of the rate constant of elimination (k_{el}). As can be seen from Table 1.5, this principle applies to the use of inhalational general anaesthetics which are eliminated from the body by exhalation. For these drugs, k_{el} is inversely proportional to the aqueous solubility (which is included in Table 1.6 as the partition coefficient between blood and air: S_b). This quantifies the amount of the drug in the plasma which is in equilibrium with one unit of the drug in the alveolar air. So, for *nitrous oxide* (with $S_b = 0.5$) of every 1.5 units reaching the pulmonary capillaries—following the cessation of anaesthesia—1.0 unit will be passed from the blood to the alveolar air (i.e. elimination of the anaesthetic from the body will be rapid). Conversely, because its S_b value is so high, the excretion of *diethyl ether* will be slow. Similar considerations govern the onset of anaesthesia with these agents: with nitrous oxide it is rapid (*c.* 2 min), with diethyl ether slow. *Halothane* is intermediate in aqueous solubility but has the possible advantage that its distribution between brain and blood (*see* Table 1.6) is greater than the other agents, so that its rate of induction of anaesthesia is not too slow.

Although the time taken to attain a plateau level of blood concentration depends entirely upon $1/k_{el}$, the *height* of the plateau reached depends upon the *concentration* of drug administered. This principle is

Table 1.6 Distribution of representative inhalational general anaesthetics between alveolar air, blood and brain

Anaesthetic gas (G) or vapour (V)	Partition coefficient blood : alveolar air*	Partition coefficient brain : blood
Diethyl ether (V)	15	1
Halothane (V)	2.5	2.5[†]
Nitrous oxide (G)	0.5	1

All figures are rounded to the nearest 0.5 for simplicity.
* Equals solubility in blood (S_b,) at body temperature.
[†] This value is contested by some workers who consider the correct value to be about 1—like most other commonly used inhalational general anaesthetics.

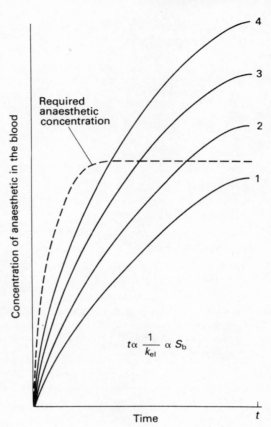

Fig. 1.8 The plateau principle as applied to the induction of general anaesthesia by inhalation. The time (t) to reach any equilibrium level is inversely proportional to the rate constant of elimination (k_{el}) for any given drug but the *height* of the plateau is dependent upon the concentration of the agent which is administered (lines 1, 2, 3 and 4 depict increasing concentrations). Therefore, a high concentration of the drug is given initially and this is lessened when a satisfactory anaesthetic level has been achieved (interrupted line). S_b, solubility in blood.

applied in practice as follows (Fig. 1.8, interrupted line). A high dosage of the agent (which would be lethal if continued) is given at first and, when the required anaesthetic depth is reached (recognised by clinical signs), the concentration is reduced to that sufficient to sustain anaesthesia.

Similar principles apply for other routes of administration, when loading doses (i.e. those necessary to attain a satisfactory therapeutic concentration of drug in the plasma rapidly) are followed by subsequent doses to maintain this level. To simplify the situation, in the following account all doses are given i.v. (for other routes, the equations would have to be modified by a factor dependent on the degree of absorption into the plasma from the relevant site).

In Fig. 1.9, the effective drug concentration (EDC) lies between 0.9 and 1 mg l^{-1}. The priming (loading) dose, assuming immediate passage into the final volume of distribution, is

$$\text{max EDC} \times V_d = D_L \text{ (loading dose)}$$

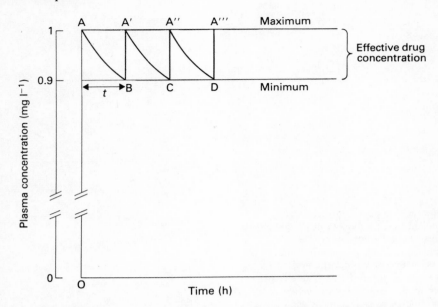

Fig. 1.9 Achievement and maintenance of an effective drug concentration in the plasma by intermittent i.v. dosage. One-compartment model. OA = priming dose (loading dose, D_L). BA′ = CA″ = DA‴, maintenance doses (D_M) each given at time t after preceding dose.

This should bring the plasma concentration of the drug from O to A in Fig. 1.9. To maintain this concentration, the rate of drug passage out of the plasma must equal that of drug into the plasma, i.e.

max EDC × clearance = maintenance dose rate

$$\text{max EDC} \times k_{el} \times V_d = Q \text{ (if given by infusion)}$$

$$= \frac{D_M}{t} \text{ (if given intermittently)}$$

where D_M is the maintenance dose and t is the dosage interval.

Let us now consider a situation (as shown in Fig. 1.9) where the EDC must not fall below 90% of the maximum value. The maintenance dose (D_M) is clearly 10% of the loading dose: in general terms

$$D_M = f \times D_L$$

where f is the fraction of the maximum EDC which has to be regained.

How frequently must the D_M be given? i.e. what is the value of t?

The general equation is: Specific example (to keep
                                            above 90%)

$$f = 1 - e^{-k_{el}\cdot t}$$
$$\therefore\ e^{-k_{el}\cdot t} = 1 - f$$
$$\therefore\ -k_{el}.t = \log_e (1 - f)$$
$$\therefore\qquad t = \frac{2.3.\log_{10}(1 - f)}{-k_{el}}\,t$$

$$f = 0.1$$
$$e^{-k_{el}\cdot t} = 0.9$$
$$-k_{el}.t = \log_e 0.9$$
$$t = \frac{2.3.\log_{10}0.9}{-k_{el}} = \frac{-0.1}{-k_{el}}$$

The same equation can be used to determine the time taken to reach a satisfactory plasma level, e.g. 90% of the maximum EDC if the drug is initially given—not as a priming dose—but at the maintenance dose rate *as an i.v. infusion*. As before, f represents the fraction of the maximum EDC value which has to be *attained*. So in the specific example

$$f = 1 - e^{-k_{el}\cdot t} = 0.9$$
$$\therefore\qquad t = \frac{2.3}{k_{el}}$$

Finally, note that, on stopping administration, most of the drug will be eliminated from the plasma in five half-lives, actually

$50 + 25 + 12.5 + 6.25 + 3.125 = $ about 97% removal.

(*see* digoxin, p. 434).

Conversely, if the drug is given by intermittent i.v. injections at intervals corresponding to its half-life, the same increments will apply so that it will achieve *c.* 97% of its plateau level in five half-lives.

1.9   Metabolism (alternative term, **biotransformation**)
This encompasses formation of more active compounds (anabolism) conversion to compounds of similar potency, and breakdown to less active substances (catabolism). It may take place in any organ or tissue of the body, and is subdivisible into special and general mechanisms.

Special mechanisms
These apply where a drug is sufficiently similar to a natural body constituent to be metabolised by a physiological enzyme system. This may be
• *synaptic*, e.g. acetylcholinesterase (2.2) hydrolyses methacholine; e.g. catechol O-methyltransferase (3.1) inactivates isoprenaline (Table 11.2)
• *in the plasma*. Butyryl ('pseudo') cholinesterase (2.2) is a relatively non-specific esterase which will hydrolyse suxamethonium, atropine, or procaine, for example
• *in most tissues*, e.g. monoamine oxidase (p. 77); e.g. amidases—which are mainly intracellular—slowly hydrolyse amides such as lignocaine (the local anaesthetic 'type substance').

Induced enzymes also constitute a special mechanism, e.g. the penicillin β-lactamases (Table 19.5) produced by resistant bacteria which inactivate the antibiotic.

General mechanisms

Some important changes are shown in Table 1.7. First, note that the products can be more, about equally or less, therapeutically active (column 4). Secondly, realise that a major centre of enzyme activity is the smooth endoplasmic reticulum (non-ribosomal part of the microsomal fraction) of *liver* cells: entry to this site appears to be enhanced by lipid solubility but is not decreased by plasma protein binding. However, metabolism does occur in non-microsomal sites and in other organs and tissues.

Once the drug has reached a metabolic site, a series of ongoing chemical reactions can take place (as depicted in Table 1.7).

1 The (so-called) *Phase I reactions*

• oxidations. These are brought about by mixed-function oxidases (monooxygenases). They require NADPH, a flavoprotein and O_2 with one of the multiple forms of cytochrome P_{450} as the terminal oxidase. An important reaction to remember is hydroxylation of a benzene ring, which will allow ionisation ($R.OH \rightleftharpoons R.O^-$, p. 6) and therefore easier removal in the urine (p. 12)

• reductions; these are relatively uncommon

• hydrolyses (*see* examples in Table 1.7).

2 The (so-called) *Phase II reactions* either replace or follow the phase I reactions. They are *conjugations* on chemical groups present naturally or produced by the preceding metabolic transformations. They almost always result in end-products which are less active and less lipid-soluble, so that they are more readily excreted especially in the urine and/or (usually to a smaller extent) in the bile. The particularly microsomal conjugations are with glucuronic acid or glutathione. A relevant example of the latter is the combination with toxic paracetamol metabolites. Normally, paracetamol is mainly excreted as the glucuronic and sulphonic conjugates; a small amount of the drug is converted to either an epoxide or N-acetyl benzoquinone imine; these are detoxified by epoxide hydrolase and by conjugation with reduced glutathione. However, in paracetamol poisoning, the glutathione available is insufficient to combine with the larger amounts of toxic metabolites formed which then react (covalently) with hepatic cells to produce (initially) nausea and vomiting, (but after 1–2 days) centrilobular necrosis. Thus a vicious circle ensues—decreased liver function leading to less toxic metabolite removal and more liver damage. Specific treatment is the *immediate* administration of N-acetyl-cysteine (acetylcysteine) which acts as a precursor for glutathione synthesis; it is useless once hepatic failure has occurred.

Table 1.7 General drug metabolism

General group	Type of reaction	Substrate	Product (**bold** = more active, *italic* = less active, therapeutically; neither = approximately equally active)	Site of reaction — Liver microsomal	Site of reaction — Non-microsomal
General group	Chemical change (N, nitrogen; O, oxygen)				
Oxidation	N-dealkylation	Imipramine	**Desmethylimipramine**	+	
		Pethidine	*Norpethidine*	+	
		Diazepam	N-desmethyl(nor)diazepam	+	
	O-dealkylation	Phenacetin	Paracetamol	+	
	Epoxide formation	Paracetamol	*Paracetamol epoxide*	+	
		Phenytoin	*Phenytoin epoxide*	+	
	Hydroxylation	Phenytoin	*p-hydroxy(phenyl) derivative**	+	
		Phenobarbitone	*p-hydroxy(phenyl) derivative**	+	
		Propranolol	p-hydroxy(phenyl) derivative†	+	
	Desulphuration	Thiopentone	Pentobarbitone (Table 1.3)	+	
	Sulphoxidation	Chlorpromazine‡	*Chlorpromazine sulphoxide*	+	
	Oxidative deamination	Tyramine	p-hydroxyphenylacetic acid		+
	Primary alcohol (via aldehyde to carboxylic acid)	Ethanol	*Acetic acid*	(+)	+
		Methanol	*Formic acid*	(+)	+
Reduction	Aldehyde to primary alcohol	Chloral hydrate	Trichlorethanol		+
	Ketone to secondary alcohol	Cortisone	**Hydrocortisone**	+	
		Prednisone	**Prednisolone**	+	
Hydrolysis	of ester	Paracetamol	*p-aminophenol*	+	+
		Aspirin	Salicylic acid §	+	+
	of amide	Lignocaine	*Xylidine*	+	+
	of glycoside	Anthraquinone purgative	**Corresponding emodin**	+	+

Continued

Table 1.7 General drug metabolism (*Cont'd*)

Type of reaction	Substrate	Product (**bold**=more active, *italic* = less active, therapeutically; neither=approximately equally active)	Site of reaction	
			Liver microsomal	Non-microsomal
Conjugation	Glucuronylation	Salicyclic acid	*Glucuronide on either .COOH or phenolic .OH*	+	+
		Paracetamol	*Glucuronide on phenolic .OH*	+	
		Morphine	*Glucuronide on either phenolic or alcoholic .OH*	+	
	Combination with glutathione	Paracetamol epoxide (*see text*)	(after series of reactions) corresponding *mercapturic acid*	+	
	Glycinylation	Salicylic acid	*Salicyluric acid*		+
	Sulphonation	Morphine	*Morphine sulphonate*		+
	N-acetylation‖	Isoniazid	*Acetylisoniazid*		+
		Sulphonamides	*N_4-acetyl derivatives*		+
	N-methylation	Histamine	*N-methylhistamine*	+	+
	O-methylation	Isoprenaline	*3-Methoxyisoprenaline*		+

+ Major site; (+) minor site.
* See p. 170.
† Some β-blocking activity but short half-life (pp. 30–1).
‡ Over 200 metabolites of chlorpromazine have been identified.
§ Less active as an analgesic, some anti-inflammatory action: weak prostaglandin cyclo-oxygenase inhibitor.
‖ Requires acetyl CoA as .COCH$_3$ donor.

Microsomal enzymes are induced gradually (over a few days) and persist for a few weeks after removal of the offending drug. Probably thousands of chemical agents—including environmental pollutants, e.g. cigarette smoke—have this potential: most, but not all, are substrates for the enzymes induced. Conversely, these enzymes are impaired by decreased liver function (e.g. chronic alcoholism) and by a few drugs (e.g. allopurinol 12.8, cimetidine, p. 319); an experimental inhibitor is proadifen (SKF 525-A).

Oxygen free radicals

A free radical is capable of an independent existence but has one or more *unpaired* electrons. Two important oxygen free radicals are *superoxide* (O_2^-) and *hydroxyl* $(OH^\bullet)$ The former is produced in many biological processes particularly in the electron transport chains of mitochondria and the endoplasmic reticulum, and also by activated phagocytes where it helps in the destruction of ingested microorganisms. However, it is not very damaging generally and is usually converted intracellularly to water via hydrogen peroxide as shown in Fig. 1.10. But if the H_2O_2 is not adequately removed, hydroxyl free radicals are formed and these are very destructive. As indicated glutathione (e.g. in the form of N-acetylcysteine—just mentioned in the detoxification of paracetamol epoxides) will again be useful by increasing peroxide breakdown.

Some corollaries

- pharmacokinetic (metabolic) tolerance, e.g. with barbiturates, p. 188
- saturation of enzymes so that first-order changes to zero-order reaction, e.g. with phenytoin, p. 20
- increased breakdown of simultaneously administered drugs, or naturally occurring steroid hormones (adrenal corticoids, oestrogens, for example)

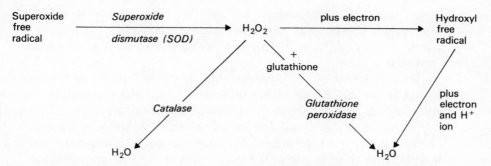

Fig. 1.10 Formation and removal of oxygen free radicals (greatly simplified).

• decreased catabolism of other therapeutic agents when the capacity of the relevant enzyme system is saturated (e.g. mutual potentiation of warfarin action with tolbutamide, Table 17.2)
• alterations in vitamin D metabolism with phenobarbitone or phenytoin, p. 170
• increased usage of folic acid as co-factor for the hydroxylation of phenobarbitone or phenytoin, resulting in megaloblastic anaemia, p. 170
• deficiency of glucuronyl transferase which can result in the 'grey baby' syndrome with chloramphenicol (p. 416) or kernicterus (if the bile pigments are not conjugated in the newborn). The latter condition can be treated with phenobarbitone—given to the mother a few days before delivery or to the infant at birth—to induce glucuronyl transferase. The dangers to the fetus or newborn infant are increased metabolism of steroid hormones and some clotting factors (e.g. prothrombin).

Further points

Enzyme induction and activity in the liver are not confined to the microsomal fraction. For example, alcohol dehydrogenase occurs in the cytoplasmic fraction where the bulk of the catabolism of ethanol and methanol (*see* Fig. 9.2) takes place. For the effect of ethanol on *microsomal* enzyme content *see* p. 386. Non-microsomal enzyme systems often occur at extrahepatic sites (e.g. the gut wall); their range of chemical transformations is shown in Table 1.7, and the extent to which they are inducible varies. Individual variation in both microsomal and non-microsomal enzyme activity and induction can differ by at least one order of magnitude and is often markedly genetically determined (1.13). Major examples of pharmacogenetics in relation to drug metabolism are shown in Table 20.4. Species differences also occur; for example, the cat is stated to have little (or no) glucuronyl transferase and the dog a deficiency of acetylating enzymes.

Finally, an important concept with respect to swallowed drugs is that of the extent of hepatic clearance of the substance on its initial passage through the liver. If the removal or inactivation on this 'first pass' is considerable (e.g. lignocaine, p. 280) then this particular route is interdicted. Conversely, sublingual administration (e.g. with glyceryl trinitrate) is rapidly maximally effective due to avoidance of the hepatic 'first pass'.

With propranolol given orally, e.g. in the treatment of essential hypertension (p. 253) or angina pectoris (p. 268), the situation is very complicated. Not only does the extent of 'first pass' liver metabolism show ethnic and individual differences but it also varies with changes in hepatic blood flow. Post-prandially, increased portal blood flow results in more absorption of the drug from the gut but less hepatic 'first pass' metabolism. Also, propranolol—with a half-life in the plasma of 2–4 hours—is partially converted (by para-hydroxylation of a benzene ring, Table 1.7, to an active metabolite which has a half-life of up to 2 hours. So, optimal therapy with propranolol is best achieved by a gradual increase in dosage *at fixed times in relation to meals* until the maximum clinical effects are obtained.

1.10 Drug excretion

Pulmonary
The expired air offers a rapid and efficient method for the removal of drugs in the gaseous or vapour states. Its major significance lies in the excretion of inhalational anaesthetics (p. 22). The exhalation of ethanol is a valid measure of intoxication although only about 1% is eliminated by this route.

Renal
By far the commonest route for the excretion of most drugs—either unchanged or as their metabolites. The general principles involved in elimination via the kidney have already been described in 1.1, namely
• *ionised compounds* are readily excreted and, in many cases, their removal is intensified by *active* acid- or base-secreting mechanisms in the proximal convoluted tubules
• *plasma protein binding* delays (passive) glomerular filtration (unless proteins are also lost in the urine, e.g. nephrotic syndrome, p. 16), but not active secretion which is, presumably, sufficiently forcible to encourage rapid dissociation from the binding
• *pH of urine* is important. This may be dietary in origin. Take the case of amphetamine: an acid-forming (carnivorous) diet will result in rapid removal of the unchanged drug, while an alkaline-forming (vegetarian) diet will result in a slower urinary excretion of one-third unchanged, one-third conjugated, and one-third converted (by para-hydroxylation) to α-methyltyramine and (by subsequent β-hydroxylation) to a-methyloctopamine (para-hydroxynorephedrine); *see* Table 3.2 and Fig. 3.3 if unsure of these chemical conversions.

Complicating circumstances arise when kidney function is diminished either by acute or chronic renal failure, or by immaturity (infants) or old age. In all these situations toxicity, e.g. of aminoglycosides (19.6) is increased.

Gastrointestinal
Biliary excretion of therapeutic agents or their metabolites is basically similar to that already described for the renal tubules: particularly, there are mechanisms for
• reabsorption (from the bile) of the more lipid-soluble components
• secretion (into the bile) of organic acids, bases and also steroids.

Thus the acids ampicillin and amoxycillin (Table 19.1) occur in high concentrations in bile (and have been used in the treatment of typhoid carriers) but, after passage into the intestine, they *can be reabsorbed* into the enterohepatic circulation and, thus, finally be *mainly* eliminated in the urine. A similar fate awaits (unchanged) rifampicin but its desacetyl derivative which is formed in the liver is not recirculated. Drugs conjugated with glucuronic acid are mainly excreted in the urine but some may pass via the bile to the faeces. As a further variation, it is possible for a biliary-excreted drug glucuronide to be hydrolysed in the gut back to its lipid-soluble precursor, which then requires further hepatic conjugation before its final removal by the kidney. But, usually the enterohepatic circulation of drugs or their derivatives is small (e.g. about 10% for phenolphthalein, p. 323).

A few substances can pass from the blood into the large intestine (e.g. active emodins derived from the anthracene purgatives, p. 323).

Other routes

Salivary
The processes involved are again similar to those occurring in the renal tubules. The amounts of drugs excreted by this route are generally insignificant in relation to removal from the body. However, for some drugs (carbamazepine, paracetamol, phenytoin, theophylline) there is a good correlation between salivary concentration and free plasma level so that measurement of the former is a non-invasive method for determining the latter. This is occasionally useful, e.g. in the very young when repeated sampling is necessary.

Sudatory
While sweat hardly contributes significantly to total excretion, the patient should be warned that it may be orange-red in colour following treatment with rifampicin.

Mammary
Here the main process is passive diffusion of non-protein-bound drugs. The major consideration is neonatal toxicity (Table 1.9 and 15.5).

1.11 Passage of drugs across the placenta
This subject is important since it closely concerns the well-being of the fetus. In general terms, the situation is similar to that at other transporting sites in the body. Thus, the extents of placental (maternal and fetal) blood flows, protein binding and drug ionisation are key factors and, while a few agents may undergo active movements or facilitated diffusion, the majority of drug transport is dependent upon

lipid solubility and concentration gradients. Occasionally, placental metabolism can take place (*compare* the *enzymatic* blood–brain barrier, p. 10). Once across the placenta, the precise distribution of a drug in specific organs of the fetus is determined by regional blood flows and uptake processes. The tissue concentrations of the drug will gradually rise unless metabolic or excretory processes, which are rudimentary in the fetus, come into play.

1.12 Overall kinetic considerations

Ideally, the physician would like to know the exact concentration of therapeutic agent attained and maintained at its site of action. This is rarely possible but the plasma drug concentration is often related to, and is a valid measure of, the required quantity. It can be quite critical with drugs that have a narrow therapeutic range, e.g. phenytoin (p. 20), lithium carbonate (p. 185), theophylline (p. 234), digoxin (p. 271), gentamicin (19.6). But exceptions occur when the drug has a delayed onset of action (e.g. antidepressants, p. 182; warfarin, Table 17.1) or an irreversible effect (e.g. organic phosphorus-containing anticholinesterases, p. 53; alkylating agents, p. 411). Therefore, in the majority of cases, the plasma half-life is the paramount determinant of dose frequency. Obviously, any of the factors shown in Fig. 1.1 may be implicated in the rise and fall of drug concentrations in the plasma. Table 1.8 shows how the volume of distribution and clearance in the urine may interact in this connection. However, for most drugs, such categories represent tendencies rather than fulfilled conditions.

Table 1.8 Plasma half-lives following the administration of single i.v. doses of four different drugs which are neither metabolised nor redistributed but excreted in the urine (70 kg human, with normal kidney function)

Drug	Volume of distribution (litres)	Renal clearance (ml min^{-1})	Plasma $t_{1/2}$ (min)*
1	Total body water (42)	c. 1 (urinary volume)	29 100 (c. 20 days)
2	Total body water (42)	c. 120 (glomerular filtration rate)	233 (c. 4 hours)
3	Total body water (42)	c. 650 (renal plasma flow)	42
4	Extracellular fluid (14)	c. 650 (renal plasma flow)	14

* Calculated from formulae in caption to Fig 1.7. V_d values from Table 1.2

$$t_{1/2} = \frac{0.693 \, V_d}{CL_p \text{ (clearance from plasma)}}$$

1.13   Factors modifying drug availability and responses

Genetic and environmental/social factors

Examples of relatively gross genetic influences of the pharmacodynamics and pharmacokinetics of several commonly used drugs are
shown in Table 20.4, but slighter genetic differences are possibly mainly
responsible for the Gaussian (normal) distribution of drug effects (Fig.
20.1). Other significant factors may be studied using monozygotic
(identical) twins in different 'environmental' situations. As mentioned
earlier (p. 29), microsomal enzyme activity is increased by cigarette
smoking and diminished by chronic alcoholism.

Age

This factor is usually allowed for when drug doses are calculated in
terms of body weight or surface area. However, neonates (especially
premature babies) and the elderly often show exaggerated responses
because they have immature or diminished active, specific processes.
Most commonly, the trend is to increase free plasma concentrations of
drugs because the majority of absorptive mechanisms are passive while
plasma protein binding and eliminatory procedures possess a higher
degree of activity and specificity. Table 1.9 shows a skeleton classification of drug differences in patients at the extremes of age—add others as
you meet them. Note that *qualitative* changes are possible, e.g. central
depressants can excite the elderly.

The suckling infant is also exposed to any agents secreted by the
mammary gland. Substances which may be contained in the milk in
high concentration are detailed in 15.5. When these drugs must be
administered to nursing mothers, the possible effects upon the baby are
the prime consideration; bottle feed if necessary.

Pathological conditions

The possibilities here are legion but a selection of salient examples
should be helpful.

Absorption from the gut is increased by constipation (greater time of
drug contact with absorptive sites) and, conversely, decreased in
diarrhoeic states (Table 20.3). Bile salt or pancreatic enzyme deficiencies result in diminished absorption of, for example, fat-soluble
vitamins (16.1).

Hepatic metabolism of drugs is appreciably lessened in cirrhosis,
and in heart failure (due to decrease in liver blood flow).

In low plasma protein states, binding is diminished which tends to
increase the 'free' concentration of an agent (1.3); however, *if the
causative condition is nephrotic syndrome*, this may be over-com-
pensated by the greater loss of protein-bound drug via the 'leaky'
glomerulus. There is a binding defect in uraemic plasma probably due
to inhibition by metabolites present in this condition.

Table 1.9 Differences of drug handling in the very young and in the old, compared with normal adult patients

Effect	In the newborn	In the elderly
Pharmacokinetic		
Absorption	Not much altered unless active processes are involved	Not much altered unless active processes are involved or senile involutionary changes or decreases in blood flow (common) occur
Hepatic function		
Plasma protein synthesis	Smaller than usual and, thus, less plasma protein binding with, for example, warfarin or phenytoin	
Clotting factor synthesis	Less, so potentiation of, for example, warfarin effects	
Enzyme production	Low, e.g. glucuronyl transferase resulting in 'grey-baby' syndrome with chloramphenicol (1.9)	Decreased, e.g. of microsomal enzymes resulting in toxicity with, for example, diazepam, propranolol or theophylline
Renal excretion		
Glomerular filtration rate	Relatively low, so increased toxicity of digoxin, aminoglycoside antibiotics, e.g. gentamicin	
Active secretion	Lessened, e.g. $t_{1/2}$ of benzylpenicillin increased	
Pharmacodynamic		
Action	Increased susceptibility to respiratory depression with morphine	*Quantitatively* increased, e.g. with warfarin there can be greater sensitivity without much change in pharmacokinetic factors. *Qualitatively* altered, e.g. CNS depressants such as barbiturates or hyoscine can produce excitement or confusion

Renal inefficiency obviously leads to difficulties with drugs that are primarily excreted by this route, e.g. gentamicin.

Central respiratory depressants (e.g. morphine, pethidine, pentazocine) should be prescribed with extreme caution in chronic bronchitic and/or asthmatic patients. The same people are also at some risk with aspirin, as a hypersensitivity reaction can cause bronchoconstriction.

Multiple drug therapy

Many examples of drug interactions will be found throughout the text, i.e. the presence of one (or more) therapeutic substances modifying the pharmacodynamic or pharmacokinetic characteristics of other agents. They are collated in 20.5.

Compliance

This connotes the extent to which the patient is reliable in taking the correct dosage of the prescribed medication regularly. Obviously this is a cardinal factor in therapy. Failure is commonest in conditions such as pulmonary tuberculosis where prolonged treatment is necessary but the patient can feel much better in a few weeks and, therefore, be tempted to stop taking the tablets. In such a case 'spot checks' of, for example, the orange-red urine produced by the rifampicin or the urinary estimation of isoniazid and its metabolites may be useful; *see also* p. 451. Patients with venereal diseases often fail to return to the clinic and so a depot preparation may be initially injected to ensure sustained treatment. Finally, for strict Muslims compliance may be erratic during Ramadan.

Placebo responses

Confidence of the patient in the doctor plays an important role in the successful outcome of a given regimen. Further, many conditions recover spontaneously or are subject to remissions. Therefore, it is not unexpected that, in clinical trials, for example, substantial improvements in a patient's health (physical as well as mental) can follow the application of an inert substance (*see* 21.3).

Part 2

Fundamental Pharmacodynamics

2 Cholinergic Peripheral Mechanisms

A drug can effect a tissue response, initially, through
- non-specific mechanisms, e.g. general anaesthetics (8.7) or
- specific mechanisms. The basic, though not necessarily the only, pharmacodynamic principle in this connection is that of a drug affecting its own particular receptors at specialised sites within the body to set in motion one or more series of effects which culminate in manifest qualitative (and quantitative) responses. Some subtleties of 'receptorology' will be discussed in Chapter 4, but these are merely variations on the straightforward actions produced in relation to the classical *peripheral* transmitter substances—acetylcholine (ACh) and noradrenaline (NA)—which will be detailed and discussed in this and the following chapter.

Criteria which should be fulfilled to identify a *post*synaptically acting transmitter are:

Content (presynaptically) of the putative transmitter or its precursor(s) plus enzymes for its synthesis. Often, also, inactivating enzymes in the vicinity of the synapse

Release following appropriate physiological stimuli, e.g. passage of nerve impulses

Application of the possible transmitter and natural activation should produce identical responses

Modification. The responses just mentioned should be similarly decreased by *specific* antagonists

increased by, for example, inhibitors of transmitter inactivation — anticholinesterases (2.6), uptake blockers (*see* 3.1).

2.1 Cholinergic and (nor)adrenergic synapses outside the CNS

The general scheme is illustrated in Fig. 2.1. All fibres shown are cholinergic, i.e. release acetylcholine, except the 'typical' sympathetic postganglionic fibres which release mainly noradrenaline (noradrenergic); conversely, in man and most other animals, the *adrenal medullary* secretion contains more adrenaline than noradrenaline. The neurotransmitters act postsynaptically (via cholino- or adrenoceptors) to produce responses and are then removed to clear the synapse for its next burst of activity. Recently, this simple picture has been complicated by

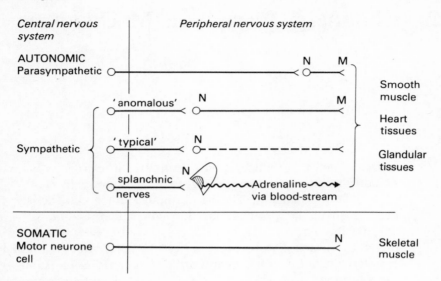

Fig. 2.1 Peripheral *motor* cholinergic and noradrenergic synapses. (Upper) Continuous lines indicate fibres which liberate acetylcholine. Postsynaptic cholinergic receptors (cholinoceptors) at ganglia, splanchnic nerve terminals in the adrenal medulla and the somatic neuromuscular junction are nicotinic (N, 2.3); while those in relation to the postganglionic fibres of all the parasympathetic system and the 'anomalous' sympathetic (e.g. to sweat glands subserving heat regulation in the human) are muscarinic (M, 2.3). Interrupted lines indicate fibres which liberate noradrenaline (plus a small percentage of adrenaline). The mammalian adrenal medulla liberates mainly adrenaline (with some noradrenaline) into the bloodstream whence it activates adrenoceptors in the autonomic effector tissues. (Lower) Presynaptic receptor types which modulate release at cholinergic and noradrenergic synapses.

the discovery that in many tissues (innervated by either system), transmitter release can be regulated via cholinoceptive and/or adrenoceptive *pre*synaptic sites. (Fig. 2.1, lower). Further, co-transmitters (p. 141), e.g. ATP, prostaglandins, enkephalins, may have modulating functions by acting at either pre- or postsynaptic receptors. The extent to which these finer details are physiologically involved is uncertain but they may have pharmacological significance in some specific situations, which will be discussed in detail as they arise.

Because acetylcholine and adrenaline/noradrenaline are so closely involved in the multifarious processes occurring at synapses (Figs 2.2 and 3.1), it is not unexpected that 'similar' synthetic molecules may partake in one or more of their activities. Thus, we may establish

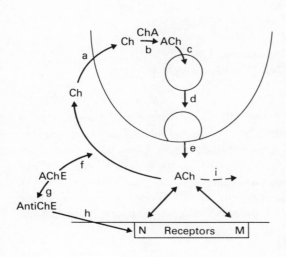

Fig. 2.2 Processes occurring at a cholinergic synapse (diagrammatic).
a, Uptake of choline (Ch);
b, Synthesis of acetylcholine (ACh), using choline acetyl(transfer)ase (ChA);
c, Storage of the transmitter in vesicles;
d, Mobilisation of vesicles preparatory to release;
e, Release of acetylcholine;
f, Breakdown of the transmitter locally by acetylcholinesterase (AChE);
g, Antagonism of the breakdown by an anticholinesterase (AntiChE);
h, An anticholinesterase also having a *direct* nicotinic action (e.g. neostigmine at the skeletal neuromuscular junction, 2.6);
i, Diffusion away (mainly significant in the presence of an AntiChE).

'*structure–activity relationships*' (i.e. show that certain chemical groupings within drug molecules can produce *specific* effects) at synapses. Such concepts have been, and are still, valuable in considering the therapeutic applications of most drugs, although they probably represent a rather crude approximation of the real picture (*see* Chapter 4, particularly p. 92). The remainder of this chapter will concentrate on drug interactions with peripheral cholinergic systems, leaving the corresponding (nor)adrenergic systems for Chapter 3.

2.2 Physiology of cholinergic synapses in the peripheral nervous system (Fig. 2.2)

Axonal transmission along the relevant nerves by the classical Hodgkin –Huxley mechanism (sodium ions in, followed by a slower passage of potassium ions out, *see* 8.2) results finally in depolarisation of the nerve terminal which opens voltage-operated calcium channels (4.10). The resultant calcium ion entry (by excitation–secretion coupling) causes release of the neurotransmitter (acetylcholine). This then activates the specific receptors ('muscarinic' or 'nicotinic', *see* 2.3), following which it is rapidly hydrolysed by acetyl('true')cholinesterase in the synaptic cleft. The main product—choline—is then largely reabsorbed by a process involving a carrier molecule into the presynaptic ending. Resynthesis to the active transmitter (using the enzyme choline acetyltransferase) is followed by storage in vesicles for subsequent nerve impulse-mediated release. This series of events is not universal: for example, at autonomic ganglia local hydrolysis is not very important, inactivation mainly taking place through diffusion from the synaptic

site and subsequent breakdown by butyryl ('pseudo', 'plasma') cholinesterase in the circulation. Thus, *anticholinesterase agents tend to have
insignificant effects upon ganglionic transmission.*

2.3   Cholinergic receptors (cholinoceptors, Fig. 2.1)
These can broadly be divided into two categories:

Muscarinic (M)
These are characterised by being stimulated selectively by muscarine or
methacholine (acetyl-β-methylcholine, *see* Table 2.1,7) and antagonised
competitively (4.4) by atropine or its allies (2.7). They occur postsynaptically in relation to all parasympathetic fibres and in 'anomalous'
sympathetic fibres, e.g. to the sweat glands subserving heat regulation in
the human. Some are also present at the predominantly nicotinic
ganglionic synapses (*see* Note on subdivision of muscarinic receptors,
p. 61 and Table 2.9).

Nicotinic (N)
These are activated selectively by N-like agents (Table 2.4). As an
alternative to competitive (non-depolarising) antagonism by ganglionic
or skeletal neuromuscular junction blocking agents, *excess* of the
natural transmitter, acetylcholine (such as that produced by anticholinesterases) or of nicotinic agonists can progress through a stimulatory
phase to blockade (depolarising or desensitising). This secondary
blocking mechanism is peculiar to nicotinic sites and has not been
shown to occur at muscarinic synapses (*see* Fig. 2.11).

Structure–activity relationships for acetylcholine-like substances

Muscarinic sites
The formula of acetylcholine is at the top of Table 2.1. Variations in the
structure—with the resultant changes in activity—are then shown and
may be taken to indicate a crude approximation (p. 90) of the optimal
structure for the muscarinic receptor (Fig. 2.3). Notice particularly the
following points:
1   Variations in the acyl group. Acetyl is the best fit; butyryl is only a
partial agonist (Table 2.2, middle column and Fig. 4.1) and valerylcholine is actually an antagonist (compare the situation at the nicotinic
receptor, *see* next section).
2   The acyl group can be replaced by an amide (e.g. carbachol) with
little loss in activity.
3   The ether and (to a lesser extent) the ketone group enhances the
agonist action—probably by combination of their partially charged
atoms with corresponding positions on the receptor (Fig. 2.3).
4   The optimal length of the chain from the charged nitrogen atom

Table 2.1 Effects of changes in the acetylcholine molecule (top) on the activity at *muscarinic* *post*synaptic site

$$
\underbrace{CH_3 \quad .CO.}_{\text{acyl group}} \quad \underbrace{\overset{\text{ether}}{O.} \quad \overset{\beta \quad \alpha}{CH_2.CH_2.} \quad \overset{+}{N}.(CH_3)_3}_{\text{choline residue}}
$$

Number in text	Modification in chemical structure		Activity*	Conclusion
1	H	.CO .(formylcholine)	+ +	acetyl gives the
	CH₃	.CO .(acetylcholine)	+ + +	optimal fit at the
	C₂H₅	.CO .(propionylcholine)	+	esteratic site
	C₃H₇	.CO .(butyrylcholine)	±	(Fig 2.3)
	C₄H₉	.CO .(valerycholine)	0	
2	NH₂.	CO.(carbamylcholine, carbachol)	+ + +	
3	CH₃	.CH₂.O.	+	ether and ketone
	CH₃	.CO .CH₂	±	groups beneficial
	CH₃	.CH₂.CH₂.	0	
4	(tetramethylammonium)	$CH_3.\overset{+}{N}.(CH_3)_3$	0	5 atom chain to $\overset{+}{N}$ essential
5		$.C.(CH_3)_3$	0	charged nitrogen atom essential
6		$\overset{+}{N}\!\!\begin{smallmatrix} \diagup H \\ —CH_3 \\ \diagdown CH_3 \end{smallmatrix}$	+	
		$\overset{+}{N}\!\!\begin{smallmatrix} \diagup H \\ —H \\ \diagdown CH_3 \end{smallmatrix}$	0	at least two methyl groups required
		$\overset{+}{N}H_3$	0	
		$\overset{+}{N}\!\!\begin{smallmatrix} \diagup C_2H_5 \\ —CH_3 \\ \diagdown CH_3 \end{smallmatrix}$	+ +	
		$\overset{+}{N}\!\!\begin{smallmatrix} \diagup C_2H_5 \\ —C_2H_5 \\ \diagdown CH_3 \end{smallmatrix}$	0	at least two methyl groups required
		$\overset{+}{N}.(C_2H_5)_3$	0	
7	S(+)-methacholine	$—\overset{\overset{\textstyle CH_3}{\textstyle \mid}}{CH}—$	+ + +	steric hindrance by β-methyl group
	R(−)-methacholine	$—\underset{\underset{\textstyle CH_3}{\textstyle \mid}}{\overset{\beta}{CH}}—$	±	when present in R(−)-configuration

*Activity in comparison to acetylcholine (approximate: varies with test tissue): + + +, equal, + +, less; +, some; ±, slight, 0, negligible.

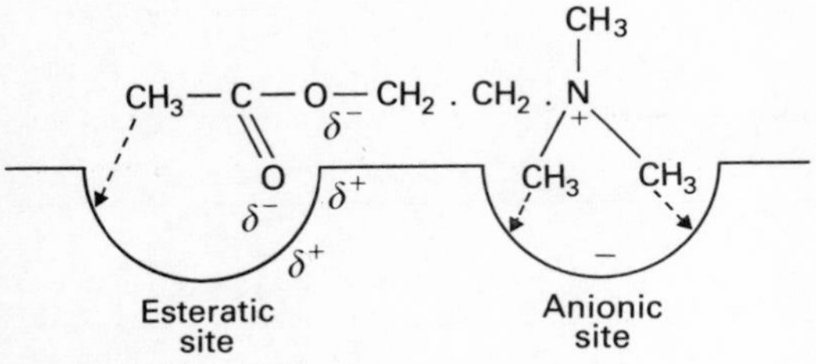

Fig. 2.3 Two-dimensional representation of the major factors involved in acceptance of an acetylcholine molecule at a postsynaptic *muscarinic* receptor. The esteratic site receives the acetyl group (optimally, Tables 2.1 and 2.2). The cationic head combines with the unit charge $(-)$ at the anionic site, δ^-, δ^+, subintegral charges; ----→ weak electrostatic bonds (*see* Chapter 4).

appears to consist of *five* atoms and activity decreases to zero when this is reduced to *one* atom (compare the autonomic ganglion nicotinic site, where tetramethylammonium is a potent agonist).

5   When the unit-charged nitrogen atom is replaced by an atom of similar size but only slightly charged (namely a carbon atom), all activity is lost indicating that the anionic site of the receptor requires a fully charged cationic head in the approaching agonist.

6   At least two of the methyl substituents on the nitrogen atom appear to be necessary for activity. This was originally interpreted as meaning that the two essential methyl groups (via van der Waals forces, Chapter 4) strengthened the ionic bond (5 above) at the anionic receptor site: but this view is not now considered to be correct.

7   Acetyl-β-methylcholine (methacholine) (a selective agonist for muscarinic receptors) is active as the S($+$)-form. Its virtual inactivity in the R($-$)-form may be attributed to the presence of the substituent group on the underside of the approaching drug molecule, preventing its usual attachment at *both* the esteratic and anionic sites simultaneously.*

Table 2.2   Effects of alteration of the acyl group of choline esters at muscarinic (M) and nicotinic (N) sites

	Relative activity* at	
Acyl substituent	M receptors	N receptors
Formyl	+ +	+ +
ACETYL	+ + +	+ + +
Propionyl	+	+ + + + +
Butyryl	±	+ + + +
Valeryl	0	+ +

*Activity in relation to acetylcholine: + + + + +, most; + + + +, more; + + +, equal; + +, less; +, some; ±, slight; 0, nil.

*Stereoisomers can be described by
• rotation of plane of polarised light: ($+$)*dextro*- or ($-$)-*laevo*rotatory
• structure in relation to a reference molecule e.g. lactic acid; D- or L-forms
• (best) the sequence rule; R- or S-forms.

Nicotinic sites

The principal differences here (using the numerical terminology employed for the muscarinic sites) are:

1 Acyl group substitution. Now (Table 2.2), propionyl provides the best fit, butyryl is stronger than acetyl and valeryl is a moderately effective agonist: indicating that the 'nicotinic' esteratic site is larger in size than that for a 'muscarinic' effect.

4 Length of intermediate chain.

At autonomic ganglia tetramethylammonium is an agonist which at higher doses (or subsequently, *see* p. 62) produces a depolarising block. Tetr*ethyl*ammonium on the other hand is a competitive (non-depolarising) antagonist at this site.

That the distance between the two essential (esteratic and anionic) receptor sites differs for the autonomic ganglionic and the skeletal neuromuscular junctional sites is suggested by the following observations

• phenyltrimethyl (vice tetramethyl) ammonium is the preferred *agonist* at the skeletal muscle junction

• consider the methonium series of compounds (Fig. 2.4). At the ganglion, optimal blocking action occurs at $n = 5$ or 6 (pentamethonium, C_5 or hexamethonium, C_6) and the effect is non-depolarising block (*see* p. 61), i.e. initial stimulation is absent. At the skeletal neuromuscular junction, the major response is at 10 carbon atoms separation (decamethonium, C_{10}) but in this case there is a depolarisation block

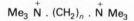

$$\overset{+}{Me_3 \, N} . (CH_2)_n . \overset{+}{N \, Me_3}$$

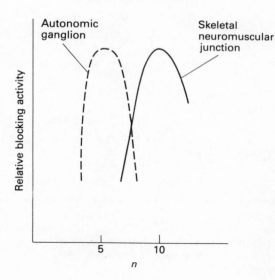

Fig. 2.4 Methonium (bistrimethyl ammonium) compounds with an intermediate polymethylene chain. General formula shown at top of figure. (Below) relative nicotinic blocking activity plotted against number (n) of methylene (CH_2) groups in the intermediate chain (schematic).

(which is preceded by stimulation), with or without subsequent receptor desensitisation (Fig. 2.17). Incidentally, there is a similar distance (about 1–1.45 nm) between the two charged nitrogen atoms of suxamethonium, D-tubocurarine and pancuronium (*see* Fig. 2.12) which also act at this site. The different mechanisms of action are compared in Fig. 2.18.

The most important actions of acetylcholine are systematised in Table 2.3, subdivided according to the two postsynaptic receptor sites. All drugs acting in relation to these situations belong to one or more of the following categories:
- muscarinic agonists ('parasympathomimetic agents')
- muscarinic antagonists

Table 2.3　Important effects mediated via peripheral, *post*synaptic cholinergic and (nor)adrenergic receptors

Site and/or function	Acetylcholine *Muscarinic*	Adrenaline α	β_1	β_2
Smooth muscle				
Bladder				
detrusor	C			R
internal sphincter		C		
Bronchial	C			R
Eye				
iris	C (sphincter pupillae)	C (dilator pupillae)		
ciliary	C			
nictitating membrane (18.1)		C		
Gut (excluding sphincters)	C	R	R	
Uterine	C	C*		R*
Vascular	R (weak)	C		R
Heart tissues				
Force of contraction			+++	
Sinus rate	− − −		+++	
Automaticity†			++ (toxic doses)	
Conduction (Table 10.5, isoprenaline)			+ (only if depressed)	
Glandular tissues				
Alimentary	+++			
Bronchial	+++			
Ciliary body (aqueous humour formation)				++

For smooth muscle: C, contraction; R, relaxation. For other functions: + + +, marked; + +, some and +, slight stimulation; − − −, marked inhibition. Absence of an entry under a heading indicates lack of therapeutically significant effect.
* Varies with species, stage of oestrus, menstrual cycle or pregnancy (Table 15.3).
† For a definition of cardiac automaticity (*see* p. 279).

- nicotinic agonists
- nicotinic antagonists

(In the last two groups, preference can be shown for either autonomic ganglionic or skeletal neuromuscular sites.)

Thus, the relevant actions can be read off from Table 2.3. These different groups of drugs and their particular properties will now be dealt with in detail.

2.4   Parasympathomimetic agents (Table 2.4)

Remember that these will also activate sympathetic cholinergic receptors (e.g. sweat glands subserving heat regulation in the human) and ganglionic muscarinic receptors (p. 61 *et seq.*).

Muscarine poisoning follows ingestion of the mushroom, *Amanita*

Table 2.3 — *Cont'd*

Site and/or function	Acetylcholine *Muscarinic*	Adrenaline α	β_1	β_2
Sweat	+++ (heat-regulating)	++ (emotional, e.g. palmar)		
Penis				
Erection	+++			
Ejaculation‡		+++		
Metabolism				
Glycogenolysis				
liver		++		+++
muscle				+++
Lipolysis			++	
Insulin release (Table 14.6)	++	− − −		
	Nicotinic			
Skeletal neuromuscular junction	+++ (excess produces blockade)			++ (tremor)
Autonomic ganglion (Fig. 2.10)				
Miscellaneous				
Capillaries§				
contraction		+++		
decreased permeability				++
K⁺ ion passage into cells‖				++
Platelets				
aggregation (17.2)		+++		− −
Kidney				
renin release (5.9)			+++¶	+++¶

‡ Also involves somatic nerves to bulbar muscles.
§ Includes small arterioles and venules.
‖ Especially into skeletal muscle, erythrocytes.
¶ Subdivision of *β*-receptors involved is uncertain.

Table 2.4 Substances which activate muscarinic (M-like) and/or nicotinic (N-like) cholinoceptors

Substance	M-like		N-like
Muscarine	+		0
Methacholine (acetyl β-methylcholine)	+	especially cardiovascular system	0
Pilocarpine	+	especially eye and glands	±
Acetylcholine	+	often at much lower dosage than for N-like effects (*see* text)	+
Carbachol	+	especially bladder and gut	+
Benzoylcholine	±		+
Dimethylphenylpiperazinium (DMPP)	0*		+
Tetramethylammonium (TMA) ⎱ lower	0*		+
Nicotine ⎰ doses			
Neostigmine† (direct at skeletal ⎱ higher	0		−
neuromuscular junction ⎰ doses			

Effects: +, present; ±, slight; 0, negligible; −, inhibition.
* Will cause M-like actions *indirectly*, by stimulation of parasympathetic ganglia but these will often be opposed by the concomitant stimulation of sympathetic ganglia (p. 49).
† Also an anticholinesterase at *both* muscarinic and nicotinic sites.

muscaria. Atropine should be given. Note: there are different kinds of poisoning induced by other mushrooms.

S(+)-*methacholine* (Table 2.1) is a muscarinic agonist which mainly affects atrial pacemakers and was once used in the treatment of supraventricular tachycardias. It is slowly hydrolysed by acetylcholinesterase but not by butyrylcholinesterase.

Pilocarpine is mainly muscarine-like: it constricts the pupil and, therefore, decreases the intraocular pressure in glaucoma (Table 18.2).

Carbachol (carbamylcholine) has both muscarinic and nicotinic agonist effects. Its main actions are on the bladder and the gut and it can be used to stimulate these organs if obstruction is absent, e.g. atonic bladder. It is not broken down by either acetyl- or butyrylcholinesterase.

Of the above, only pilocarpine has significant clinical usage.

Following the i.v. injection of acetylcholine in many animal experiments (e.g. cat blood pressure) the muscarinic effects of vasodilation and bradycárdia resulting in hypotension occur at a much lower concentration—about a thousandth—than is necessary for the hypertensive effect generated via nicotinic receptors. This rise in blood pressure is due to sympathetic ganglion stimulation reinforced by adrenal medullary secretion resulting in vasoconstriction and positive inotropic and chronotropic effects (opposed by parasympathetic ganglion activation mainly of a negative chronotropic response). But, in the therapeutic situation, acetylcholine (given exogenously) is ineffective due to its rapid inactivation by acetyl- and butyryl-cholinesterases. However, by preventing breakdown of the transmitter, anticholinesterases are used to produce muscarinic effects or, when these are blocked by atropine, they can manifest nicotinic actions and they are the preferred drugs for both of these sites as described in 2.6.

2.5   Nicotinic agonists

From Table 2.4, it can be seen that dimethylphenylpiperazinium (DMPP) is useful experimentally in this connection as is benzoylcholine (which also, however, shows some direct muscarinic effects). Substances like tetramethylammonium and nicotine itself (with time or increased dosage) pass through the stimulant phase to that of depolarising blockade.

Nicotine is only of toxicological significance. Even then the exact course of its lethal effects is difficult to prophesy, being the result of a multiplicity of actions which are often mutually antagonistic. These include initial stimulation (sometimes absent) followed by depression in relation to either the peripheral nervous systems or the CNS.

Peripheral nervous systems
• skeletal neuromuscular junction (*see* Fig. 2.11)
• autonomic ganglia (both parasympathetic and sympathetic). In many tissues, one or other of the two branches of the autonomic nervous system provides the major control of tone (Table 2.3) and so the actions upon this particular branch of the system will predominate (e.g. parasympathetic *increasing* gut secretions, sympathetic *vasoconstricting* blood vessels and *strengthening cardiac force*). On the heart rate (during the stimulatory phase of nicotinic action) the vagal bradycardia *opposes the sympathetic quickening; the latter usually predominates*
• adrenal medulla and chromaffin tissue (release of catecholamines). The extent of most of this contribution to any final effect (upon rises in blood pressure, for example) can be determined by the responses before and after ligation of the adrenal vessels.

Central nervous system
Stimulation/depression here may be on many centres either directly or reflexly (especially from the carotid and aortic chemoreceptors, on the

controlling areas for respiration and circulation). Two conditions are worthy of note:

1   Acute nicotine poisoning (e.g. from insecticides) which culminates in peripheral respiratory paralysis. This is due to a depolarising block of the relevant skeletal neuromuscular junctions for which there is no antidote (p. 69); treatment is with intermittent positive pressure respiration plus general measures to control fits and blood pressure changes.

2   Smoking. The initiate may experience nausea and vomiting, dizziness and palpitations but tolerance to these effects develops quite rapidly: *see* Table 7.9 for dependence liability. Chronic smokers with concomitant pathology or pregnancy expose themselves to the dangerous effects listed in Table 2.5; drug interactions are more common due to the induction of liver microsomal enzymes (p. 29) and there is an increased incidence of cancer (Fig. 20.3), particularly bronchial.

2.6   Anticholinesterases

Figure 2.5 represents the acetylcholine molecule undergoing hydrolysis at the surface of the acetylcholinesterase locally present at the synapse. The ionic bond formed between the quaternary nitrogen ion of acetylcholine and the anionic site of the enzyme is weaker than the covalent bond via a serine residue at the esteratic site, so that the latter is more persistent. Thus the breakdown of acetylcholine proceeds as shown in Table 2.6, i.e. attachment to both sites of the enzyme, hydrolysis (at A in Fig. 2.5) of the enzyme-substrate compound, the spontaneous dissociation of the weaker bond (the removal of choline from the anionic site) leaving the acetylated enzyme which, as the final step, is rapidly deacetylated. Variations on this theme are produced by the three groups of anticholinesterases also depicted in Table 2.6.

For the actions of anticholinesterases go down the list in Table 2.3, noting cholinergic effects at all muscarinic sites and nicotinic receptors at the skeletal neuromuscular junction (but negligible changes at autonomic ganglia where local acetylcholine hydrolysis is not the major inactivating mechanism — *see* p. 42).

Edrophonium only attaches itself significantly to the anionic site and, as it is rapidly both redistributed to inactive sites and renally excreted, its action is brief. This is ideal for its two indications—as a diagnostic test for myasthenia gravis and to distinguish between a myasthenic and a cholinergic crisis (it relieves the former and intensifies the latter). Edrophonium contains a quaternary nitrogen ion, like acetylcholine, and it also has a direct agonistic action (h, Fig. 2.2) on the receptors of the skeletal neuromuscular junction but (unknown why) *not* at ganglia or muscarinic sites.

Carbamates attach to both sites of the enzyme (Table 2.6). The carbamate end of the anticholinesterase molecule occupies the esteratic site in all cases and the anionic site receives one of the following

Table 2.5 When smoking should be stopped

| Condition | Deleterious effects due to | |
	Nicotine	Other tobacco substances
Angina pectoris	Increased heart work due to increase in rate and force of contraction; increased fatty acid levels in blood (sympathetic stimulation/ adrenaline release—*see* Fig. 14.3)	Carbon monoxide forming carboxyhaemoglobin ⟶ decreased oxygen carriage ⟶ increased heart work
Intermittent claudication (obliterative vascular disease)	Vasoconstriction of leg blood vessels	
Chronic bronchitis		(Unspecified) irritant: lowered ciliary activity
Peptic ulcer	Increased secretion of gastric acid: ? increased output of adrenal glucocorticoids (*see* p. 320)	(Unspecified) irritant
Tobacco amblyopia (18.4)		Cyanide: give hydroxocobalamin to chelate (Table 20.5)
Pregnancy	Vasoconstriction of blood vessels leading to greater incidence of pre-eclampsia	(Unspecified) increased risk of still-birth or neonatal mortality

Fig. 2.5 Hydrolysis of acetylcholine (ACh) by acetylcholinesterase (AChE)—diagrammatic. The ester group of the substrate attaches to a serine .OH group at the esteratic site of the enzyme by a strong (covalent) bond. The cationic head of acetylcholine interacts less strongly (ionic bond, wavy line) with the anionic site. Thus, following hydrolysis (at A), the cationic end of the split molecule (choline) is rapidly released, leaving the acetylated enzyme. This, in turn, is hydrolysed to reactivate the acetylcholinesterase. Anticholinesterases interfere with one or more of these processes and therefore allow the transmitter to exert a more prolonged effect.

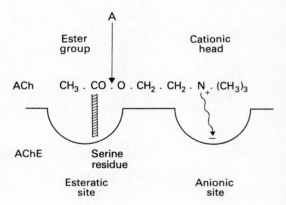

Table 2.6 Stages of interaction with acetylcholinesterase for acetylcholine and three groups of anticholinesterases, and additional effects of these latter at the skeletal neuromuscular junction

	Acetylcholine	Edrophonium	Carbamates, e.g. physostigmine†, neostigmine, pyridostigmine	Organophosphorus compounds, e.g. dyflos (DFP)
Attachment site	Anionic and esteratic	Anionic mainly*	Anionic and esteratic	Esteratic only
Hydrolysis of enzyme–substrate compound	+	0	+	+
Dissociation of bond at anionic site	+	+	+	0
Form of enzyme at this stage	Acetylated	Regenerated	Carbamylated	Phosphorylated
Hydrolysis to regenerate the enzyme	Deacetylation very rapid	0	Decarbamylation: slow (see text)	Dephosphorylation: negligible spontaneously (see text)
Duration of action		Short (few min)	Moderate (several hours)	Prolonged (few weeks)
Direct nicotinic action at skeletal neuromuscular junction		+	Physostigmine 0 Neostigmine + Pyridostigmine +	0

+, present; 0, absent.
* Edrophonium does bind weakly at the esteratic site but this bond dissociates at least as quickly as that at the anionic site.
† Also called eserine.

- a tertiary nitrogen group, which must be protonated (i.e. receive an H^+ ion) before it is capable of forming the necessary ionic bond, e.g. physostigmine (eserine). With a pK_a of 8, it does have, at pH 7.4, a predominance of the charged form
- a quaternary N^+ ion, e.g. neostigmine, pyridostigmine.

Following this attachment at both sites (Table 2.6), hydrolysis occurs (analogous to that at position A in Fig. 2.5) and the group remaining at the anionic site (analogous to choline) is released, leaving the carbamylated enzyme. Decarbamylation is very much slower (millions of times) than deacetylation and therefore *all* the 'local' (acetyl)cholinesterase is effectively bound so that the natural transmitter is free to exert prolonged agonist actions. Additionally the carbamates which contain a quaternary nitrogen ion exert (like edrophonium) a *direct* action at the *skeletal neuromuscular junction* and thus are more effective at this site. So, neostigmine is the drug of choice as an antagonist to competitive inhibitors (e.g. post-operatively to reverse the effects of D-tubocurarine) or in the treatment of myasthenia gravis — a chronic skeletal muscle weakness due to an autoimmune-induced loss of acetylcholine receptors (p. 93). In this latter condition, *oral* pyridostigmine is often preferred as it is longer-lasting. If these drugs have to be *injected*, it is rational to add atropine (ideally, given 5 minutes earlier, *see* next section) to prevent unwanted muscarinic side-effects but in myasthenia this has the disadvantage that it will nullify an important sign of overdose (cholinergic crisis), namely pupillary constriction. When carbamate anticholinesterases are required to act at a muscarinic site, neostigmine does not have the advantage of any direct action and in fact physostigmine (which is less charged and so crosses the blood–brain barrier more readily) is preferred for an effect upon the CNS, e.g. in the treatment of atropine poisoning (*see* next section) and Huntington's chorea (7.2). Physostigmine is also used for its muscarinic effects on the eye—in glaucoma or to reverse homatropine (p. 391).

Organophosphorus compounds (type substance, dyflos) were developed during World War II as 'nerve gases' and some (e.g. malathion—which is selectively inactivated by humans) are widely used as insecticides. As shown in Table 2.6, they attach only to the esteratic site. The bond there is initially reversible but subsequently it assumes an 'aged' (dealkylated) form which is irreversible either spontaneously or by use of an antidote (*see* later): it is therefore vital to give the antidote immediately. When untreated, the duration of action of this group of anticholinesterases can be very protracted (up to a few weeks). This could be beneficial in chronic diseases such as myasthenia gravis and glaucoma, to obviate the necessity of daily therapy, but unfortunately the organophosphorus anticholinesterases, have not been successful in practice for three reasons:

1 Lack of specificity: because they attach to the enzyme at a serine

group (Fig. 2.5), they inhibit other serine esterases (hydrolases), e.g. trypsin, thrombin.

2   The development of tolerance due to decreased acetylcholine release and receptor subsensitivity.

3   Nerve demyelination in the long term due to inhibition of a neuropathy target ('neurotoxic') esterase.

Consequently, their significance is toxicological rather than therapeutic. A variant—ecothiopate (an organophosphorus derivative of thiocholine and thus attaching at both sites of acetylcholinesterase)—is sometimes used in glaucoma (p. 391). Long term there is a danger of cataract.

During the reversible phase, organophosphorus anticholinesterases can be antagonised (Fig. 2.6). Pralidoxime (which has a quaternary nitrogen ion) attaches to the *unoccupied* anionic site and its free oxime end 'attracts' the phosphorus atom from the esteratic site of the enzyme: the oxime-phosphonate then detaches from the anionic site leaving the reactivated cholinesterase. But as pralidoxime is a charged compound it will not cross the blood–brain barrier, and is therefore useless against the CNS manifestations of anticholinesterase poisoning. Further, it needs to attach to the anionic site of the enzyme, and, accordingly, is less effective as an antidote to the carbamate anticholinesterases where that site is not free: in excess it can act as an anticholinesterase itself.

Other oximes are available, e.g. obidoxime (which is more potent) and, e.g. diacetylmonoxime (DAM). The latter antidote lacks a quaternary nitrogen ion so that it combines mainly with organophosphorus compounds free in the body fluids—rather than those bound to a cholinesterase—and is, therefore, less effective; but, it can cross the blood–brain barrier.

Deaths from poisoning by the organophosphorus anticholinesterases result from three main mechanisms.

1   Excessive muscarinic stimulation peripherally, resulting in bronchoconstriction and bronchorrhoea: antagonised by atropine/pralidoxime.

2   Progressive nicotinic excitation peripherally, leading to a depolarising block at all skeletal neuromuscular junctions. The lethal manifestation is a peripheral respiratory paralysis: treat with intermittent positive pressure (because of the accompanying bronchoconstriction) respiration and pralidoxime.

3   CNS effects due to an excess of acetylcholine. These will be more severe the greater the lipid solubility of the poison, as it will then enter the neuraxis more readily. Dyflos is extremely lipid-soluble and it produces protean CNS effects: these are to some extent reversible with atropine; diazepam is useful against convulsive phases. Also use DAM.

2.7   Muscarinic antagonists (antimuscarinic agents)

All useful ones are competitive in type. Valerylcholine, as shown earlier (Table 2.1), can attach to the anionic site of the receptor but (due to its

Fig. 2.6 How pralidoxime (pyridine 2-aldoxime methiodide, P2AM) reactivates cholinesterase reversibly bound by an organic phosphorus-containing compound (R.P at the esteratic site). The antidote attaches to the vacant anionic site and its free oxime group is situated at just the right distance to combine with the P atom and break its bond (a) with the esteratic site (interrupted lines). The resultant oximephosphorus compound is then liberated from the anionic site to regenerate the enzyme.

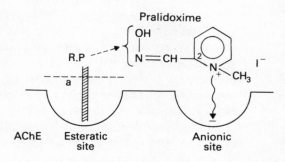

size) is unable to combine with the esteratic site and, thereby, effectively hinders combination of transmitter acetylcholine with that vital position. Many other choline derivatives with large groups at the acyl end of the molecule similarly act as antagonists. Some illustrative formulae are shown in Fig. 2.7. Both benzilylcholine and lachesine (and atropine, *see* below) act as reversible, competitive antagonists. The formation of a corresponding nitrogen mustard produces an *irreversible* antagonist, e.g. benzilylcholine nitrogen mustard. For note on subdivision of muscarinic receptors *see* p. 61 and Table 2.9.

Atropine (given as the racemate which is, chemically, DL-hyoscyamine) has a structural formula which is less easily visualised as

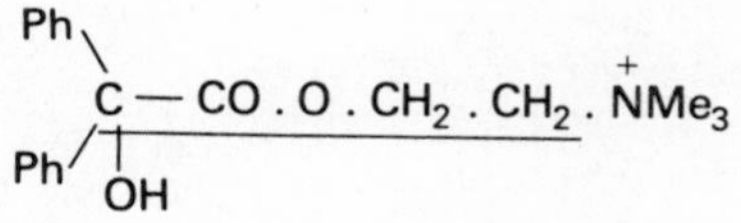

Benzilylcholine

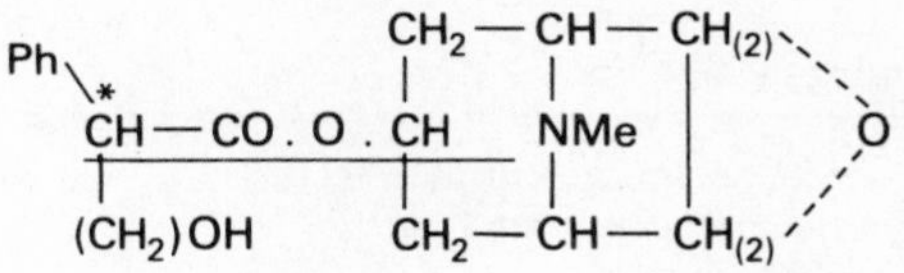

Atropine

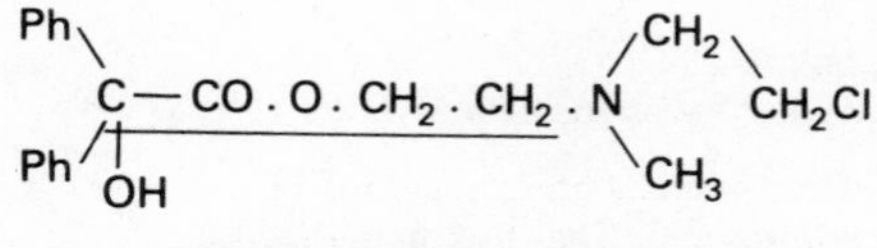

Benzilylcholine mustard

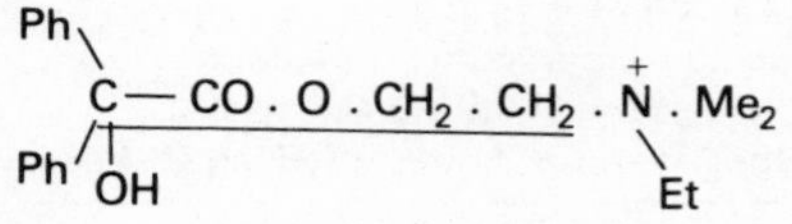

Fig. 2.7 Antimuscarinic agents—illustrative formulae. Ph = phenyl. Underlined segments indicate approximation to five atom rule (p. 43, **4**). In the atropine formula: *indicates the asymmetric carbon atom; interrupted lines indicate formation of corresponding epoxide, hyoscine; removal of bracketed methylene (CH_2) group forms next lower *hom*ologue, *hom*atropine.

Lachesine

providing antagonistic properties at the muscarinic receptor; but it is the type substance in this connection. Its actions may conveniently be divided into those normally occurring at therapeutic concentrations and those of toxicological significance (Table 2.7). The therapeutically useful actions are practically all antimuscarinic and can be determined by reference to Table 2.3. These effects are particularly shown in organs which are normally in strong parasympathetic tone, e.g. eye, heart, salivary glands, but will affect others *either* if in spasm, e.g. gut (colic), bronchioles (asthma) *or* if only marginally functional, e.g. hesitant micturition or impotence in older males. Tachycardia is characteristic. However, this may be absent in infants and the elderly, due to their minimal vagal tone to the heart. It may also be preceded by bradycardia, caused by stimulation of the cardioinhibitory centre (Fig. 10.7), which action has a shorter latency than the peripheral vagal blockade. This effect is evanescent and is only significant in practice if other vagal stimulation is simultaneously present. Thus, if neostigmine has to be *injected* in the treatment of myasthenia gravis (2.6) or post-operatively to antagonise a non-depolarising, skeletal neuromuscular blocker (e.g. D-tubocurarine), atropine should be administered 5 minutes previously, so that the vagal effects do not summate to produce a dangerous degree of bradycardia.

Apart from this one CNS effect and its original use against parkinsonism (7.2), the central effects of atropine are only produced by

Table 2.7   The actions of atropine

Therapeutic dose or 'full' atropinisation prior to operation	Toxicological (higher) dose, e.g Belladonna poisoning

Peripheral antimuscarinic effects particularly manifested as:
  pupil dilation
  loss of accommodation for near vision
  tachycardia
  dry mouth (decreased salivary
  secretions)
	The same effects to a greater degree resulting in:
	  widely dilated pupil
	  blurring of near vision
	  racing pulse: palpitations
	  difficulty in swallowing
	
	  dry, hot skin
	  (decreased sweat secretion)

CNS stimulation only significant on the cardioinhibitory centre to produce (not always) a slight, evanescent, initial bradycardia (*see* text)	CNS effects marked and consisting of initial stimulant actions (hallucinations, delirium, convulsions) leading, subsequently, to coma and CNS paralysis with terminal respiratory depression
	Peripheral vasodilation by a direct action (possibly due to the prevention of passage of calcium ions through the blood vessel walls) resulting in, for example, a reddened skin

overdose (Table 2.7). This should be treated with physostigmine (an anticholinesterase which enters the CNS) plus diazepam if convulsions are a prominent feature.

Toxic doses also cause flushing of the skin due to direct peripheral vasodilation (Table 2.7).

Hyoscine is the epoxide of atropine (Fig. 2.7) and is usually prescribed as the S($-$)L-form (US: scopolamine). It has antimuscarinic actions which are qualitatively identical to those of atropine, though (quantitatively) hyoscine is rather more potent on the eye and bronchial secretion but produces less gut relaxation and tachycardia than atropine. In contrast, its CNS effects occur at similar (*not higher*) doses and are *predominantly depressant*, including amnesia. Therefore, hyoscine is generally preferred if central sedative actions are required (e.g. motion sickness, 13.4) or in pre-operative medication, except in children and the elderly where decreased CNS activity may not be desirable. Like atropine, however, hyoscine *in overdose* produces stimulation and this can occur with therapeutic doses, especially in the presence of pain or in the elderly to cause confusion.

Homatropine, is an antimuscarinic drug, which is, chemically, the next lower homologue of atropine (Fig. 2.7). It is usefully applied to the eye where (*see* Table 2.8) its actions are both weaker (and therefore less likely to precipitate glaucoma in susceptible patients) and of shorter duration than those of atropine. This makes it preferable as a short-term cycloplegic and mydriatic in ophthalmological investigations, especially as the effects can be more readily reversed with physostigmine, (but see footnote [†] to Table 2.8). However, if the sphincter pupillae is in spasm, as in acute (irido)cyclitis, the more potent atropine is mandatory and its *prolonged* dilation of the pupil is also advantageous.

Table 2.8 Comparison of the effects of atropine and homatropine upon the eye (applied as drops into the conjunctival sac)

	Atropine	Homatropine
Potency	*c.* 10	1
Duration of		
cycloplegia	2–3 days	$\frac{1}{2}$–1 day
mydriasis	1–2 weeks	1–2 days
Reversibility with physostigmine	Difficult: only partial*	Easy
Clinical indication(s)	Acute iridocyclitis	General mydriatic and cycloplegic[†]

* Although in theory complete reversal should be feasible, in practice it is not, possibly due to difficulty in achieving an adequate concentration of the antidote at the site.
[†] *See* p. 392, replaced by tropicamide—which has an even shorter action—for routine retinoscopy.

Pirenzepine is a selective antagonist at M_1 muscarinic receptors (Table 2.9) which is used in the treatment of peptic ulcer (p. 319) with fewer peripheral side-effects than atropine. It also has negligible CNS actions due to insignificant passage across the blood–brain barrier.

A number of commonly used drugs have peripheral antimuscarinic side-effects, particularly chlorpromazine (Table 7.6), imipramine (Table 7.8), pethidine (7.12) and many anti-(H_1)histamines (Table 5.5).

Therapeutic uses of antimuscarinic substances

Atropine and its allies are very important drugs, not only because of their effectiveness but also due to their wide range of uses, as follows:

1 *Peripheral* (go down the list in Table 2.3, omitting irrelevant headings)

a Smooth muscle

• bladder. Vesicular spasm, e.g. accompanying infection (care in prostatism)

• bronchial. Asthma: not primarily used as tends to thicken the secretions (p. 291); ipratropium inhalation might have less of this disadvantage

• eye. For routine dilation of the pupil and cycoplegia. Acute irido-cyclitis

• gut. Spastic colon.

b Heart tissues

Against bradycardia following myocardial infarction or induced by the general anaesthetic, halothane (Table 8.7). Halothane also enhances the production of (nor)adrenergic ventricular dysrhythmias, which are accentuated in the presence of vagal slowing (*see* p. 282) and are thus minimised by the use of atropine. This is the main reason for giving it as pre-operative medication nowadays (8.6).

c Glands

Alimentary (gastric): *see* peptic ulcer treatment, p. 319

d All peripheral tissues

With neostigmine (to offset its muscarinic side-effects) in the antagonism of D-tubocurarine postoperatively or in the treatment of myasthenia gravis (but note caveat, p. 56).

2 *Peripheral and central*

• parkinsonism (p. 173). As well as correcting the dopaminergic/cholinergic imbalance in the CNS (caudate nucleus), antimuscarinic drugs (e.g. benzhexol, orphenadrine, Table 6.2), also decrease hypersalivation which sometimes occurs in the condition

• poisoning with *Amanita muscaria* (pp. 47–8) or anticholinesterases

• pre-operative medication (in all but the young and the very old, hyoscine can be used, p. 220).

3   Central

Antimuscarinic substances are used as anti-emetics (e.g. hyoscine (p. 317). In this they overlap greatly with H_1 (histamine)-antagonists.

2.8   Drugs which block ganglionic cholinergic synapses

'*A drug is stated to be a ganglion-blocking agent. How would you determine its exact site and mode of action?*'

A suitable preparation is the superior cervical ganglion (Fig. 2.8). Experiments to perform (in successive order) are as follows:

I Stimulate alternately (at 10-second intervals) pre- and postsynaptically: then, after a control period, give the test drug intra-arterially. Subsequent loss of the response to pre- but not to postsynaptic stimulation confirms that the drug is a specific ganglion-blocking agent. If both routes of stimulation are now ineffectual, the conclusion is that the agent is a local anaesthetic, preventing conduction along all nerves.
II The next stage is to determine whether the block is pre- or postsynaptic. The simplest method is to inject acetylcholine intra-arterially before and after the effect of the blocking drug on the response to presynaptic nerve stimulation has been produced. If the response to acetylcholine is unaffected by administration of the drug, the latter is exerting its blocking action *pre*synaptically, e.g. hemicholinium-3 in

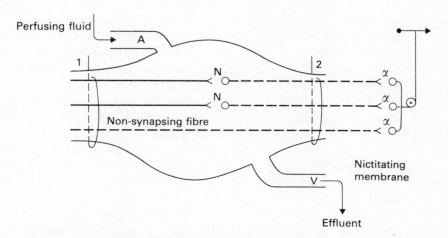

Fig. 2.8 Superior cervical ganglion (diagrammatic). Effects produced at the nicotinic junctions (N) of *synapsing* fibres can be monitored by observing the contractions (via postsynaptic noradrenergic fibres — interrupted lines — and α-adrenoceptors; *see* Chapter 3) of the nictitating membrane. 1 and 2 indicate, respectively, pre- and postganglionic stimulation sites. Vascular perfusion is achieved via the appropriate artery (A) with collection of the effluent from the corresponding vein (V).

Fig. 2.9. However, if the response to acetylcholine decreases similarly to that of nerve stimulation in the presence of the blocking agent, there is a *post*synaptic element in the latter's action, e.g. D-tubocurarine in Fig. 2.14a.

III A *pre*synaptic action can be further analysed (Fig. 2.2) by remembering the mnemonic 'USSR', indicating changes in:

Uptake of choline (blocked by hemicholinium-3, triethylcholine)

Synthesis of acetylcholine (choline acetylase inhibited by diphenylbutyl acetate, for example)

Storage of the transmitter (opposed by black widow spider—*Latrodectus*—venom: the active ingredient is α-latrotoxin)

Release (decreased by botulinum toxin).

Synthesis block is readily detected by an appropriate biochemical experiment to show any diminution in choline acetyltransferase activity. Storage prevention is indicated by an initial increase in output of the transmitter followed by the loss of vesicles and complete disorganisation of the junction as shown on an electron micrograph a few days later (α-latrotoxin produces similar effects at noradrenergic presynaptic terminals).

Thus, the analysis finally involves a separation of, for example, the effects of hemicholinium-3 from those of botulinum toxin. The former has three characteristic distinguishing features (most easily shown at the skeletal neuromuscular junction, Fig. 2.9) namely

• the block produced is frequency-dependent, i.e. the faster the nerve is stimulated the more intense is the effect as the acetylcholine synthesis progressively fails to match its release (not shown by botulinum toxin which is merely stopping release of preformed transmitter)

• the block is reversible by choline (that due to botulinum toxin is not)

• *during the development of the block*, with hemicholinium-3 the miniature end-plate potentials (mepps) decrease in size but not in frequency (whereas with botulinum toxin there is a decrease in frequency but not in size). With complete block, of course, there are no mepps. Hemicholinium block also has a slow onset (not shown in Fig. 2.9) because preformed acetylcholine stores have first to be depleted.

IV If experiment **II** indicated a *post*synaptic action of the drug this could be particularised as follows. Consider the postsynaptic receptors present at an autonomic ganglion. Transmission is normally nicotinic but, *if the nicotinic element is almost eliminated* by D-tubocurarine, other processes can be revealed as manifested in the ganglion potential recorded postsynaptically following preganglionic stimulation.

As shown in Fig. 2.10 there are three main phases, namely:

1 An initial depolarisation mediated by activation of the nicotinic receptors which are normally primarily involved in ganglionic transmission.

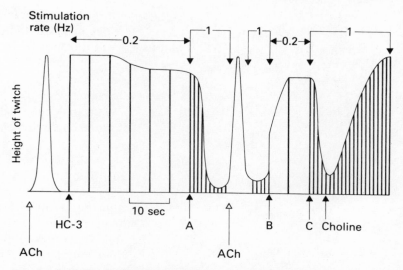

Fig. 2.9 Distinguishing features of the block produced by *hemicholinium-3 (HC-3)* at the mammalian skeletal neuromuscular junction (schematic). Lack of effect on the response to intra-arterial injection of acetylcholine (ACh) indicates a *pre*synaptic site of action. Frequency-dependence is shown by intensification of the block when the rate of stimulation is increased from 0.2 to 1 Hz (A,C) and vice versa (B). Choline relieves the paralysis. *Note*: In subsequent similar diagrams, simplification may be achieved by replacing individual twitches by the response profile.

2 A subsequent hyperpolarisation via M_2-muscarinic cholinoceptors.*
3 A delayed depolarisation via M_1-muscarinic cholinoceptors.*

Phases **2** and **3**, however, are not normally significantly concerned in the transganglionic passage of the nerve impulse, so that any immediate postganglionic blockade may simply be considered in terms of nicotinic receptors. As stated earlier, there are two possible mechanisms of postsynaptic block.

1 *A non-depolarising block* which manifests itself by lack of initial stimulation. This may be a reversible, competitive antagonism, e.g. with tetraethylammonium (p. 45). However, in the cases of hexamethonium, pentamethonium and D-tubocurarine the site of blockade is not

---

*Note on subdivision of muscarinic receptors: Determinations of the molecular structures of muscarinic receptors (p. 104) indicate at least four subtypes, and functional studies should soon enable a rational subdivision to be made. The present classification, based on selective binding of the antagonist, pirenzepine (p. 58), and the agonist, McN-A-343, to M_1 receptors, is unsatisfactory. A provisional subclassification is given in Table 2.9. Apart from pirenzepine, all the *commonly used* muscarinic antagonists are non-selective on this basis.

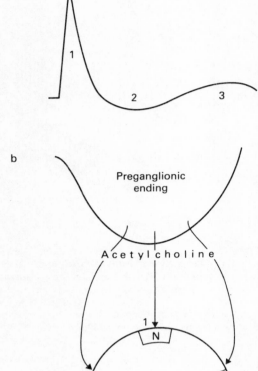

Fig. 2.10 Transmission processes occurring at an autonomic ganglion (*see* text). a, Postsynaptic potential registered in a *partially curarised* ganglion, showing phases **1**, **2** and **3**. b, Interpretation of the processes involved in a. The acetylcholine released acts on either nicotinic (N) or muscarinic (M_1 or M_2) cholinoceptors.

the acetylcholine receptor but its associated channel: so that they are *not* competitive antagonists whose inhibition can be overcome by increasing the agonist concentration. In fact the block which produces D-tubocurarine is *use-dependent*, i.e. the more frequently the channel is opened by the agonist the greater the degree of block, and increased by hyperpolarisation which enhances negativity at channel sites so that the cationic drug binds more effectively. The antagonism produced by hexamethonium also shows this latter property but is not use-dependent.

2   *Depolarisation block*, e.g. with tetramethylammonium (p. 45) or nicotine. This effect is preceded by an initial stimulation of the postsynaptic soma but then excess of the transmitter, or one of these

Table 2.9 A provisional subdivision of muscarinic cholinoceptors

	M_1	M_2	M_3
Selective agonist	McN-A-343	Pilocarpine	?
Selective antagonist	Pirenzepine	AF-DX 116 Gallamine*	4-DAMP†
Site and effect	Postsynaptic delayed depolarisation at autonomic ganglia (Fig. 2.10)	Atrial actions (Table 10.5) Presynaptic inhibition of acetylcholine release (Fig. 2.1, lower)	Glandular secretions (e.g. alimentary) increased Some smooth muscle actions, e.g. bronchoconstriction (Fig. 11.1)

* Also 'curare-like' at the skeletal neuromuscular junction (Table 2.10, p. 67).
† 4-DAMP, 4-*d*iphenyl*a*cetoxy-N-*m*ethyl*p*iperidine methiodide. Other drugs with abbreviated titles are not acronyms.

similarly acting agents, results in an inactivation of the synapse (for possible mechanisms *see* 2.10) *which cannot be relieved by increasing the agonist concentration.*

Ganglion-blocking agents of the non-depolarising type were once used in the treatment of hypertension but abandoned because of their unacceptable side-effects. See if you can work out their actions, using Table 2.3. Here is a start:

1 Block of sympathetic ganglia. Therapeutic action: to lower a raised blood pressure. Side-effects: postural hypotension (Fig. 10.6), loss of ejaculation.
2 Block of parasympathetic ganglia. Side-effects similar to those to atropine (Table 2.7) although exerted more proximally.

Notes on the release of catecholamines from the adrenal medulla
1 By splanchnic nerve stimulation. Classically the terminals release acetylcholine which interacts with nicotinic receptors on the adrenal medullary cells (Fig. 2.1): recently, however, some excitatory postsynaptic muscarinic receptors have been characterised, *which are not predominant* but can be evoked under specific circumstances. The immediate analogy which springs to mind is that of postsynaptic receptors at the autonomic ganglion, but a more pertinent similarity is that of the Renshaw cell (6.2) where both nicotinic and muscarinic postsynaptic receptors are excitatory with the former predominant. Additionally, at *low-frequency* stimulation (0.5 Hz), significant catecholamine secretion still occurs in the presence of combined nicotinic and muscarinic receptor block, which is attributed to the liberation of an

excitatory co-transmitter (p. 141). NB An enkephalin is also released at this site (p. 167).

2   By autacoids, e.g. histamine (p. 131), 5-hydroxytryptamine (p. 132). Low concentrations of histamine cause release by a direct (H_1-receptor) action on adrenal medullary cells but at higher concentrations there is additional catecholamine secretion which is dependent upon an intact innervation.

2.9   Cholinergic synapses (excluding presynaptic receptors)

Figure 2.11 illustrates major sites and types of drug actions. The central part of the diagram represents the autonomic ganglion discussed in the previous section. As can be seen, at both the muscarinic (postsynaptic) junctions and the skeletal neuromuscular synapses, the drugs acting *pre*synaptically exert effects similar to those shown for the ganglion, but the *post*synaptically acting agents differ—particularly with respect to blocking mechanisms. At the purely muscarinic synapses only competitive antagonism is possible. At the skeletal neuromuscular junction, even more complicated processes than those occurring in the ganglion can be involved (*see* section 2.10).

2.10   Skeletal neuromuscular junction block

Presynaptic

Similar to the ganglion except for the addition of an extra stage (between storage and release in Fig. 2.11), of mobilisation, i.e. the passage of acetylcholine-containing vesicles from their usual (central) site in the nerve terminals to fusion with the terminal membrane prior to the ejection of the transmitter by exocytosis. This process is opposed by aminoglycoside antibiotics (e.g. gentamicin, 19.6) which prevent calcium ion entry into the nerve terminal (p. 41).

Postsynaptic

There are five mechanisms of blockade here but it is simplest initially to concentrate on the two types which yield the only therapeutically useful agents. These are

● non-depolarising (competitive, reversible) blockers, e.g. D-tubocurarine

● depolarising (non-competitive) antagonists, e.g. suxamethonium

A comparison of these substances is made in Table 2.10. Note (as shown in Fig. 2.12) the separation of their two charged nitrogen groups by the 'skeletal neuromuscular' distance of 1–1.45 nm. Obviously, such highly ionised substances are inactive by mouth and to produce the rapid effects for which they are used, they are given intravenously.

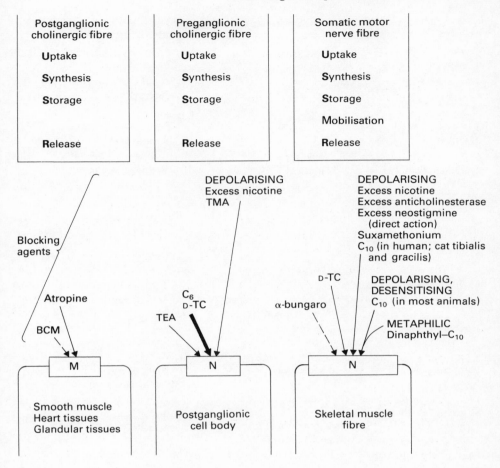

Fig. 2.11 Possible sites of drug interaction at cholinergic synapses; muscarinic (M), at a postganglionic ending (left); mainly nicotinic (N), autonomic ganglion (centre) and skeletal neuromuscular junction (N, right). *Presynaptically*, the three situations are similar with identical agents working upon the processes of uptake of choline (U), synthesis of acetylcholine (S), its storage (S) and release (R). *Postsynaptically*, blocking agents are exemplified. Non-depolarising drugs are shown approaching each receptor on *the left* at all synapses: thin, continuous lines if competitive reversible, e.g. atropine, TEA (tetraethylammonium), D-Tc (D-tubocurarine) at the skeletal neuromuscular junction); interrupted lines if competitive irreversible, e.g. BCM benzilycholine mustard: α-bungaro (toxin); the thick, continuous line indicates non-depolarising drugs which do not *act* competitively, e.g. C_6 (hexamethonium), D-TC at the autonomic ganglion. At the M junction these are the only types of blocker; at the ganglion, depolarising blockade may additionally occur; at the skeletal neuromuscular synapse, even further mechanisms of antagonism may be involved, e.g. desensitisation, metaphilic block. Examples of drugs acting in relation to depolarising mechanisms (*see* p. 62 and Fig. 2.18) are indicated as approaching the relevant receptor on *the right*. TMA, tetramethylammonium; C_{10}, decamethonium.

Table 2.10 A comparison between curare and suxamethonium

Pharmacopoeial name	D-tubocurarine	Suxamethonium
Correct chemical name	D-tubocurarine	Succinyldicholine
Other synonyms	Curare	Scoline®; US: succinylcholine
Route of administration	i.v.	i.v.
Inactivation/excretion	Hepatic metabolism and unchanged via kidney	Rapidly hydrolysed by plasma cholinesterase
Duration of paralytic action	10–30 minutes	1–3 minutes
Actions 1. Skeletal neuromuscular junction		
(a) Focally innervated (twitch) muscle, e.g. mammalian		
Initial stimulation	Absent	Present but lasts less than a minute
Paralysis due to	Non-depolarising (competitive, reversible) antagonism	Depolarising block: can be followed by desensitisation (*see* text)
End-plate potential	Decreased to zero	High; falls to zero in desensitisation phase
Block relieved by (experimentally) (in the clinical situation)	Application of cathode Stimulation of motor nerve Anticholinesterases (e.g. neostigmine, 2.6)	Application of anode D-tubocurarine No antidote (*see* text)
During the development of the block tetanus post-tetanic potentiation	 Poorly maintained Present	 Well-maintained Absent
(b) Multiply innervated (contracture) muscle, e.g. frog rectus	Negligible effect	Contracture
(c) Avian muscle, e.g. chick biventer	Flaccid paralysis	Spastic paralysis
2. Autonomic ganglion	Non-depolarising (channel) block *see* pp. 61–62	(Weak) initial stimulation followed by depolarising block
3. Histamine release	Often marked	Uncommon/slight
Pharmacogenetic effects	Not significant	(Table 20.4) prolonged apnoea in the presence of low affinity plasma cholinesterase (1A): malignant

Table 2.10 — *Cont'd*

Drugs acting in a similar fashion at the neuromuscular junction	Pancuronium, atracurium, vecuronium, gallamine; benzoquinonium and hemicholinium-3 (*see* Table 2.11); halothane (p. 220); α-bungarotoxin (irreversible: used as a ligand, Table 4.3)	hyperthermia (8) Anticholinesterases, e.g. excess of neostigmine in the treatment of myasthenia gravis (2.6). Decamethonium in human and a few cat muscles, e.g. tibialis, gracilis (Fig. 2.17a)
Uses	Relaxation (e.g. of the abdominal muscles during surgery)	Relaxation of larynx prior to intubation; with electroconvulsive therapy; to decrease muscle spasm prior to reduction of a fracture or dislocation

$$(CH_3)_3 . \overset{+}{N} \underline{\hspace{5cm}} (CH_2)_{10} \underline{\hspace{5cm}} \overset{+}{N}(CH_3)_3$$

Decamethonium

$$(CH_3)_3 . \overset{+}{N} \cdot CH_2 . CH_2 . O . CO . CH_2 . CH_2 . CO . O . CH_2 . CH_2 . \overset{+}{N}(CH_3)_3$$

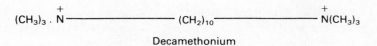

Choline residue   1   Succinic acid residue   2   Choline residue

Suxamethonium (succinyldicholine)

$(CH_3)_2 . \overset{+}{N}$ $\overset{CH_3}{\underset{H}{\overset{+}{N}}}$ Protonated

D-tubocurarine

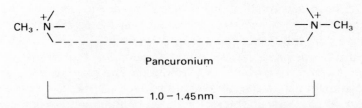

$CH_3 . \overset{+}{N} —$ $— \overset{+}{N} — CH_3$

Pancuronium

|— 1.0 – 1.45 nm —|

Fig. 2.12 Illustrative skeleton formulae of some drugs acting to block the skeletal neuromuscular junction. Suxamethonium breakdown by *plasma* cholinesterase takes place successively at sites 1 and 2. *See also* Fig. 2.4.

Suxamethonium is destroyed by plasma (but not acetyl-) cholines-terase via succinyl monocholine to choline (sites 1 and 2 in Fig. 2.12) in a few minutes—except in patients with diminished plasma cholinester-ase either due to anticholinesterase poisoning (2.6) or to idiosyncrasy (1A, Table 20.4). Conversely, and very uncommonly, patients with a more potent plasma cholinesterase (idiosyncrasy 1B, Table 20.4), re-main unaffected by suxamethonium.

There is insignificant absorption of D-tubocurarine from the gut. Hunters who use this arrow poison know that, after paralysis of the animal and its respiratory failure or clubbing to death, they may safely eat the prey—unless they have a cut inside the mouth through which the agent would gain immediate access to the circulation. D-tubocurarine given intravenously is partly broken down in the liver and partly excreted unchanged in the urine; however, its duration of action of 10–30 minutes (depending on the dose) is probably mainly determined by redistribution.

The paralysis produced by D-tubocurarine on mammalian (focally innervated) skeletal muscle occurs almost immediately and is due to the antagonist molecules occupying the postsynaptic receptors, decreasing the frequency of channel opening and, thus, preventing the develop-ment of the end-plate potential. So the latter decays to zero and an action potential cannot be generated in the muscle fibre. This situation may be reversed (i.e. the block relieved) by mechanisms which depolarise the end-plate region: experimentally by the application of a cathode or motor nerve stimulation; in the intact animal by the administration of neostigmine.

With *suxamethonium*, there is initially muscle stimulation (fascicu-lations: which can cause post-operative pain: mechanism uncertain) but this is evanescent and depolarising block ensues within a minute. There are a number of explanations for this unusual phenomenon; one is shown in Fig. 2.13. Depolarisation produces the propagated action potential (a) but, due to the continued presence of the depolarising agent at the end-plate, repolarisation of the adjacent muscle membranes is incomplete (d). While the *h* gates of their sodium channels are mainly open at full repolarisation (say, -90 mV—see Fig. 8.1, lower, and *caveat* in caption), they are 100% closed at -50 mV. Thus, some further action potentials (b, c) are generated. Subsequently, the end-plate held at such 'high' (less negative) potentials that the *h* gates of the sodium channels are fully inactivated (Fig. 8.2) and it is impossible to achieve the brief depolarisations necessary to generate action potentials: i.e. there is a 'zone of inexcitability' round the end-plate region preventing activation of the muscle fibres. Another idea ascribes the repolarisation defect to the loss of internal potassium ions consequent upon the sustained depolarisation of the junction, which results in a less negative

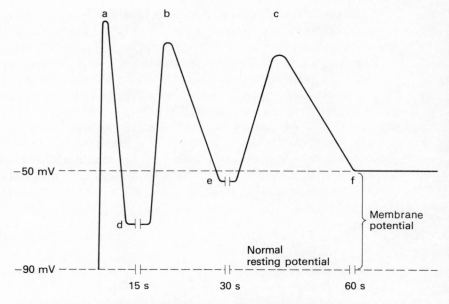

Fig. 2.13 One explanation of the onset of depolarisation block in a focally innervated skeletal muscle (schematic). a, b and c represent propagated muscle fibre action potentials (at 0, 15 and 30 s after suxamethonium) which are initially generated (*see* Fig. 2.14b) as the membrane potential gradually builds up to a depolarisation of 40 mV. At 60 s this latter value is reached, the voltage-sensitive sodium channels become completely inactivated and the muscle is paralysed to nerve stimulation. d, e and f indicate incomplete repolarisations.

resting potential. Whatever the precise explanation of the paralysis, it is obviously made worse by neostigmine which, in addition to intensifying the depolarisation, also prolongs the effect by preventing the breakdown of suxamethonium. Under *experimental* conditions such a depolarising block can be reversed by processes which decrease the endplate potential, e.g. the application of an anode or D-tubocurarine. In practice, the latter is unsatisfactory as an antidote for the following reasons. First, imagine that a patient is paralysed with a depolarising neuromuscular blocking agent: a dose of D-tubocurarine is given and the paralysis persists. There is now no *simple* way of deciding whether the antidotal treatment has been inadequate or whether it has been excessive and produced a competitive blockade. Of course, the distinction can readily be made in the experimental animal by motor nerve stimulation or injecting neostigmine (*see* Table 2.10). But, in the patient, use of ulnar nerve stimulation to see if the tetanus (e.g. in the adductor pollicis) wanes or a test injection of edrophonium is not always diagnostic. *Secondly*, there is evidence that suxamethonium blockade may contain a desensitisation element (p. 75) which would not be reversible by D-tubocurarine. Thus, for practical purposes, there are not any antidotes to depolarising drugs.

Further differences between D-tubocurarine and suxamethonium are shown by nerve stimulation at a rate sufficient to produce tetanus of the muscle (indirect tetanic stimulation) (Table 2.10 and Fig. 2.14) *during the development of the block*. The competitive antagonist shows a poorly maintained tetanus and post-tetanic potentiation while the depolarising blocker gives a well-maintained tetanus but no post-tetanic potentiation. Whereas most of Fig. 2.14 shows the drug effects upon a focally innervated muscle (e.g. cat tibialis) indirectly stimulated once every 10 seconds with a pulse duration of a few ms, the tetanic

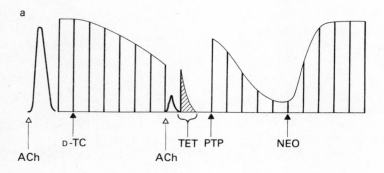

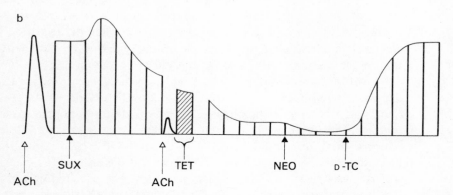

Fig. 2.14 Characteristics of mammalian skeletal neuromuscular blockade by: a, *D-tubocurarine (D-Tc)*, a competitive, reversible antagonist, showing lack of initial stimulation, poorly maintained tetanus (TET), post-tetanic potentiation (PTP) and reversal by neostigmine (NEO).

b, *Suxamethonium (SUX)*, a predominantly depolarising agent, showing initial stimulation, well-maintained tetanus, no post-tetanic potentiation, made worse by neostigmine (*see* text) and reversal by D-tubocurarine. *See* note to Fig. 2.9 for reference to response profile. Note that both drugs act *post*synaptically as shown by the decreased responses to local (close) arterial injections of acetylcholine (ACh).

stimulation consists of about a hundred pulses (of similar duration) every second for 10 seconds. Increased synaptic usage enhances excitation-secretion coupling which during the tetanus is offset by massive release. But for a time after the tetanus there is increased transmitter release *per twitch stimulus* which partially relieves the D-tubocurarine block i.e. produces post-tetanic potentiation. Conversely, the arrival of more transmitter at the receptor sites following tetanic stimulation will tend to intensify the suxamethonium block, so there is no post-tetanic potentiation.

One explanation (probably a considerable over-simplification) of the degree of *maintenance* of the tetanus is as follows. In Fig. 2.15 it can be seen that the amount of the transmitter released during tetanic stimulation falls off with time as release is exceeding synthesis. Due to the occupation by D-tubocurarine of postsynaptic receptor sites, the threshold amount of transmitter required to generate sufficient end-plate potential to activate a twitch is raised (to 2) so that the tetanic contraction is short-lived. Additionally, there is recent evidence that *during tetanic stimulation* D-tubocurarine can significantly decrease release of acetylcholine possibly by the blockade of *pre*synaptic facilitatory nicotinic cholinoceptors. (Fig. 2.1, lower). These explanations (and other suggestions) for the poorly maintained tetanus with D-tubocurarine may be rationalised as producing an unfavourable imbalance between the number of transmitter molecules necessary and those available at the motor end-plate. On the other hand with *suxamethonium, during the development of the block* there is an all-or-none response (i.e. each individual motor unit is either completely blocked or unblocked) *with a normal threshold* (Fig. 2.15), so that there is an adequate 'safety-factor' to maintain the tetanus. Additionally, the incomplete repolarisation (d, e, Fig. 2.13) means that fewer acetylcholine molecules are required to attain threshold depolarisation.

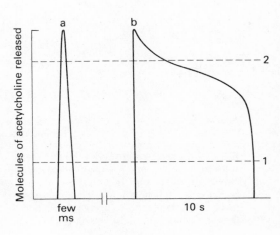

Fig. 2.15 Mammalian skeletal neuromuscular junction. Time course of release of acetylcholine during: a, twitch; b, tetanus. Threshold amounts of transmitter for activation of postsynaptic impulse along muscle fibres: 1, normal; 2, in the presence of D-tubocurarine (schematic).

A second type of skeletal muscle is multiply innervated (e.g. frog rectus, leech muscle). In this case the whole surface of the muscle is equally sensitive to the transmitter and the amplitude of the resultant contracture (a relatively slow contraction like that normally developed in most smooth muscles) is proportional to the magnitude of the end-plate potential which is generated. So, multiply innervated tissues provide a further distinction, as suxamethonium will elicit a marked contracture whereas D-tubocurarine will not.

A third type of skeletal neuromuscular activation is present in some avian muscle (e.g. chick biventer), which consists of a mixture of the previous two types. As shown in Fig. 2.16a, nerve stimulation produces twitches which are superimposed upon a contracture if a depolarising drug is simultaneously present. D-tubocurarine blocks both twitches and contracture (Fig. 2.16b) resulting in flaccid paralysis whereas suxamethonium only eliminates the twitches so that the contracture still occurs, i.e. it induces spastic paralysis (Fig. 2.16c).

At *autonomic ganglia*, D-tubocurarine is a non-depolarising antagonist (p. 61); suxamethonium has little effect but, if anything, tends to stimulate prior to producing a depolarising block. The other major action of D-tubocurarine is to cause *histamine release*. It is interesting that its three actions (in humans) all tend to decrease the blood pressure: skeletal muscle paralysis (resulting in less venous return and, therefore, diminished cardiac output), autonomic ganglionic block which is depressor (Table 10.2), and histamine release which is

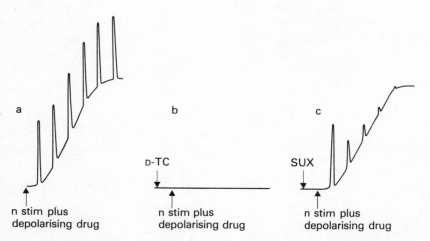

Fig. 2.16 Chick biventer cervicis muscle preparation (diagrammatic). a, repetitive stimulation of the motor nerve (n stim) causes twitches superimposed upon a contracture elicited by the simultaneous application of a depolarising drug; b, in the presence of D-tubocurarine (D-Tc) both responses are blocked resulting in a flaccid paralysis of the muscle; c, suxamethonium (SUX) eliminates the twitches but not the contracture (spastic paralysis).

hypotensive in man (5.5). The latter two effects are negligible with, for example, pancuronium, vecuronium: atracurium may release histamine but is useful if there is liver insufficiency because its breakdown is spontaneous, i.e. non-enzymatic, *in vivo* (pH 7.4, 37° C). These agents have largely replaced D-tubocurarine.

Multiple sites and mechanisms of action
Some substances act at more than one site at the skeletal neuromuscular junction. Such overlap is shown in Table 2.11 and will now be particularised.

Hemicholinium-3. The presynaptic actions and their analysis have already been described (2.8) but, at high doses, it is curare-like, with the appropriate properties, so that choline will not then reverse its action (compare Fig. 2.9).

Benzoquinonium. This, in addition to its D-tubocurarine-like effect, is also an anticholinesterase so that it manifests all the characteristics of a competitive blockade (Fig. 2.14a) except that its paralytic actions are not reversible by anticholinesterase administration.

Neostigmine. As well as its anticholinesterase effect this has a direct depolarising effect at the neuromuscular junction (Tables 2.4 and 2.6). The direct action can be shown experimentally by the fact that neostigmine will produce a twitch response after synaptic acetylcholinesterase removal either with the irreversible antagonist, dyflos, or following denervation and a lapse of 10 days to allow degeneration of the motor nerve.

Table 2.11 Some drugs which act significantly at more than one site at the skeletal neuromuscular junction

Drug	Presynaptic uptake of choline inhibited	Postsynaptic		
		Competitive block	Depolarising stimulation with subsequent block (direct)	As an anticholinesterase
Hemicholinium-3	+	+ (higher doses)		
Benzoquinonium		+		+
Neostigmine			+	+

+, effective.

a
Depolarisation
Muscular
paralysis
t
C_{10}
b
Muscular
paralysis
Depolarisation
t
C_{10}

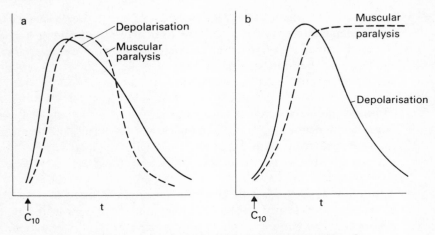

Fig. 2.17 Types of depolarisation block produced by decamethonium, C_{10} (diagrammatic): a, cat tibialis — here the depolarisation and muscle paralysis follow essentially similar time courses; b, frog sartorius — in this case the depolarisation initially produces paralysis which, however, persists after the resting potential has returned to its usual value, i.e. desensitisation of the receptors has then occurred.

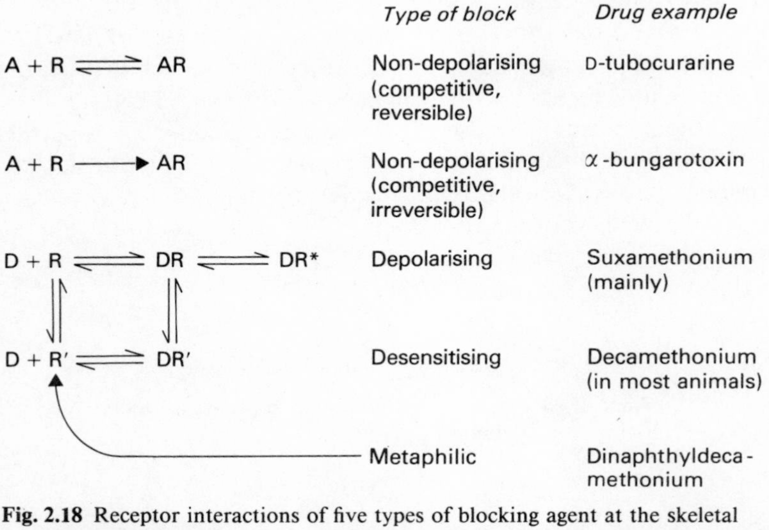

Type of block
Drug example
A + R ⇌ AR
Non-depolarising (competitive, reversible)
D-tubocurarine
A + R → AR
Non-depolarising (competitive, irreversible)
α-bungarotoxin
D + R ⇌ DR ⇌ DR*
Depolarising
Suxamethonium (mainly)
D + R′ ⇌ DR′
Desensitising
Decamethonium (in most animals)
Metaphilic
Dinaphthyldeca-methonium

Fig. 2.18 Receptor interactions of five types of blocking agent at the skeletal neuromuscular junction. A, antagonist; D, drug (agonist). Receptors: R, normal; R*, activated; R′, desensitised.

In addition to the competitive, reversible and depolarising block-ades described above, the skeletal neuromuscular junction can be blocked competitively but irreversibly by α-bungarotoxin. Further it is unusual (e.g. compared with the autonomic ganglion) in that other 'nicotinic' paralysing effects are possible. As indicated in Fig. 2.11 decamethonium in, for example, cat tibialis, produces a fairly pure depolarising block, i.e. the paralysis (Fig. 2.17a) is approximately synchronous with the depolarisation. However, if the effect of this drug on the frog sartorius muscle is observed (Fig. 2.17b), it can be seen that initially a depolarising block is produced but later that there is no depolarisation (i.e. the potential at the end-plate returns to its normal resting value) yet the paralysis persists. This is ascribed to *desensitisation* of the receptors (Fig. 2.18; *see* also p. 104), which can now only regenerate slowly to normally active receptors. Probably most depolar-ising drugs (e.g. nicotine, suxamethonium, anticholinesterases) produce some degree of desensitisation. Finally, a class of substances has been found (e.g. dinaphthyldecamethonium, DN-C_{10}), which will only com-bine with the *desensitised* form of the receptor. Therefore, these drugs have no effect if given alone but, in the presence of decamethonium (which produces desensitised receptors), they will intensify the block: this is termed *metaphilic antagonism* (Gk: *meta*, after—with connota-tion of change; *philein*, to love).

For final synopsis, *see* Fig. 2.18.

3 Noradrenergic Peripheral Mechanisms

3.1 Physiology of adrenergic synapses in the peripheral nervous system

The peripheral (nor)adrenergic system (*see* Fig. 2.1) includes most of the postganglionic sympathetic synapses reinforced by the blood-borne activity of the adrenal medullary secretion (which in the human is predominantly adrenaline). The receptors are divisible into three major categories, which can be separated as shown in Table 3.1.

The typical presynaptic sympathetic impulse (via calcium excitation –secretion coupling, 4.10) releases noradrenaline (Fig. 3.1) which, after receptor interaction, is removed from the synaptic cleft by any combination of the following three processes.

a *Uptake₁ (neuronal uptake, U_1)*

An active mechanism showing stereospecificity (e.g. $R(-) > S(+)$-noradrenaline) and limited capacity which is used, and therefore can be saturated by many drugs in relation to (nor)adrenergic synapses;

Table 3.1 Agents used to classify adrenoceptors

Adrenoceptor	Agonists	Antagonists
α	NA $\geqslant$ A > ISOP	Phentolamine (reversible)
	Phenylephrine	Phenoxybenzamine (irreversible)
β_1	NA $\approx$ A < ISOP	Atenolol
β_2	NA << A <	} Propranolol
	ISOP	Butoxamine
	Salbutamol (US: albuterol)	

Interpret the chart as follows (> means at least three times more).

At the α-receptor, the effects of noradrenaline (NA) are greater than or approximately equal to those of adrenaline (A), and greater than those of isoprenaline (ISOP) which are usually negligible; phenylephrine is an almost pure (p. 84)—though weaker (Table 3.2)—agonist; all these actions are blocked by either phentolamine or phenoxybenzamine. For subdivision of α-adrenoceptors, *see* Table 3.5.

At the β_1-receptor, ISOP has greater activity than A or NA whose effects are approximately equal; atenolol is a β_1-selective antagonist.

At the β_2-receptor, ISOP has greater potency than A which, at this site, has much greater agonist activity than NA; salbutamol is a β_2-selective stimulant. Butoxamine is a β_2 selective antagonist but it is not very potent and therefore, actions at these receptors are considered proven if they are antagonised by propranolol (which blocks both β_1 and β_2-receptors) but not by atenolol.

Fig. 3.1 Processes occurring at a noradrenergic synapse (*see* text). a, uptake$_1$; b, uptake$_2$, followed by metabolism (COMT and MAO); c, diffusion away from the synapse; d, vesicular uptake from the cytosol. The vesicles contain granules in which the transmitter is present together with specific proteins (chromogranins) and ATP; e, reserpine interferes with vesicular uptake so that the transmitter is deaminated by mitochondrial MAO and passed out of the ending as an inactive compound; f, an *indirectly acting* sympathomimetic agent which enters the terminal via uptake$_1$ (a) and releases the transmitter; g, a *directly acting* sympathomimetic agent activates the receptors point-blank; h, a 'mixed' sympathomimetic agent which acts partly directly and partly indirectly; i, block of transmitter release.

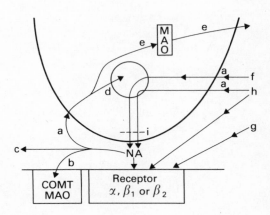

isoprenaline is a notable exception. Three potent blockers of this re-uptake mechanism are desmethylimipramine, imipramine and cocaine (in that order); *see also* phenoxybenzamine (3.6).

b *Uptake$_2$ (extraneuronal uptake, U_2)*
This process differs from U_1 in being much less selective and less readily saturable. Uptake$_2$ is followed by metabolism by COMT and/or MAO if these are applicable (*see* structure–activity relationships, Table 3.2). Blockers of this uptake process include metanephrine, phenoxybenzamine (3.6), and adrenal glucocorticoids (11.5).

Note on metabolism (see Fig 3.2)
• COMT (*c*atechol-*o*xygen-*m*ethyl*t*ransferase) acts on catecholamines to convert the phenolic hydroxyl group on the R_2 (meta) position (Table 3.2) to a methoxyl group, producing (nor)metanephrine from (nor)adrenaline
• MAO (*m*ono*a*mine *o*xidase). Here, a number of isoenzymes are involved but the fundamental reaction is removal of the amino-group with subsequent oxidation of the residual side-chain to the aldehyde which is further oxidised to the corresponding carboxylic acid (more commonly) or reduced to the primary alcohol (a glycol).

The combined effect of both these enzymes on either noradrenaline or adrenaline produces 3-methoxy-4-hydroxymandelic acid (also called vanillylmandelic acid, VMA).

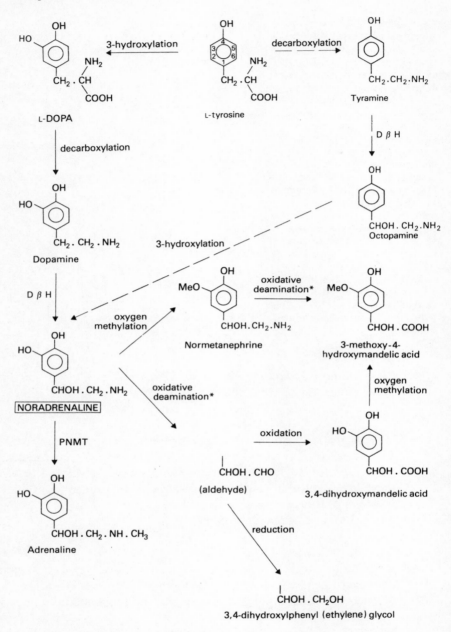

Fig. 3.2 Synthesis and breakdown of noradrenaline (dopamine and adrenaline undergo corresponding catabolic reactions). For enzymes involved *see* Fig. 3.3 and text. DβH = dopamine β-hydroxylase. Interrupted lines indicate *one* minor pathway. For oxidative deamination (*), the intermediate aldehyde stage and primary alcohol (glycol) product are shown for the lower but not the upper pathway. PNMT *p*henylethanolamine-*n*itrogen-*m*ethyl*t*ransferase) is present in chromaffin tissue and converts noradrenaline to adrenaline.

c *Diffusion*

Diffusion of the transmitter away from the synaptic site (c in Fig. 3.1) is followed by inactivation by MAO in the liver or excretion either unchanged or conjugated with glycuronate or sulphate in the urine. Such urinary excretion is especially marked when large amounts of naturally occurring catecholamines enter the circulation (e.g. in phaeochromocytoma).

The relative contribution of these particular processes to inactivation of any transmitter or drug varies with
● the site, e.g. rat heart, (−)-noradrenaline: U_1, 70%; U_2, 25%, diffusion away, 5%. Conversely, in the peripheral vasculature, diffusion is the major inactivating factor
● the agent, e.g. rat heart, U_1: (−)-noradrenaline, 70%; (−)-adrenaline, 50%; isoprenaline 0%.

Thus, using the rat heart, U_1 inhibitors (such as desmethylimipramine) potentiate noradrenaline slightly more than adrenaline without any effect upon isoprenaline actions. Conversely, because MAO is rarely the major factor in the removal of these catecholamines from their peripheral postsynaptic sites, inhibition of the enzyme does not usually modify the agonist responses. The case may be different within the central nervous system. Also, when MAO inhibitors (e.g. phenelzine) are given for CNS effects, they allow any sympathomimetic agents in the diet which are normally destroyed in the gut wall and liver by MAO (e.g. tyramine in some cheeses) to gain access to sympathetic terminals and produce a hypertensive attack (p. 184).

3.2 Drugs acting on presynaptic processes

These may be classified (similarly to those affecting the corresponding cholinergic synapses, p. 60) as influencing one or more of the following stages

Uptake of noradrenaline (as just described)

Synthesis (*see* later). Necessary only to 'top up' the content in tissues with appreciable U_1 of the transmitter

Storage ⎫
Release ⎭ (*see* below).

Storage

Following U_1, the noradrenaline in the cytosol is vulnerable to the MAO in the presynaptic mitochondria (which thereby control transmitter content) and, therefore, vesicular uptake (another active process—d, Fig. 3.1) is essential. Reserpine is the type substance of drugs which interfere with this mechanism. Given over a few days it gradually depletes the nerve ending of transmitter which is eliminated from the nerve terminal as the inactive (deaminated) metabolite (e, Fig. 3.1).

However, the use of such a drug would be extremely dangerous if MAO inhibitors were simultaneously present because, then, massive amounts of noradrenaline would be released into the general circulation. Reserpine invariably causes diarrhoea, due to unopposed activity of the parasympathetic system on the gut musculature.

Release

Release of noradrenaline can be triggered either by a nerve impulse (associated with calcium ion entry at the nerve terminal—as for the cholinergic system, p. 41) or by a drug (e.g. amphetamine, tyramine, *see* Table 3.2) which, in contradistinction to reserpine, causes the liberation of noradrenaline. These drugs might displace noradrenaline from vesicular to cytosolic sites where the transmitter is not significantly deaminated—because these agents are monoamine oxidase inhibitors —and so could be liberated from the nerve ending. Additionally, because they need to be taken into the nerve ending by U_1 to produce their action, they act as U_1 inhibitors and thus potentiate the effects of the noradrenaline which they release. Such substances are termed *indirectly acting* sympathomimetic agents in contrast to drugs (e.g. noradrenaline, adrenaline, isoprenaline) which naturally or when given exogenously act directly on adrenoceptors (g, Fig. 3.1). Intermediate forms—*'mixed'* sympathomimetic agents (h, Fig. 3.1)—act partly directly and partly indirectly (e.g. ephedrine, Table 3.2). Release of the active transmitter can be prevented (i, Fig. 3.1) with bretylium which concentrates in noradrenergic rather then cholinergic synapses, due to its preferential absorption by U_1. However, this drug is obsolete therapeutically because it can produce unexpected hypertensive episodes due to the sporadic development of tolerance. Guanethidine has a similar action at this site but its overall effect is complicated by other manifestations (*see* later).

Synthesis

Because much of the transmitter is returned unchanged (via U_1 and vesicular uptake) into the presynaptic stores in many tissues, *de novo* synthesis is only necessary to replenish the noradrenaline content. The stages for the *main* pathway are illustrated in Figs 3.2 and 3.3. The enzyme necessary to convert noradrenaline to adrenaline (phenylethanolamine-N-methyltransferase) is only present (outside the central nervous system) in chromaffin tissue—mainly the adrenal medulla—so that the small percentage of adrenaline released at the sympathetic nerve terminals has come from the blood via U_1. The first step is the rate-limiting one and is normally controlled by end-product (noradrenaline) feed-back. However, inhibition of tyrosine hydroxylase, e.g. with α-methyl(para)tyrosine, is normally ineffective in depleting noradrenaline content *in vivo* because the prospective block is (naturally) overcome both by increased tyrosine production in the body and

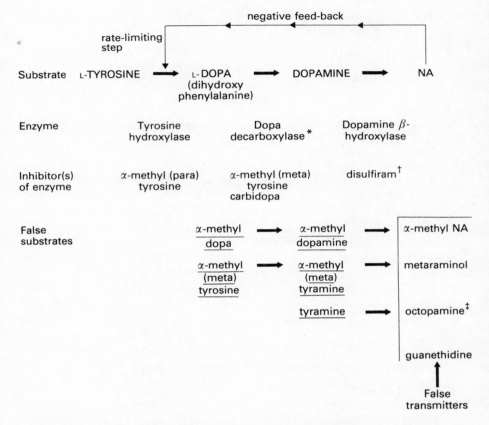

Fig. 3.3 Synthetic processes occurring inside a noradrenergic (NA) terminal: one minor pathway is shown in Fig. 3.2. Drugs acting as false substrates are underlined and false transmitters shown in the lower right-hand column.
*More correctly termed 'aromatic L-amino acid decarboxylase.
†After conversion to diethyldithiocarbamic acid which chelates the Cu^{2+} co-factor of the enzyme.
‡Originally extracted from salivary glands of an octopus.

bypassing of the main route of synthesis by the use of alternative (normally minor) pathways. Carbidopa is an important dopa decarboxylase inhibitor (*see* 7.2). The inhibition of dopamine-β-hydroxylase by disulfiram is interesting in connection with the effects of this drug upon ethanol metabolism (9.2). As shown in Fig. 3.3, a drug (e.g. α-methyldopa, itself a dopa decarboxylase inhibitor) or a dietary constituent (e.g. tyramine) can enter this synthetic pathway and thereby produce a 'false transmitter': this may be a full agonist or a partial agonist. *See also* guanethidine (below).

Multiple actions
Since noradrenaline participates in most of the processes already mentioned, it is not surprising that many drugs have multiple sites of

Table 3.2 Structure–activity relationships of some illustrative sympathomimetic agents (substituted ethylamines)

	R_1	R_2	β R_3	α R_4	R_5	
Noradrenaline (US: norepinephrine, levarterenol)	OH	OH	OH			directly acting
Adrenaline (US: epinephrine)	OH	OH	OH		CH_3	
Isoprenaline (US: isoproterenol)	OH	OH	OH		Isopropyl	
Dopamine*	OH	OH				
Phenylephrine		OH	OH		CH_3	'mixed'
Metaraminol		OH	OH	CH_3		
Ephedrine		OH	OH	CH_3	CH_3	
Octopamine	OH		OH			
Tyramine†	OH					indirectly acting
Amphetamine				CH_3		

For clarity, all substituents which are hydrogen atoms are omitted.

GENERAL RULES

1. If *both* R_1 and R_2 are hydroxyl groups (*catechol*amines) there are strong *direct* sympathomimetic effects.

2. If R_3 is a hydroxyl group and *in the R(—)-configuration*, there are moderate *direct* sympathomimetic actions. Thus, dopamine is a weaker agonist than noradrenaline.

3. *In the noradrenaline series*, the R_5 group determines which receptors are maximally activated. The larger the substituent (up to isopropyl) the more β-agonist action.

4. If R_1 and R_2 are unsubstituted and R_4 is a methyl group, the compound gains in lipid solubility so that it can cross the blood–brain barrier and exert stimulant effects upon the CNS—more marked with the *dextro*-configuration at R_4, i.e. (+) > (—)-amphetamine: the isomers of ephedrine are less active.

5. COMT will only attack catechol (i.e. both R_1 and R_2 being hydroxyl groups) derivatives and, therefore, only noradrenaline, adrenaline, isoprenaline and dopamine of the drugs depicted.

6. MAO acts at the amine end of the molecule but will not accept as substrates compounds either with a large group (e.g. isopropyl) on R_5 or methyl on R_4. Thus isoprenaline, ephedrine and amphetamine can be administered orally as they are not inactivated by MAO in the gut wall and the liver. Conversely, tyramine contained in food (e.g. some cheeses) will, if an MAO inhibitor is present, reach the sympathetic nerve endings and release noradrenaline causing a hypertensive crisis.

*Can also liberate noradrenaline, e.g. in the heart.

†Also weak direct action on a few tissues, e.g. rabbit ear artery.

action. Thus *phenoxybenzamine*, as well as blocking α-receptors, also inhibits both U_1 and U_2 (*see* p. 88); while *guanethidine* acts as an adrenergic neurone-blocking agent (Table 10.2) by several mechanisms:
Uptake$_1$ block—preventing noradrenaline retrieval
Storage block (like reserpine and, similarly, causing diarrhoea).
   Also, by replacing noradrenaline in the vesicles, it becomes a 'false transmitter' (Fig. 3.3); however, as it has negligible agonist action, purists call it a 'non-transmitter'
Release block. But, if given i.v., there may be a paradoxical initial enhancement of *nerve-stimulated* noradrenaline release.

   Guanethidine is used in thyrotoxicosis to relieve lid retraction (p. 337) and in glaucoma (p. 390). Large and repeated doses can result in destruction of adrenergic fibres (chemical sympathectomy)—an effect more easily attained by the use of 6-hydroxydopamine, *see* p. 156. A method for peripheral *immuno*sympathectomy using nerve growth factor antibodies is described on p. 106.

   Finally, as in the corresponding cholinergic systems, *presynaptic receptors* may also be involved (3.6).

3.3   Sympathomimetic agents
From a large number of these, a selection of theoretically—and therapeutically—important drugs is shown in Table 3.2 to illustrate the structure–activity relationships with respect to certain key properties. Attachment to the receptor appears to be via the following groups
*   the basic amine, R_5 (ionic bond)
*   the alcoholic hydroxyl, R_3 (hydrogen bond)
*   the two phenolic hydroxyls, R_1 and R_2 (chelate formation with receptor). When R_1 and R_2 are ortho to each other in the 3 and 4 benzene ring positions, the compound is a *catechol*amine.

   It must be emphasised that the rules below the table, while correct for the compounds tabulated, are not immutable. Means of separating directly, 'mixed' and indirectly acting sympathomimetic agents are shown in Table 3.3. These tests are also valuable insofar as they may be used in reverse, e.g. a U_1 blocker, a depleter of noradrenaline vesicular content or a preventer of transmitter release will antagonise the postsynaptic responses to tyramine while potentiating those of adrenaline and noradrenaline.

   Many of the uses and toxic effects of sympathomimetic drugs are cardiovascular and are discussed in Chapter 10. Their employment in the treatment of bronchial asthma is described in 11.5. For other significant actions, go down the list in Table 2.3 and *see* below.

Bladder
The main function of the sympathetic innervation is to keep the internal sphincter closed during filling. Thus ephedrine has been used in

Table 3.3 Separation of directly, 'mixed' and indirectly acting sympathomimetic amines in terms of responses to their application

Factor involved or modified	Directly acting	'Mixed'	Indirectly acting
Dose required	Small	Intermediate	Large
Delay	Slight ($c.10s$)	Intermediate	Longer ($c.1$ min)
Tachyphylaxis*	Nil	Some	Marked
After uptake$_1$ block (e.g. with desmethylimipramine)	Potentiation† (i.e. an increased response)	Neither potentiation nor inhibiton	Inhibition (i.e. a lessened response)
After depletion with reserpine for 3 successive days previously	Potentiation	Neither potentiation nor inhibition	Inhibition, restored temporarily by noradrenaline infusion‡
After depletion by sympathectomy 10 days earlier	Potentiation	Neither potentiation nor inhibition	Inhibition, not restored by nor-adrenaline infusion‡
After prevention of noradrenaline release with, for example, guanethidine	Potentiation	Neither potentiation nor inhibition	Inhibition
Change in the release of ^{3}H-noradrenaline from nerve endings or noradrenaline from splenic nerve granules (ox)§	Nil	Some increase	Marked increase

*Tachyphylaxis indicates a diminished response to the drug on repeated application (e.g. every 2–3 min).
†An exception is isoprenaline which is not affected by uptake$_1$ (3.1).
‡A (20 min) noradrenaline infusion will *temporarily* restore the response when the vesicles are intact, (e.g. after reserpine normally — but high doses will disrupt the vesicles), but not after sympathectomy.
§Granules containing noradrenaline (and adrenaline) can be squeezed from the ox splenic nerve and they release the catecholamines spontaneously into the bathing fluid.

noctural enuresis but, more importantly, the longer-acting agents (such as ephedrine and amphetamine, which are not broken down by either COMT or MAO) can precipitate acute urinary retention in patients liable to prostatism.

Eye (18.2)
Phenylephrine is an almost pure α-agonist (it has a slight effect on β-receptors due to a weak indirect action releasing noradrenaline) and is sometimes used to dilate the pupil. As the ciliary muscle has no sympathetic innervation, accommodation for near vision is minimally

affected (slightly attenuated, reflexly, due to the pupillary dilation, *see* p. 390). Cocaine was once used both to dilate the pupil (produced by block of U_1) and to exert a local anaesthetic effect in eye operations.

Uterus
The relaxation of this organ is mediated via β_2-adrenoceptors and so a selective agonist such as salbutamol (Table 3.1) can be used as a uterine relaxant in premature labour (p. 361).

Metabolism
Injections of adrenaline were once used as temporary measures in the emergency treatment of hypoglycaemic coma but endogenous release is occurring anyway and exogenous glucose or glucagon is much more effective (p. 347).

3.4 Alpha-adrenoceptor antagonists (α-blockers)

These do not show any obvious structure–activity relationship, although they are predominantly hydrophilic, and consist of a heterogeneous collection of chemical compounds. This in turn means that they lack postsynaptic specificity and therefore have multiple, different side-effects. The type substance is phentolamine (which does not show α_1 or α_2-selectivity, *see* Table 3.5). Its side-effects *due to α-block* are mainly the result of vascular dilation, e.g. postural hypotension with reflex bradycardia, nasal stuffiness, red sclerae. Alpha-blocking agents alone are useful pharmacologically for the demonstration of 'adrenaline reversal' (p. 242) and in the treatment of some cases of peripheral vascular disease (e.g. Raynaud's phenomenon) and of hypertension (*see* prazosin, Table 10.3). However, they find their main therapeutic applications in combination with a β-blocking agent in situations where there is an excess of circulating adrenaline and/or noradrenaline (e.g. phaeochromocytoma or tyramine/MAO inhibitor interaction).

Some drugs have incidental α-blocking activity (e.g. chlorpromazine, which may contribute to its hypotensive side-effect, Table 7.6). There is a marked overlap between α-adrenoceptor and many 5-hydroxytryptamine antagonists (5.8). Some agents possess both α- and β-adrenoceptor blocking activity (e.g. labetalol, Tables 10.2, 10.13).

3.5 Beta-adrenoceptor antagonists (β-blockers)

These have a well-defined structure–activity relationship (fundamentally being related to isoprenaline) and, further, there are good chemical rules to separate β_1 from β_2-selectivity. These drugs manifest (as shown in Table 3.4) different proportions of the following:
1 Beta-adrenoceptor antagonism which is particularly marked under conditions of *high* sympathetic (β) tone. A drug may show selectivity,

Table 3.4   Relative properties of illustrative β-adrenoceptor blocking agents

Drug	β-antagonism	Membrane stabilisation*	Partial agonist activity	Lipid solubility
Pindolol	+++	+	++	Intermediate
Oxprenolol	++	+	+	Intermediate
Propranolol R(−)	++	+	0	High
S(+)†	0	+	0	−
Timolol	+++	0	0	Intermediate
Atenolol	++ (β₁-selective)	0	0	Low
Sotalol	+	0	0	Low

+++, strong; ++, moderate; +, present; 0, negligible.
*Experimental method: frog sciatic nerve preparation (Table 8.2).
†Can be used to separate β-antagonism from membrane stabilisation.

but not specificity, toward one subdivision of these receptors. For example, atenolol is normally β_1-selective but at higher dosage it can also antagonise actions at the β_2-receptors.

2   Membrane-stabilising (local anaesthetic) activity: may be a useful ancillary action in the treatment of cardiac dysrhythmias (10.13); although probably only significant at high doses.

3   Beta-adrenoceptor stimulation (partial agonist activity—p. 95—or intrinsic sympathomimetic action, ISA). This property is stated to result in diminished side-effects (specifically bronchoconstriction, cardiodepression and cold extremities, *see* below); and can be visualised as predominating in situations of *low* sympathetic (β) tone—the opposite to **1** above.

Uses
These agents are much more important therapeutically than the α-adrenoceptor antagonists and have a wide range of uses, including some very common conditions.

Cardiovascular
- hypertension (p. 253)—mechanism of action still uncertain
- angina pectoris (p. 267)—prophylactic use to decrease cardiac activity, especially on exercise or excitement during rest
- heart dysrhythmias (p. 280)
- to minimise sympathetic effects accompanying hyperthyroidism (p. 337) or psychiatric conditions (7.4 and 7.5)
- in combination with an α-adrenoceptor blocking agent (or use labetalol), as detailed in the preceding section
- glaucoma—decreased production of aqueous humour at the ciliary body (Table 2.3, *see also* p. 390).

Voluntary muscle. To decrease tremor, which is a β_2-effect (Table 2.3).

Side-effects
These are obvious from Table 2.3.

Smooth muscle
Bronchoconstriction, especially dangerous in asthmatic patients (p. 286) although less likely to occur with β_1-selective antagonists (e.g. atenolol) or with partial agonists.

Vascular side-effects such as cold extremities (p. 254) due to reflex α-adrenoceptor vasoconstriction may be worsened if there is concomitant block of any β_2-adrenoceptor-mediated vasodilation (reported to be less with partial agonists or β_1-selective blockers).

Heart tissues
Force of cardiac contraction. In incipient heart failure there is increased (reflex) sympathetic tone to the myocardium (Fig. 10.11) and, if this is inhibited, complete failure may be precipitated; this occurs less often than might be anticipated but appears to be less common if a β-blocker with significant partial agonist activity is used. Sinus rate is a useful measure of degree of block. (Maximum therapeutic effect at 55–60 beats min^{-1}; dangerous below this range.) Conduction of the cardiac impulse may be slowed, thus accentuating any tendency to heart block.

Metabolic
When a diabetic patient takes insulin, the therapeutic lowering of the blood sugar level is opposed by liver and muscle glycogenolysis, which are predominantly β-sympathetic actions (Table 2.3). Therefore, if β-blockers are simultaneously present, there may be a phase of insulin hypoglycaemia unannounced by the typically sympathetically mediated symptoms of tachycardia or tremor. Diabetics should be warned of this possibility (p. 347).

The original β_1-selective blocking agent—practolol—unfortunately resulted in fibroses in eye, pleural, pericardial and retroperitoneal tissues, inner ear and skin (oculomucocutaneous syndrome). These were unpredictable and only occurred in a small minority of patients, sometimes after the discontinuance of therapy. The reactions were most likely immunological in origin but have not been reported for any other β-blocking agent. Finally, β-blockers which are highly lipid-soluble (e.g. propranolol, Table 3.4) are metabolised — in the liver — most quickly and can cross the blood–brain barrier in sufficient concentration to produce CNS side-effects (e.g. nightmares). Agents of low lipid solubility, e.g. atenolol, are mainly excreted unchanged in the urine slowly and, therefore, only need be given once (or twice) daily.

3.6   Presynaptic (nor)adrenergic receptors

Catecholaminergic receptors have been reported at presynaptic sites on both adrenergic and cholinergic postganglionic fibres in a number of tissues. Those most extensively studied at peripheral presynaptic noradrenergic endings are a subtype of the postsynaptic α_1-adrenoceptors, termed α_2. Stimulation of these (Fig. 2.1, lower) results in a decreased release of the transmitter and, conversely, blockade produces an increased outflow. Certain α-adrenoceptor agonists and antagonists are considered to be more α_2- than α_1-orientated and vice versa—a classification is shown in Table 3.5: their use reveals that α_1- and α_2-receptors are present both pre- and postsynaptically. The *physiological* significance of presynaptic receptors is uncertain but they may be important in particular *pharmacological* situations, which will be indicated as they arise. One example is phenoxybenzamine which blocks both α_1- and α_2-adrenoceptors as well as U_1 and U_2. On an α-mediated response (e.g. contraction of the nictitating membrane or vascular smooth muscle) postsynaptic antagonism of sympathomimetic effects predominates and is competitive irreversible (Fig. 4.2, Ib). Conversely, on β-innervated tissues (e.g. myocardium) phenoxybenzamine potentiates sympathomimetic actions by prevention of breakdown plus increased release of transmitter.

Recently, β_2-presynaptic receptors (considered to increase noradrenaline release) have been implicated in the antihypertensive effect of some β-adrenoceptor blocking agents (p. 254).

Table 3.5   A subclassification of α-adrenoceptors

	α_1	$\alpha_1 + \alpha_2$	α_2
Sites	Peripheral post- and presynaptic noradrenergic Central postsynaptic catecholaminergic		Peripheral pre- and postsynaptic noradrenergic Central pre- and postsynaptic catecholaminergic
Agonists*	Phenylephrine Methoxamine	Noradrenaline Adrenaline	Clonidine α-Methylnoradrenaline
Antagonists*	Prazosin Labetalol†	Phentolamine	Yohimbine Piperoxan
Mechanisms (Table 4.6)	Increased phosphatidyl inositol diphosphate hydrolysis		Decreased cyclic AMP formation

*The drugs indicated are stated to show selectivity (not specificity) in favour of the particular subtype.
†Also β-blocker.

3.7 Dopamine receptors

The classical receptors, i.e. acetylcholine and adrenaline/noradrenaline, were originally characterised in the (simpler) peripheral nervous system and subsequently found within the CNS; unlike these, specific dopamine receptors were first discovered in the caudate nucleus (Table 6.1) When the blood pressure responses to dopamine (which are species-variable) are subjected to complete α- and β-adrenoceptor blockade (10.2), a depressor element remains which can be shown to be due to peripheral vasodilation (particularly in the renal, mesenteric and possibly, coronary vessels) and can be blocked by drugs known to antagonise *central* dopamine receptors (e.g. haloperidol or α-flupenthixol, Table 6.4), also weakly by ergometrine (Table 15.5). Note that dopamine stimulates the heart both directly via β_1-adrenoceptors and indirectly via noradrenaline release (See footnote, Table 3.2).

3.8 (Nor)adrenergic co-transmitters

See p. 141 and Fig. 10.4.

4 Receptors and Responses

Receptors are specific cellular structures with which drugs and body substances interact, binding by complementarity (and using a variety of chemical forces) to trigger changes in activity which result in the final (observed) effects. Some properties of the more common bonds are shown in Table 4.1.

Covalent bonds
These arise when two valency electrons are shared by two atoms: if the latter are of different elements, the electrons will be shared unequally and a dipole (between subintegral charges, δ^+ and δ^-) thus induced. These bonds are relatively uncommon in drug–receptor interactions, unless a chemical change has to occur (e.g. hydrolysis of acetylcholine, 2.6). For coordinate covalency, *see* Table 4.1.

Electrostatic bonds
These result from the attraction of oppositely charged atoms.

Table 4.1 Bonds between drug molecules and/or biological components

Type of bond	Subgroup	Energy of bond (kcal mol^{-1})	Dipole	Drug example(s)
Covalent	Same atoms } Different atoms	40–150	Absent / Present	Organic phosphorus-containing anticholinesterases (2.6) Alkylating agents (p. 411)
	Coordinate (one atom supplies both electrons)	*c.* 40	Large	Chelating agents (20.9)
Electrostatic	Ionic	5–10		
	Ionic-dipole	2–5		
	Dipole-dipole	1–4		Most drugs
	Hydrogen bond	2–5		
	Induced dipole	0.1–1		
Hydrophobic (*see* text)				

Ionic. If both charges are integral; otherwise, ionic–dipole or dipole–dipole.

Hydrogen. When a proton bridges two electron donors (e.g. O, N, S).

Induced dipole. When atoms come very close together (but outside the distance at which their nuclei repel each other) distortion of their electron clouds produces weak dipoles (e.g. van der Waals forces).

Such bonds are extremely important in drug–receptor combinations. While the ionic bonds are often instrumental in the initial alignment of drug and receptor molecules, their continued propinquity is frequently assured by the multiplicity of relatively weak bonds exerted over quite short distances. The orientation of associated water molecules may play an additional important role especially with respect to electrostatic bonds.

Hydrophobic bonds
The aggregation of hydrophobic groups will expel some water molecules from their vicinity, as in the lipid bilayer of the cell membrane (Fig. 1.2). Such lipophilic bonds are usually weak but may assume importance, for example in relation to the mechanisms of action of general anaesthetics (8.7).

The final drug-receptor interaction is determined
• *spatially*, by the algebraic sum of all the attractive bonds and repulsive forces. If the total bonding energy cannot be achieved immediately, the combination can occur in stages (like the closure of a zip-fastener, e.g. 'zipper model', glucagon binding (Table 14.7)
• *temporally*, by the relative rates of association (affinity constant, 4.4) and of dissociation. To dissociate from a receptor, a molecule has to acquire a kinetic energy greater than its bonding energy. The average kinetic energy due to thermal agitation at 37°C is 0.37 kcal mol^{-1} and there is a 50% chance of achieving a higher kinetic energy. The possibility shows a negative exponential variation, such that there is less than 1 in a million likelihood of attaining 10 kcal mol^{-1}, and a coordinate bond of 40 kcal mol^{-1} is, in effect, irreversible spontaneously.

4.1 Receptors (*see* Fig. 4.5)
These may be extracellular or intracellular. They are *extra*cellular if, for example, microiontophoretic application of acetylcholine is made to a single skeletal neuromuscular junction, the dose of transmitter required to produce a standard response decreases to a minimum as the surface of the end-plate is approached, but the transmitter is ineffective once the micropipette has pierced the cellular membrane (*see also* insulin,

glucagon, Table 14.7). The classical example of *intra*cellular receptors is that of the steroid hormones (e.g. oestrogens, adrenal glucocorticoids) which enter the target cell and combine with a receptor protein associated with nuclear chromatin. The binding induces or represses genes which modify protein production and, thereby, cause changes in the structure or function of target tissues.

The initial recognition is usually much more complicated than was originally envisaged in the simple 'lock-and-key' analogy, derived from structure–activity relationships such as those shown in Tables 2.1 and 3.2. When the two-dimensional formulae (e.g. Fig. 2.3) are replaced by three-dimensional models, a truer picture is obtained; however even when this is shown to fit a complementary wooden block—representing the receptor—there are serious deficiencies. To begin with, the drug molecule *in vivo* approaches the receptor, not in air, but in an aqueous medium within which there is usually continuous rotation round many of its bonds resulting in a continually changing drug profile. However, a few drugs are conformationally restricted, e.g. muscarine, *see* Table 2.4. Next, structured water molecules in relation to hydrophobic areas in the drug or receptor (*see* clathrates, 8.7) may need to be modified before drug–receptor interaction can occur. Further, many receptors exist in different affinity states (*see also* two-state model, Fig. 4.3). Also, the receptor is often dynamic so that moulding both of the drug and of its receptor area can occur as interaction progresses: the latter might reflect drug-induced allosteric modification by non-receptor membrane constituents.

Finally, surface receptors are continually being formed intracellularly, inserted into the plasma membrane ('externalisation'), taken back into the cell interior ('internalisation') and, then, either degraded or recycled. This series of events can be modulated by nervous activity (*see* below), hormonal environment (p. 106), receptor activation (for example, insulin receptors p. 344) or pathological conditions (heart failure p. 273), and result in 'up' or 'down regulation'.

4.2   Drug–receptor combination
The simple combination of a drug with its specific receptor to produce the eventual response is further complicated by upward or downward modification of the initial reaction. Table 4.2 shows a general outline.

An *increased* effect may result from:
1 *Persistence of transmitter* (or similar compound) in the synaptic cleft, e.g. acetylcholine in the presence of an anticholinesterase (2.6), e.g. noradrenaline or another directly acting sympathomimetic amine (not isoprenaline) in the presence of an $uptake_1$ blocker (*see* Table 3.3).
2 *Persistence plus increased transmitter release*, e.g. phenoxybenzamine potentiates the cardiac effects of sympathetic nerve stimulation (due to U_1 and U_2 block plus presynaptic α_2–adrenoceptor antagonism, p. 88).

Table 4.2   Some mechanisms influencing receptor responses

Factor involved	Increased response	Decreased response
Transmitter concentration	More release Greater persistence	Less release (acutely)
Receptor availability	Increased number ('up regulation') Decreased spontaneous occupation	Decreased number ('down regulation')
Receptor sensitivity	Supersensitivity	Desensitisation

For examples, *see* text.

3 *Increased transmitter release*, for example release of dopamine (possibly associated with enhanced postsynaptic sensitivity), causing tardive dyskinesia with chlorpromazine, p. 180).
4 *More receptors available*. This may be a result of
• an absolute increase in number, e.g. at the skeletal neuromuscular junction, the end-plate region is normally thousands of times more sensitive to the iontophoresis of acetylcholine than the rest of the muscle membrane; however, following denervation, all parts become equally sensitive. It appears that latent receptors become accessible possibly due to loss of inhibitory trophic factors and/or production of activating factors by nerve degeneration: *see also* 'up regulation' of insulin receptors with sulphonylureas (p. 349), and of hepatic LDL receptors with, for example, clofibrate (Table 13.3).
• decreased spontaneous occupancy. The potentiation of directly acting sympathomimetic agonists (*see* Table 3.3) following appropriate pretreatment with drugs which block vesicular uptake or release of noradrenaline *may* belong to this category.
5 *Receptors being more sensitive*, e.g. abstinence syndrome in a morphine addict (7.10).

A *decreased* effect (hyposensitivity) is termed tachyphylaxis, if immediate, and tolerance, if delayed (*see also* p. 187 and note on theory of morphine tolerance, 7.10). It may be produced by:
1 *Lessened transmitter release* due to the inability of synthesis to match usage acutely. This is the cardinal sign of indirectly acting agents when they are given at short intervals, e.g. tyramine at noradrenergic synapses (Table 3.3).
2 *Loss of receptors*, e.g. a plasma antibody decreases the available skeletal muscle nicotinic receptors in myasthenia gravis patients; e.g. available insulin receptors in target tissues are inversely related to the amount of hormone secreted—thus older persons who overeat, hyper-secrete insulin and can develop non-insulin dependent diabetes mellitus by 'down regulation' and negative cooperativity (*see* p. 344); e.g. β_1-adrenoceptor 'down regulation' in heart failure (p. 273).

3 *Decreased receptor sensitivity*, e.g. desensitisation (Fig. 2.18 and *see* p. 104).

See also cooperativity (4.5), other points concerning receptors (4.7) and, for post-receptor factors affecting the response, 4.8 *et seq.*

4.3   Qualitative aspects

Receptor types are usually originally defined in terms of responses to specific agonists and specific antagonists (as in 2.3 and Table 3.1). This is useful, especially when considering therapeutic applications of drugs but, even here, it must be remembered that absolute specificity is rarely attained: most drugs are selective rather than specific, e.g. atenolol (3.5); salbutamol (11.4). From a pharmacological point of view, it is probably wise to regard subtyping of receptors (e.g. α-, β_1- and β_2-adrenoceptors) as representing artificial divisions separating groups in a spectrum which runs from (almost) pure α-adrenoceptor-containing tissue (? nictitating membrane of cat), through mainly β_1- receptor-containing organs, to (almost) wholly β_2-adrenoceptor tissues. Most organs contain a mixture of these receptor types but usually one is predominant, as indicated in Table 2.3. Unusually, there are considerable numbers of more than one subtype subserving the same response (e.g. the gut muscle contains significant amounts of α- and β_1 adrenoceptors, both of which cause relaxation).

A similar caveat applies to subtyping of all other receptors.

4.4   Quantitative considerations

The classical pharmacological approach is to plot dose–response curves (DRCs) for agonists both alone and in the presence of different concentrations of antagonists. Let us consider the former first. The curve, obtained from a range of doses separated by adequate wash-out periods, is sigmoidal (acetylcholine, Fig. 4.1) if the responses are plotted against the *logarithms* of the doses (concentrations in the organ bath, usually); under these conditions, the graph between 30% and 70% of the maximum effect can be considered to be a straight line. A similar result may be obtained more expeditiously by not washing the drug out between each dose but merely adding sufficient to achieve the next-higher required concentration and recording the *total* response on each occasion, until the maximum effect is attained for two consecutive concentrations (*cumulative* DRC).

When DRCs are plotted for the acyl derivatives of choline at *muscarinic* receptors (Table 2.2), as in Fig. 4.1, it becomes clear that acetyl > formyl > propionyl are 'full' agonists because (at sufficient concentrations) they can produce maximal responses; that butyryl never achieves the maximum (and is termed a 'partial' agonist at these receptors); and that valeryl has no agonist activity. Acetylcholine is the

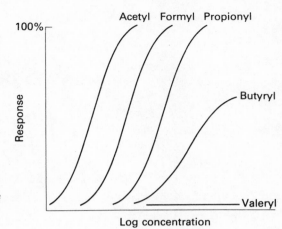

Fig. 4.1 Dose–response curves
(diagrammatic) for a series of choline
esters on a tissue containing
muscarinic receptors.

most effective agonist because it needs to occupy fewest receptors to achieve any given response. At the maximum response, unoccupied specific sites are called *spare receptors* and their number (in relation to that of the necessarily occupied receptors) is the *spare-receptor ratio*. Partial agonists—acting alone—produce attenuated effects but, in the presence of a full agonist, they can act as antagonists by less effectually occupying receptors vital to the full agonist action (i.e. encroaching beyond the spare-receptor limit).

Antagonists
Antagonists acting at or in close proximity to receptor sites fall into three main categories (Fig. 4.2)
a Competitive reversible. These show a parallel displacement of the DRC to the right with increasing concentrations of antagonist (Fig. 4.2, Ia).
b Competitive irreversible. Here, the combination of the antagonist with the receptor is covalent, so that breakdown is slow. Therefore, with increasing antagonist concentrations, the agonist DRCs move in a parallel manner to the right until insufficient receptors are available, when the maximum of the DRCs declines. Fig. 4.2, Ib enables a computation of the number of spare receptors as follows: the X on each DRC indicates 50% of the maximum response at that particular concentration of the antagonist. If these mid-points are joined by two straight lines, the intersection represents the 50% response of the most-displaced DRC at which a maximum response would be obtained: therefore, the displacement D_1 to D_{3a} represents the spare-receptor ratio. Thus, if its value (in log units) were 2, this would indicate that only 1 in 101 of the total receptor population need be available for the agonist in question to achieve a maximal response.

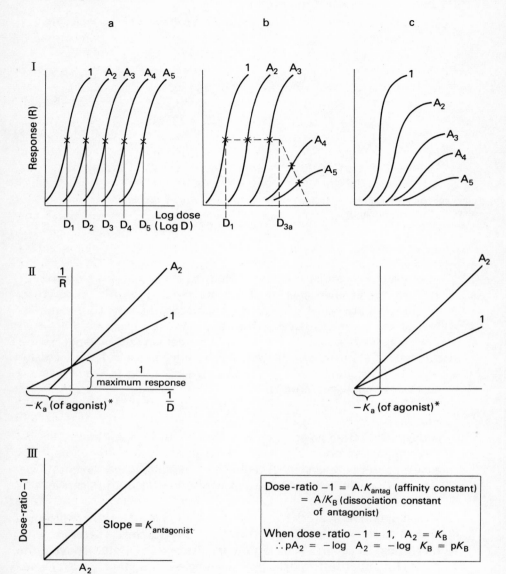

Fig. 4.2 I Dose–response curves (DRCs) for agonist alone (1) and in the presence of increasing concentrations (2, 3, 4, 5) of the following types of antagonist (A): a, competitive reversible; b, competitive irreversible; c, non-competitive.
II Reciprocal plots for similar data. *assuming no spare receptors.
III Dose-ratio plot (*see* text). Dose-ratio $- 1 = A.K_{antag(onist)}$.

c Non-competitive. This implies that the antagonist is not working at the same site as the agonist but that, by modifying an adjoining part of the tissue surface (allosteric site; Gk: *allos*, other), it is preventing agonist–receptor interaction. This usually (but not inevitably) results in an immediate decline in the maximum response (Fig. 4.2, Ic).

One way of separating competitive from non-competitive antagonists is to perform a double-reciprocal plot. This is analogous to a Lineweaver–Burk graph in enzyme kinetics. The reciprocals of the responses in the absence and in the presence of a given concentration of the antagonist are plotted against the reciprocals of the corresponding doses (*not* log doses). If the graphs intersect on the *y*-axis, (Fig. 4.2, IIa— indicating similar maximum responses as already shown in Fig. 4.2, Ia) the antagonism is competitive (though competitive irreversible antagonists do not *always* produce such a result): if the graphs intersect on the *x*-axis (Fig. 4.2, IIc), there is a decreased maximum response in the presence of the antagonist and the antagonism is non-competitive. In either case the affinity constant of the *agonist* (K_a) is given as shown in Fig. 4.2, II. When the law of mass action is applied to a simple drug–receptor interaction

$$D + R \underset{k_2}{\overset{k_1}{\rightleftharpoons}} DR \tag{1}$$

the affinity constant of the agonist, $K_a (k_1/k_2)^*$, is found to be the reciprocal of the drug concentration which achieves occupancy of 50% of the receptors (i.e. $1/D_1$ in Fig. 4.2, Ib). However, this usually produces an affinity constant which is far too high—both in terms of the maximum possible rate of diffusion to the site and compared with the values obtained using other methods of measuring this constant. The fallacy is obvious. In many tissues it is not necessary for 100% of the receptors to be occupied to achieve the maximum response and, when the spare-receptor ratio is taken into account and the reciprocal of D_{3a} (Fig. 4.2, Ib) is used, a reasonable K_a for the agonist is obtained.

The affinity constant of the *antagonist* (K_{antag}) is a more significant value because it is clearly a measure of combination of the antagonist with the receptor ($A + R \rightleftharpoons AR$, analogous to equation (1) above); whereas in the case of an agonist, the affinity constant is only an imperfect measure because of subsequent events in the reaction sequence–equation (2), p. 99. K_{antag} is readily obtained from Fig. 4.2, Ia as follows. Considering DRCs 1 and A_2 it can be shown that the dose-ratio (dose necessary for 50% response in the presence of the antagonist compared with that of the agonist alone, i.e. D_2/D_1) minus one equals

---

*The dissociation constant K_d ($= k_2/k_1$) is the reciprocal of K_a.

$A_2 . K_{antag}$ (where A_2 = antagonist concentration). Similarly, D_3/D_1 minus one equals $A_3 . K_{antag}$ (where A_3 = antagonist concentration in $DRCA_3$) and so on. This enables Fig. 4.2, IIIa to be drawn in which, by plotting dose-ratio minus 1 against antagonist concentration, the slope of the line is K_{antag}. This computation is also valid in Fig. 4.2, Ib *as long as the curves reach the maximum response*, i.e. for DRCs 1, A_2 and A_3.

The potency of a competitive reversible antagonist can be expressed as a pA_2 value. This is the negative logarithm of the concentration (A_2) of the antagonist which reduces the response of twice the dose of the agonist to that of a single (unit) dose. The required value of A_2 is obtained as shown in Fig. 4.2, III and, as explained alongside, is equal to the dissociation constant of the antagonist (K_B). The higher the pA_2 (pK_B) the greater the effectiveness of the antagonist.

In Fig. 4.2, Ia and Ib represent 'ideal' results. In practice the 'irreversible' DRCs may only tail off at very high antagonist concentrations (e.g. if there are a large number of spare receptors). Conversely, the 'reversible' DRCs may, under similar circumstances, fail to achieve a maximum response. This is due to the fact that, whereas agonists combine with and are released from receptors with half-lives of microseconds, antagonists—showing less fit—often take several seconds (or even minutes) to perform the same cycle. Therefore, at the limit of the spare-receptor ratio, even reversible antagonists appear to be combining for prolonged periods, i.e. to be 'irreversible' in comparison with agonists. In equivocal cases a separation of reversible and irreversible antagonists can be made by varying the time during which the tissue is exposed to the antagonist before the exhibition of the agonist. Consider Figs. 4.2, Ia and Ib. In the former, if the antagonist concentration used in $DRCA_2$ was given originally 1 minute previously, it would still produce the same curve following a pre-incubation of 2 minutes. The reason is that, during the extra minutes, antagonist molecules will associate with and dissociate from the receptor approximately equally. However, with the irreversible antagonist, during the extra minute of pre-incubation more molecules of antagonist combine *permanently* with the receptor so that the DRC will be shifted to the right (e.g. from $DRCA_2$ to $DRCA_3$ in Fig. 4.2, Ib).

Synergists

Synergism (Gk: *syn*, together; *ergon*, work) is the converse of antagonism. It indicates that two (or more) drugs are acting to produce the same effect. If the combined response equals the sum of the individual actions, it is called *addition*: if it is greater, the term used is *potentiation*. For examples, *see* p. 439. *Note*: In the presence of a synergist the DRC of the original agonist is displaced *to the left*.

4.5   Theories of drug–receptor interaction in relation to response

Occupation theories
The original hypothesis postulated that the intensity of drug response was proportional to the number of specific receptors in a particular tissue or organ with which the drug combined. This simple 'occupation theory' was found to be deficient in a number of respects (e.g. lack of cognisance of spare receptors in many tissues) and so was modified to become an 'occupation theory with spare receptors'. On occupation theory, agonists of different potencies (as illustrated in Fig. 4.1) could vary in either
- *affinity*, i.e. capacity to bind to the receptor or
- *efficacy*, i.e. ability to activate the receptor (DR*) and produce the observed response, viz.

$$D + R \overset{\text{affinity}}{\rightleftharpoons} DR \overset{\text{efficacy}}{\longrightarrow} DR^* \longrightarrow \text{effect} \tag{2}$$

Thus, on muscarinic receptors, the efficacy of acetylcholine could be greater than that of formylcholine which, in turn, exceeded that of propionylcholine. The butyryl derivative could have such a low efficacy that it would require more than 100% of receptors to be present to achieve the maximum response. Such a partial agonist might, for example, induce only a brief channel open time and/or low ionic conductance (*see* 4.8).

Two-state model
Alternatively, the partial agonist effectiveness may be better explained in terms of a model in which the receptor is postulated to exist in two configurations which preferentially combine with the agonist and the antagonist, respectively ('two-state model', Fig. 4.3).

Another major difficulty with occupation theories is seen when acetylcholine combines with its specific receptors in skeletal muscle and in the electric organs of the eel (*Electrophorus*) or ray (*Torpedo*), namely *positive cooperativity*. This means that the interaction of one agonist molecule favours binding of subsequent agonist molecules to the same

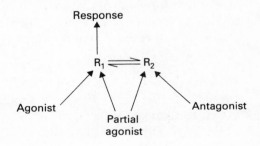

Fig. 4.3 Two-state model. For explanation, *see* text.

receptor. A similar phenomenon is also found in enzyme biochemistry where one explanation has been the two-state model. This may be applied to drug–receptor interaction as shown in Fig. 4.3. The receptor exists in two interchangeable states, R_1 which preferentially binds the agonist *to produce a response*, and R_2, to which the antagonist binds more readily. Efficacy may be equated with the extent of R_1 compared with R_2 binding. Also, when an agonist combines with R_1, more R_2 receptors change to the R_1 configuration, thus providing an explanation for positive cooperativity. Conversely, when R_2 sites are occupied by antagonist molecules, the equilibrum is moved in the opposite direction so that fewer R_1 sites are available and, therefore, a greater concentration of agonist is required to produce an effect equal to that obtained in the absence of antagonist, i.e. displacement of the DRC to the right by the antagonist (Fig. 4.2, Ia). The two-state model also provides a satisfactory explanation of *partial agonist* action for (as shown in Fig. 4.3) such drugs can combine with either receptor. Given alone, they interact with R_1 sites and produce an agonist response; however, in the presence of a full agonist, they tend to interfere with its action both by competing for R_1 receptors and, by binding with the R_2 site, causing more receptors to change configuration from R_1 to R_2.

An occupation theory assumes that agonist and antagonist interact with the same receptor sites. For the most fully characterised receptor (nicotinic acetylcholine, a glycoprotein of pentameric structure, p. 104) the agonists and antagonists are considered to combine with the same subunit(s). However, this does not impugn the validity of the two-state model which is not a two-site model. On both occupation theory and the two-state model, *overall* affinity constants both for agonists and for antagonists are indistinguishable, and, in either case, desensitisation of receptors can be accommodated by the addition of a further configurational change so that a diminished affinity (or efficacy) results (Fig. 2.18).

In conclusion, the 'occupation theory with spare receptors' and the 'two-state model' represent concepts which were valuable in the initial development of receptor pharmacology but are relatively naïve in that they are too static and too immutable. They fail to take account of the dynamic nature both of the approaching drug and its receptor(s) (p. 92), and of the several factors (4.7) which can modify this first link in the chain of drug–response relationships.

4.6   Selective ligands
Ligands (L*: *ligare*, to bind) are molecular entities which selectively attach to tissue sites, in particular to specific receptor configurations (Table 4.3). They have two main uses.

---

*L, Latin

Table 4.3 Selective ligands for some common receptors*

Receptor type	Ligand	Agonist or antagonist
Acetylcholine		
muscarinic	^{3}H-atropine	Antagonist
nicotinic	^{3}H-α-bungarotoxin	Antagonist
Adrenaline		
α	^{3}H-phenoxybenzamine	Antagonist
β	$(-)^3$H-dihydroalprenolol	Antagonist
Histamine		
H$_1$	^{3}H-mepyramine (US: pyrilamine)	Antagonist
H$_2$	^{3}H-cimetidine	Antagonist
Opiate†		
δ	^{3}H-*D*-ala, D-leu-enkephalin	Agonist
κ	^{3}H-*k*etocyclazocine	Agonist
μ	^{3}H-*m*orphine	Agonist
σ	^{3}H-*S*KF 10047 (N-allylnorphenazocine)	Agonist
GABA$_A$ (Table 6.7)	^{3}H-muscimol	Agonist

*This list is only meant as a guide: discovery of even more specific ligands is a continuing process, especially as receptor types become subdivided ever further.
†Initial letters of prototype ligands (italicised)—converted to the Gk. equivalent—indicates the bizarre origin of opiate receptor terminology.

Affinity determination

When radioactively labelled, ligands can be used on whole or broken cell preparations (e.g. synaptosomes, p. 149) to determine the amount of binding, i.e. the affinity of either an agonist or an antagonist. It must be realised that most drugs—if in sufficient concentration and especially if charged—will bind to oppositely charged, exposed, cell constituents. Therefore, the essential requisites for a suitable *selective* molecule are:

- high specificity (including stereospecificity, if applicable)
- high affinity
- inhibition by specific agents (if an agonist)
- displacement by similarly selective agents (for either agonists or antagonists).

Fig. 4.4a illustrates a typical experiment in which a particular tissue is exposed to different ambient concentrations of radioactively labelled agonist or antagonist (abscissa) and, after a standard time, the total amount of the ligand which has become bound to the tissue is determined and plotted as ordinate (OA). A line (OB) is then determined experimentally by measuring the amount of radioactive binding in the presence of a large excess of the non-radiolabelled form of the same or a similarly bound drug. Because there is only a limited number of *specific* (receptor) sites compared to a relatively unlimited number of non-specific sites, the large excess of the non-radiolabelled form effectively excludes the radiolabelled moiety from the specific, *saturable* sites. Therefore, OB represents combination with the non-specific, non-saturable components and subtraction of the OB values from those of OA results in the curve OC. This indicates the specific, saturable, component—the total number of available sites (B_{max}, binding maximum) being indicated by the intercept on the ordinate, and the affinity constant (by similar reasoning to that given in 4.4) by the reciprocal of the concentration of ligand necessary to achieve 50% of the total specific binding.

This method is unsatisfactory if the curve OC never achieves a constant value and the *preferable*, alternative method is illustrated in Fig. 4.4b. Here, a double-reciprocal plot is made: the ordinate is the reciprocal of the *specific* binding (difference between that in the absence and that in the presence of a large excess of the same (or a similarly binding) drug which is not radioactively labelled). Now, the affinity constant for the specific binding of the radioactive drug is given by minus the *x*-intercept and the total number of specific binding sites (B_{max}) by the reciprocal of the *y*-intercept. A third possibility is a Scatchard plot (*see* Fig. 4.4c which is self-explanatory): a straight line usually indicates homogeneity of binding sites; conversely, discontinuities or curves indicate multiple binding sites and/or cooperative effects.

When a competing ligand—agonist or antagonist—is introduced, the amount of the original ligand specifically bound will decrease. The affinity constant of the displacing ligand (K_2) can be determined under two conditions as follows.

1 When the displacing ligand is in a constant concentration (i), use a double–reciprocal plot (Fig. 4.4b, line D)
Then

$$K_2 = \frac{\dfrac{K_a}{x} - 1}{i}$$

2 When the displacing ligand is varying in concentration, plot as in Fig. 4.4d and determine the concentration (A) of the displacing ligand which reduces the specific binding of the original ligand to 50% of its initial value. Then

$$K_2 = \frac{1 + DK_1}{A}$$

where D and K_1 are, respectively, the concentration and the affinity constant of the original ligand.

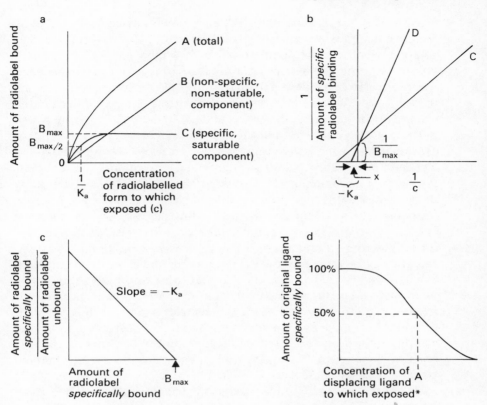

Fig. 4.4 Methods for obtaining affinity constants from binding experiments (*see* text for details). For a single ligand: a, simple plot; b, double-reciprocal plot (line C); c, Scatchard plot. For a displacing ligand: *at constant concentration*, b (line D); *at varying concentration*, d, (*log scale often preferable).

Calculations of affinity constants by these methods agree well with those determined by classical methods (e.g. DRCs, 4.4). They also show adequate differential effects between active (strongly binding) and less active (weakly binding) stereoisomers, such as $S(+)$- and $R(-)$-methacholine at muscarinic receptors (Table 2.1).

Caveat. It is vital to appreciate that, while many agents show extremely selective affinity for (presumably) specific areas in particular tissues, such results are only relevant pharmacologically if it can be demonstrated that affinity is related to *an effect* (in the case of an agonist) or to prevention of a response (in the case of an antagonist).

Receptor isolation (and analysis of function at a molecular level)
The commonest technique is *affinity chromatography*. In this, a specific ligand attached to the chromatography column retains the receptor

fraction when a solubilised membrane extract is passed through it. The receptor material is then eluted by the passage of a specific ligand solution which is subsequently removed by dialysis.

Further processes in the determination of receptor mechanisms at the molecular level are well exemplified by the intensively-studied nicotinic acetylcholine receptor. This is present in large amount in the electric organs of the ray (*Torpedo*) and eel (*Electrophorus*) from which it was originally extracted and shown to consist of four subunits (α, β, γ, δ) arranged—when viewed from the outer surface of the membrane—as a pentameric (e.g. α, β, α, γ, δ) rosette. When inserted into a lipid bilayer, the receptor orientated itself as an integral protein (Fig. 1.2) protruding on both sides of the membrane and thus able to act both as the receptor (responsive to *two* agonist molecules binding successively at *two* α-sites) and *also as the associated ion channel* (allowing sodium ions to pass inwards) across the membrane. Analysis of each subunit of the (protein) receptor revealed their amino acid sequences and enabled complementary DNAs (cDNAs) to be cloned so that receptors could be manufactured (in *Xenopus* oocytes). Mutagenesis of these clones at specific sites allowed the determination of the exact site(s) on the α-subunits which received the agonist and detailed models of the whole receptor–channel complex to be proposed. Further, single-channel recordings (*see* p. 108) enabled kinetic properties—opening and closing times, conductances—to be evaluated.

Nicotinic acetylcholine receptors isolated from the skeletal neuromuscular junctions of several vertebrate species show a high degree of amino acid sequence homology with that of the *Torpedo* receptor. Greater differences are found between nicotinic muscular and ganglionic receptors which could account, for example, for the different antagonists at skeletal neuromuscular and autonomic ganglionic sites (p. 41). Central nervous system nicotinic acetylcholine receptors also appear to be heterogeneous.

While the fine details of structure and function are being evaluated for the nicotinic acetylcholine receptor, other well-characterised receptors—in terms of function, e.g. β-adrenoceptors, muscarinic cholinoceptors—are being isolated and analysed with regard to structure and molecular function. No doubt in the future similar rigorous criteria will be demanded as the final proof for any specific receptor.

4.7   Other points concerning receptors

Receptor regulation (*see also* 4.2)

The phenomenon of *desensitisation* of the nicotinic acetylcholine receptor, which has been briefly described on p. 75, now appears to be of much more general significance than was originally thought. It can occur over a range of time scales and via a number of mechanisms (not all of which need apply to a particular receptor) which can be systematised as follows.

Autoregulatory ('homosynaptic', 'homologous') control implies that the agonist receptor sites are responsible for the effect. For example, in the case of the *nicotinic* acetylcholine receptor successive binding of two agonist molecules to two α-subunit sites not only opens the ionic channel but also (over a longer time interval) converts the receptor protein to a non-channel-forming configuration.

Heteroregulatory ('heterosynaptic', 'heterologous') control occurs when the desensitisation is caused by a second substance (e.g. co-transmitter, autacoid, hormone, drug) which does not act primarily on the receptors. The effect commonly appears to involve the production of a protein kinase (4.9) which phosphorylates the cytoplasmic portion of the original receptor, e.g. application of cAMP analogues or forskolin (Fig. 4.6) can both phosphorylate *and* desensitise nicotinic cholinoceptors in muscle cell cultures.

Conversely, similar but *positive* (reinforcing) feedback mechanisms may be responsible for receptor sensitisation. Physiologically, desensitisation and sensitisation can be visualised as modulating influences which allow finer control of responses: therapeutically, they suggest caution when drugs are used chronically.

Innervation

While, for example, prostaglandin receptors are present in many tissues in the absence of pure prostaglandinergic nerves, and histamine receptors are mostly non-innervated, it is sometimes difficult to realise that, for example, β_2-adrenoceptors subserving vasodilation in the peripheral circulation (Fig. 10.7) are independent of an efferent nerve supply. This illustrates an important distinction between physiological neurotransmitters and pharmacological agents: for the latter the *receptor*, rather than the nerve supply, is paramount. For example, the umbilical vessels are not innervated but respond to many transmitters and autacoids. Even the formation of subsequently innervated receptors can be initially independent of nerve supply (e.g. 4-day-old chick embryo heart cells produce positive inotropic responses to catecholamines in the absence of innervation). Similarly, embryonic (non-innervated) skeletal muscles respond to acetylcholine along the whole surface of the muscle fibre (compare denervation, 4.2) whereas, when the nerve supply is established, the end-plate region shows selective sensitivity (4.2). Thus, nervous activity can undoubtedly affect receptor distribution.

It also has an important role to play as a trophic agent. In normally innervated tissues, denervation results (within periods varying from days to months) in complete degeneration of the motor junction. Initially, the relevant tissue shows hypersensitivity (4.2) to directly applied drugs but later these responses may become attenuated due to the chronic absence of tissue receptor trophic factors. A further example of the latter is nerve growth factor (NGF) which is produced by effector organs and transported retrogradely to sympathetic and sensory nerve cell bodies. It is necessary, particularly in neonatal animals, for correct growth of the *peripheral* sympathetic and sensory systems. An antibody to NGF, given experimentally, causes degeneration (in order of importance) of sympathetic ganglia, sensory neurones, and sympathetic neurones.

Hormonal milieu
This can affect receptors
• quantitatively, e.g. cardiac β-adrenoceptors increase in hyperthyroidism and decrease in hypothyroidism (p. 282)
• qualitatively, e.g. the balance of adrenoceptors in uterine muscle. In many species they are predominantly β_2 (causing relaxation, Table 2.3): oestrogen pretreatment can increase the number of α-receptor sites (producing contraction) but the simultaneous administration of a progestogen restores the β_2 predominance. Similar considerations may explain some sex differences in drug responses.

RECEPTOR–RESPONSE LINKING
(Synopsis, Fig. 4.5. Details, for extracellular receptors, Figs 4.6–4.9) For intracellular receptors, *see* pp. 91–92.

For extracellular receptors there are two main *primary* mechanisms which result in cellular responses, namely
• ion-flux changes across the cell membrane
• enzyme modifications.
There is often considerable interplay between these two processes, e.g. enzyme modifications in the cell membrane (Figs. 4.8 and 4.9) generate intracellular enzymes which modulate Ca^{2+} ion channel entry and thus alter the activity of Ca^{2+}-calmodulin (dependent) protein kinases.

4.8   Ion-flux changes
These may be evoked *either* by receptor activation/inactivation (receptor-operated channels, ROC), e.g. at synapses; *or* by voltage changes (voltage-operated channels, VOC), e.g. transmission along nerve, muscle or cardiac conducting tissue membranes. In both cases, the ionic flow at a given voltage depends upon the number of channels open, their conductances and the lengths of time during which they are open. Originally, the *mean* channel lifetime and conductance were determined by Fourier analysis of the small fluctuations in membrane

1. EXTRACELLULAR RECEPTORS

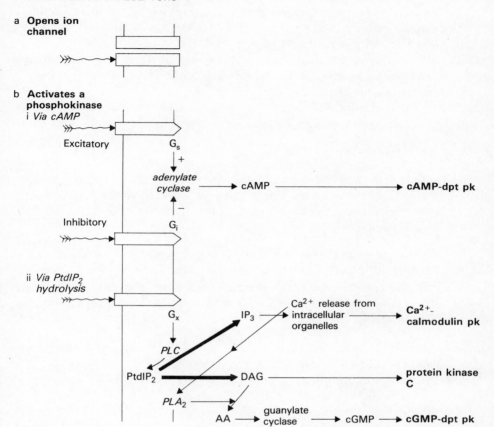

a **Opens ion channel**

b **Activates a phosphokinase**
  i *Via cAMP*

Excitatory — G_s

adenylate cyclase → cAMP → **cAMP-dpt pk**

Inhibitory — G_i

  ii *Via PtdIP$_2$ hydrolysis*

G_x — IP$_3$ → Ca^{2+} release from intracellular organelles → **Ca^{2+}-calmodulin pk**

PLC

PtdIP$_2$ → DAG → **protein kinase C**

PLA$_2$

AA → guanylate cyclase → cGMP → **cGMP-dpt pk**

2. INTRACELLULAR RECEPTOR

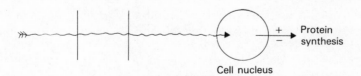

+/− Protein synthesis

Cell nucleus

Fig. 4.5 Synopsis of main mechanisms of receptor–response linking.
1. Extracellular (for details, *see* Figs. 4.6–4.9): a, receptor acts as an ion channel when activated by the agonist (or may open an ion channel via a G protein, *see* muscarinic agonist on heart muscle, Fig. 10.13); b, drug–receptor binding activates enzymes in the cell membrane which produce intermediate messengers which in turn activate specific phosphokinases, i. via cyclic AMP—either excitatory or inhibitory, ii. via phosphatidyl inositol diphosphate (PtdIP$_2$) hydrolysis.
2. Intracellular (pp. 91–2): lipid-soluble drug enters the cell nucleus and combines with receptors which modulate specific new protein production.
Dpt, dependent; pk, protein kinase. For other abbreviations *see* following diagrams.

current ('noise')—due to asynchronous opening and closure of a large number of channels—recorded following drug application. Nowadays single channel recording using the patch-clamp (gigohm-seal) technique allows *direct* measurement of

- the membrane current evoked by the drug at a given voltage (clamped) and thus allows calculation of the channel conductance—from equation (1), p. 213
- the mean times during which the channel is open *and closed*.

Examples of major channel types follow.

Sodium channels

Voltage-operated. See pp. 211–19; blocked by, for example, tetrodotoxin, local anaesthetics. For binding agents used in the isolation and characterisation of voltage-dependent sodium ion channels *see* p. 219 and Table 8.6.

Receptor-operated. At the skeletal neuromuscular junction, successive binding of two agonist molecules to two α-subunits of a nicotinic receptor converts the receptor *which itself forms the channel across the membrane* from the closed to the open state, so that sodium ions enter the end-plate region and cause depolarisation (the end-plate potential).

Potassium channels
See 4.14 and Table 4.9.

Calcium channels
See 4.10.

Chloride channels

Receptor-operated. At many inhibitory synapses, especially those involving $GABA_A$ (Fig. 7.2) or glycine receptors (pp. 163–4), a specific increase in chloride conductance is produced which results in hyperpolarisation of the postsynaptic membrane.

Note on the production and maintenance of ionic gradients across membranes. This is achieved by active processes which usually involve a carrier molecule. Many such exist but it is convenient at this juncture to exemplify their physiological and pharmacological importance by describing some relevant properties of *sodium, potassium, (magnesium)-activated adenosine triphosphatase:* $Na^+, K^+, (Mg^{2+})$-ATPase; 'sodium pump'. The physiological function of this membrane-bound enzyme is to act as an ionophore actively transporting Na^+ and K^+ ions against their concentration gradients which, for example, results in

- the maintenance of the resting potential in excitable tissues (dependent on K^+ ion gradient and permeability: nerve, 8.2; heart muscle, 10.12)

- the passage of potassium ions into, for example, skeletal muscle, erythrocytes (Table 2.3, footnote ||)
- the absorption of sodium ions and, hence, for example, water, glucose and amino acids from the renal tubular fluid (Fig. 12.3) or the alimentary canal (13.1).

This enzyme is stimulated by (nor)adrenaline, phenytoin (p. 170, p. 284), lower concentrations of digoxin (p. 271), and aldosterone (Fig. 12.3). It is depressed by higher concentrations of digoxin which thereby increase intracellular Na^+ in cardiac tissue and allow calcium ion entry (Fig. 10.12).

4.9 Enzyme modifications

Basically the responses elicited are mediated by protein phosphorylations produced by the actions of a variety of *protein kinases which are serine and threonine specific* and are generated via three main systems (see also *tyrosine* kinase, Fig. 14.6)*

- cyclic AMP formation
- membrane phospholipid transformations. The most important of these is phosphatidyl inositol diphosphate hydrolysis
- calcium ion entry or release from intracellular organelles.

Each of these will now be discussed in detail but, as can be seen from Figs 4.8 and 4.9, in practice there is considerable overlapping of their *intermediate messenger* processes.

Responses are terminated both by receptor inactivation and by protein *de*phosphorylation (with phosphatases 1, 2A, 2B and 2C).

Cyclic adenosine 3,5-monophosphate (cAMP) formation
This nucleotide is an extremely common intermediate messenger (especially for many polypeptide hormones and some neurotransmitters) which can both amplify the signal and trigger a wide variety of subsequent events. The fundamental arrangement is illustrated in Fig. 4.6.

An *activating* agent attaches to a receptor exposed on the outer surface of a cell and is considered to induce the following train of events:

1 The receptor is modified so that it combines with a *stimulatory* guanine nucleotide-binding regulatory protein, G_s (which in the inactive state has three subunits α, β and γ, with GDP attached to the α-subunit) to release GDP (guanosine diphosphate).

2 $G_{s\alpha}$ then combines with GTP, separates from the $\beta\gamma$ subunits and stimulates the catalytic unit of adenylate cyclase to increase the production of cAMP.

---

* Because the kinases phosphorylate hydroxyl (.OH) groups of proteins, they can only interact with amino acid residues containing .OH groups namely serine, threonine and tyrosine.

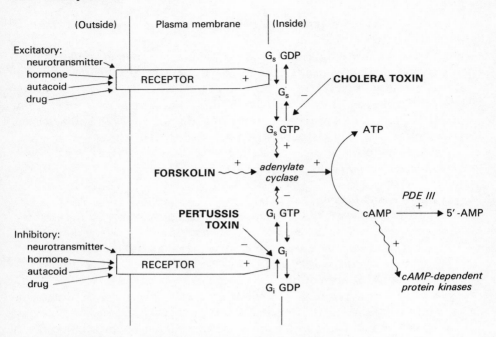

Fig. 4.6 The formation and inactivation of CAMP (diagrammatic). G_s guanine nucleotide-binding regulatory protein, stimulatory; G_i guanine nucleotide-binding regulatory protein, inhibitory. GD(T)P, guanosine di-(tri-)phosphate. PDE III, phosphodiesterase III. For mechanisms of substances shown in bold type viz. forskolin, cholera toxin, pertussis toxin, *see* text. +, excitatory; −, inhibitory. Wavy arrows indicate activation/inactivation of enzymes (italicised).

3   There is a resting level of cAMP formation and the system returns to this as
• $G_{s\alpha}$ (acting as a GTPase) loses GTP by hydrolysis, recombines with the $\beta\gamma$ subunits and then reassociates with GDP
• cAMP is broken down (particularly by phosphodiesterase III, PDE III) to inactive 5'-AMP.
Note the actions of two analytical agents: *forskolin*, which activates adenylate cyclase independently of the guanine nucleotide stage, and *cholera toxin* which ADP-ribosylates $G_{s\alpha}$ and prevents the hydrolysis of $G_{s\alpha}$ GTP so that there is a continued raised level of cAMP.

An *inhibitory* agent induces a corresponding train of reactions via an *inhibitory* guanine nucleotide-binding regulatory protein, G_i, the final effect of which is to lessen the intracellular concentration of cAMP. An analytical tool here is *pertussis toxin* which ADP-ribosylates G_i and prevents the combination of the activated receptor with G_i, so that there is not a fall in cAMP.

The involvement of cAMP is considered to be proved when the criteria in Table 4.4 (analogous to those on p. 39) are fulfilled. The most

Table 4.4 Criteria to show cAMP involvement in the production of a response

1 Activation of adenylate cyclase (shown on whole or isolated plasma membrane preparations)
2 Increased tissue concentration of cAMP, *which must precede the response*
3 Production of a similar response by *either* 8-bromo-cAMP *or* forskolin (which activates adenylate cyclase independently of the stimulatory guanine nucleotide-binding regulatory protein, Fig. 4.6): effect blocked by N-ethylmaleimide, an alkylating agent (p. 411) which irreversibly inactivates adenylate cyclase.
4 Effect
   (a) potentiated by phosphodiesterase *(PDE) inhibitors, e.g. theophylline (1,3-dimethylxanthine, p. 235), IBMX (3-isobutyl-1-methylxanthine).
   (b) antagonised by PDE activators, e.g. imidazole, N-methyl imidazole.

*Cyclic nucleotide phosphodiesterases inactivate cAMP and cGMP. There are three major isoenzymes: of these, PDE III is the one which shows marked selectivity and high affinity for cAMP. An example of a PDE III selective inhibitor is SK&F 94120; theophylline and IBMX are non-selective.

common initial molecular mechanism is activation (by binding to a regulatory subunit) of a cAMP-dependent kinase which then phosphorylates a serine or threonine residue of a protein (e.g. glucagon action, Fig. 14.6), however this can lead to a very wide repertoire of effects as can be seen from the representative examples shown in Tables 4.5 and 4.6. The corollary is that particular tissues and organs contain different adenylate cyclases which respond selectively to different

Table 4.5 Some important hormonal effects mediated via cAMP

Body constituent	Effect	Agonist hormone	Antagonist hormone
Carbohydrate	Liver glycogenolysis	Glucagon Adrenaline Somatotrophin	Insulin
Fat	Lipolysis	Adrenaline Somatotrophin	Insulin
Protein	Gluconeogenesis	Adrenal glucocorticoids Corticotrophin	Insulin
	Enzyme production for synthesis of adrenal gluco- and sex corticoids		
Calcium	Calcium release from bone	Parathyroid hormone	Calcitonin
Water	Increased permeability of distal convoluted tubules and collecting ducts of kidney	Vasopressin	

Table 4.6 Neurotransmitter receptor subtypes considered to act through the intermediation of *either* cyclic AMP *or* phosphatidyl inositol diphosphate (PtdIP$_2$) hydrolysis

Neurotransmitter	Receptor type		
	Increasing cAMP	Decreasing cAMP*	PtdIP$_2$ hydrolysis
Acetylcholine[1]		muscarinic	muscarinic
(Nor)adrenaline[2]	β	α_2	α_1
Histamine[3]	H$_2$		H$_1$

For actions: 1 and 2, *see* Table 2.3; for 3, *see* Table 5.2.
*Usually only if cAMP increased first.

(specific) stimuli. A closely studied example is the interaction of adrenaline with β_1-adrenoceptors in heart muscle which activate cAMP and produce a positive inotropic effect (PIE). A similar response can be achieved by glucagon, forskolin (which increases cardiac adenylate cyclase activity directly) or by prevention of cAMP breakdown, particularly with phosphodiesterase III inhibitors (*see* footnote to Table 4.4 and Fig. 10.13).

As shown in Table 4.5 some hormones act by opposing cAMP activity, particularly insulin (Fig. 14.6) and calcitonin.

Membrane phospholipid transformations
Figure 4.7 shows the sites of action for different phospholipases.

Phosphatidyl inositol diphosphate hydrolysis
As shown in Fig. 4.8, agonist combination with a receptor via a guanine nucleotide-binding regulatory protein, G$_x$, activates a specific phosphatidyl inositol phospholipase C to break down the membrane lipid, phosphatidyl inositol 4,5-diphosphate, into D-inositol 1,4,5-triphosphate (IP$_3$) and 1,2-diacylglycerol (DAG). These intermediate messengers then generate protein kinases which greatly affect calcium ion entry into cells and release from intracellular stores—note the negative feedback of protein kinase C on the latter.

Analytical agents are *phorbol esters*, which are analogues of DAG and can themselves activate protein kinase C: and *haemoglobin*, which inhibits cytoplasmic (soluble) guanylate cyclase by competing for sites normally occupied by the haem moiety of the enzyme. *Lithium* (p. 185) inhibits IP$_2$ breakdown.

A growing number of specific receptors are considered to be linked to this system. Important examples (Table 4.6) are muscarinic receptors (also decrease cAMP—if tissue levels are initially increased), α_1-adrenoceptors (*see* Table 3.5) and H$_1$-histamine receptors (Table 5.2).

a *Phosphatidyl inositol diphosphate hydrolyses*

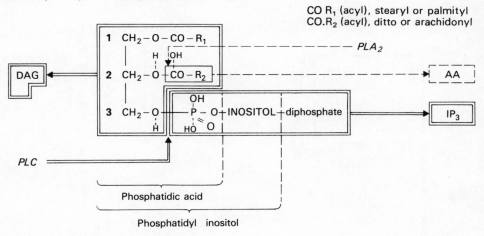

b *Formation of platelet activating factor (PAF)*

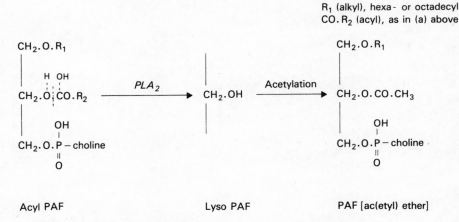

Fig. 4.7 Phospholipid hydrolyses. a, phosphatidyl inositol breakdown by *phospholipase C (PLC)* which produces inositol triphosphate (IP$_3$) and diacylglycerol (DAG): the latter can be further hydrolysed by *phospholipase A$_2$* to arachidonic acid (AA). For actions of these breakdown products *see* Figs 4.8 and 4.9. Note that phosphorylation of DAG results in the phosphatidic acid necessary for the synthesis of PtdIP$_3$ (Fig. 4.8); and that AA can be produced by the action of PLA$_2$ on the unhydrolysed phospholipid (Fig. 5.6). b, generation of platelet activating factor [acetyl ether] (PAF[acether], p. 146). *Note* that arachidonic acid can also be produced from PAF.

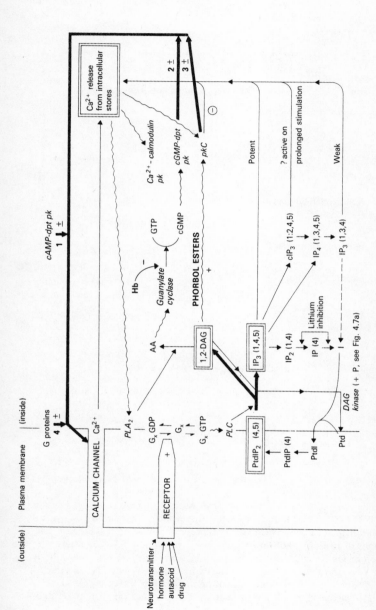

Fig. 4.8 How receptor-activated mechanisms acting *via* the phosphatidyl inositol system modify calcium release from intracellular stores and entry from the extracellular fluid (diagrammatic). Receptor stimulation, *via* a guanine-nucleotide regulatory protein (G_x), activates a phospholipase C (PLC)—specifically phosphatidylinositidase C—to hydrolyse phosphatidyl inositol diphosphate (PtdIP$_2$) with the formation of inositol triphosphate (IP$_3$) and 1,2-diacylglycerol (DAG). These two intermediate messengers then affect release of calcium from intracellular stores (−, inhibition) and the resultant formation of three phosphokinases (pks) namely Ca^{2+}-calmodulin, cyclic GMP-dependent (cGMP-dpt) and protein kinase C (pkC). Thick lines indicate receptor-operated factors (labelled 1–4 here and in Fig. 4.9) affecting calcium channels (+/−, opening or closing depending upon the tissue involved). For actions of haemoglobin (Hb), phorbol esters and lithium, *see* text. AA, arachidonic acid; cIP$_3$, cyclic inositol triphosphate; PLA$_2$, phospholipase A$_2$; Ptd, phosphatidic acid. Bracketed numbers after P groups indicate points of attachment to the inositol ring. Wavy lines indicate activations of *enzymes* (italicised); interrupted line indicates multi-stage process.

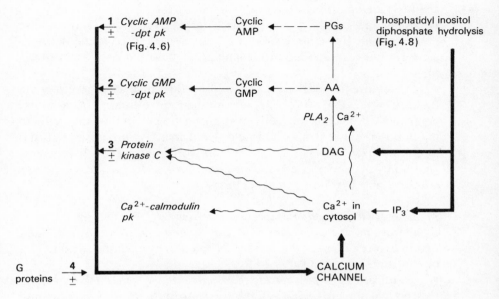

Phosphorylation
mechanisms
(protein kinases, pk)

Fig. 4.9 Genesis of protein phosphorylation mechanisms (*all those shown are serine and threonine specific*) and their importance (1–4) in relation to calcium channel activation ($+/-$ opens or closes depending on the particular tissue involved)—*see also* Fig 4.8.
PGs, prostaglandins (Fig. 5.6); other abbreviations as in Fig. 4.8.
Note: While mechanism 1 acts by phosphorylating channel proteins, mechanisms 2 and 3 work less directly, probably by the phosphorylation of regulatory units associated with the channel protein. The mode of action of mechanism 4 is unknown at present.

Further subtleties are still being discovered in the system. For instance, the production of inositol *cyclic* 1:2, 4, 5-triphosphate—cIP_3 (1:2, 4, 5)—is normally slight but on prolonged stimulation it accumulates due to slower breakdown than IP_3. Additionally, further feedback and feed-forward mechanisms are coming to light.

Finally, note the mechanisms by which *calcium* channels (discussed in 4.10) may be modified. These are numbered 1–4 in Figs 4.8 and 4.9. Similar modulating influences can affect calcium-activated *potassium* channels (Table 4.9).

4.10 Calcium

In addition to its structural functions (including membrane stabilisation, Table 8.1) and importance in thrombin formation (see Fig. 17.4), this ion occupies a central role as an intermediate messenger. A

simplified diagram of its distribution in various body compartments is shown in Fig. 4.10 from which it is obvious that the ion
• will pass into cells down a concentration gradient (when calcium channels are open)
• will be in a constant state of flux between a number of intracellular pools, such as free cytoplasmic (the active agent in coupling mechanisms, *see* later) and bound intracellular (e.g. in sarcoplasmic reticulum, mitochondria)
• will require (in addition to the sodium–calcium exchange, either via the cell wall, Fig. 10.12 or membranes surrounding intracellular organelles) a mechanism actively transporting it out of the cell—to maintain the concentration gradient—and an active process to return it to intracellular organelles, i.e. calcium ion pumps (which are most commonly dependent upon magnesium ions and *blocked by vanadate*), namely Ca^{2+}, Mg^{2+}-activated ATPases.

Methods for the detection of calcium involvement
• alterations in the *extracellular Ca^{2+} ion concentration* by the addition of extra calcium or the removal of calcium by chelation with EGTA or trisodium edetate (Table 20.5)
• modifications of *passage along selective calcium channels* by activators, e.g. calcimycin (A 23187), BAY K 8644, or blockers, e.g. verapamil (*see* 4.11)
• *free cytoplasmic Ca^{2+} ions* concentrations can be monitored by the quantitative measurement of fluorescent indicators such as fura-2 or aequorin: these concentrations can be *in*creased experimentally by flash-photolysis of cells preloaded with a photolabile calcium chelator, for example nitr-5
• prevention of *calcium release from intracellular stores* by ryanodine.

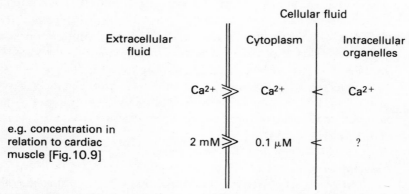

Fig. 4.10 Calcium ion distribution in relation to intermediate messenger function. ?, variable concentration (depending on organelle) but greater than in cytosol.

Table 4.7 Processes involving the Ca^{2+} ion as an intermediate messenger

Excitation–contraction coupling (examples in text)	Excitation–secretion coupling	
	Process	Example(s)
Skeletal muscle contraction	Neurotransmitter release	Acetylcholine (2.2) Noradrenaline (3.2)
Cardiac muscle contraction	Autacoid release Exocrine secretion	Mast cell contents (5.3) GI tract secretions
Smooth muscle contraction	Endocrine secretion	Insulin (14.4)

Note a similar effect of dantrolene (Table 7.3) in the treatment of skeletal muscle spasticity or malignant hyperthermia (p. 442).

The relationship between Ca^{2+} and Mg^{2+} ions at receptor sites is complicated. In some situations (e.g. skeletal neuromuscular junction) their effects are antagonistic, so that $MgCl_2$ can produce paralysis rapidly reversible by an equimolar amount of $CaCl_2$. However, in other cases, the actions of the two ions are synergistic, e.g. Ca^{2+}, Mg^{2+}-activated ATPase.

Calcium ions act as intermediate messengers in two main situations (Table 4.7)
1 Excitation–contraction (E–C) coupling in skeletal, cardiac (10.7) and smooth muscle, p. 243.
2 Excitation–secretion (E–S) coupling in neurotransmitter or autacoid release and in most exocrine and endocrine secretions.
To show the broad principles underlying most coupling reactions involving calcium ions, take a simple well-known case. In *skeletal muscle*, the action potential depolarises the T-tubules which results in the release of Ca^{2+} ions from the sarcoplasmic reticulum into the cytosol. These calcium ions combine with troponin C to produce a conformational change in tropomyosin which exposes a reactive part of the actin filament: this interacts with the myosin head, inducing both movement and myosin ATPase activity.

Methods for the generation of increased levels of cytoplasmic Ca^{2+} ions
There may be
● direct release, i.e. the stimulus opens channels which allow calcium ions to enter the cell, or liberates sarcoplasmic reticulum stores
● indirect release, i.e. the stimulus acts via intermediate messengers to cause calcium ion entry or the mobilisation of free cytoplasmic ions from intracellular reservoirs (Figs 4.8 and 4.9).

Direct release. This is brought about by depolarisation of the cell membrane and is well exemplified by the slow inward current in the nodal pacemaker tissues of the heart (Fig. 10.14) which is usually activated at a membrane potential between -60 and -45 mV. Thus calcium ions enter the cell via *voltage-operated channels* (VOCs) which have the additional property of slow inactivation. These particular channels are now designated as L(ong-lasting) channels, are activated by the 1,4-dihydropyridine (BAY K 8644) and have several binding sites for calcium channel blockers which might be important in the final subdivision of the latter (*see* 4.11).

Two other voltage-operated calcium channels have been described, neither of which is significantly blocked by the drugs just mentioned.

1 T(ransient) channels. These transmit *small* currents which are of brief duration due to rapid inactivation. As they are activated at slightly more negative membrane potentials than the L-channel currents they can precede the latter, e.g. in cardiac pacemaker tissues (p. 278). They are specifically blocked by nickel ions.

2 N(euronal) channels. These pass a larger current and occur in nervous tissues. L and T channels have also been identified in neurones.

Indirect release. Receptor activation of either the cyclic nucleotide or phosphatidyl inositol system modulates calcium channel availability as shown in Fig. 4.9. The channels involved may be

• voltage-dependent (VOCs), for example β_1-adrenoceptor activation of cardiac tissues generates cAMP which activates voltage-operated calcium channels (Fig. 10.13)

• voltage-independent. These are termed *receptor-operated channels* (ROCs): whether they are specific for calcium ions or are non-specific cation channels is unclear. In most smooth muscles they are not blocked by calcium channel blockers: but they are in vascular smooth muscle (*see* below).

Excitation–contraction coupling may be summarised as follows

• *skeletal muscle, see* earlier

• *cardiac muscle, see* Fig. 10.9 and accompanying text

• *smooth muscle, e.g. gut, uterus.* There are both voltage-operated channels (inactivated by calcium channel blocking drugs) and receptor-operated channels (not blocked by drugs)

• *smooth muscle, e.g. vascular* (Fig. 10.4). Depolarisation occurring naturally or experimentally induced by the application of a 'high', e.g. 20–80 mM, KCl solution to the cellular surface) results in an influx of calcium ions into the cells via voltage-operated channels which produces a contraction preventable by the prior administration of calcium channel blockers.

Noradrenaline application (Fig. 10.4) commonly results in

• an initial rapid ('phasic') contraction due to the mobilisation of calcium ions from intracellular stores (via α_1-adrenoceptors triggering phosphatidyl inositol diphosphate hydrolysis—Fig. 4.8); this grades into

• a more sustained ('tonic') contraction produced by entry of Ca^{2+} ions into the smooth muscle cell via *voltage-operated channels* (prevented by calcium channel blockers) and/or *receptor-operated channels* (these show a wide variation in their sensitivity to calcium channel blockers in different vascular tissues).

Similar principles may be applied to other calcium-dependent cellular processes.

Envoi

The most important calcium current is that mediated via L(long-lasting) voltage-operated channels and prevented by the classical calcium-channel blockers, e.g. verapamil. These channels can also be activated indirectly, e.g. by β_1-adrenoceptor agonists on cardiac tissues (Fig. 10.13).

4.11 Calcium channel blocking agents (also termed Ca^{2+} antagonists)

These can be defined as producing

• selective block of, for example, myocardial ('slow') calcium channels without significant effects on ('fast') sodium channels

• antagonism of the effects of calcium channel agonists (facilitators), such as BAY K 8644 (which is a dihydropyridine).

More specifically, the channels involved are voltage-operated L-type, and binding studies indicate three groups of blocking agents (as shown in Table 4.8) which attach to different stereoselective sites within the channel and allosterically affect each other. The calcium channel blocking agents move the steady state inactivation curve for the L-channels to the left (which is similar to the action of lowered extracellular Ca^{2+} ion concentration on the *h*-gate curve for sodium channels—*see* Fig. 8.5). Thus, at any given membrane potential there are less calcium channels available for activation. Further, the action of verapamil is frequency-dependent and also delays channel recovery from inactivation, which indicates binding of the blocker to the *inactivated* form of the channel (state-dependence).

Note, however, that in *vascular* smooth muscle, *receptor*-operated channels are also inactivated by these blocking agents.

Therapeutically, an important difference is that nifedipine is more potent on vascular smooth muscle (producing vasodilation) whereas *verapamil* is more effective on the heart. Thus, the latter is used as an antidysrhythmic agent (against supraventricular tachycardias, p. 283) but will cause more depression of heart muscle contraction (negative inotropy) and bradycardia (negative chronotropy), and so must be used

Table 4.8 Sub-groups of calcium channel blocking agents

Type substance	Nifedipine	Verapamil	Diltiazem
Chemical class*	1, 4-Dihydropyridines	Phenylalkylamines	Benzothiazepines
Block of calcium channels in:			
Cardiac tissues			
Sinu-atrial and atrioventricular nodes	+	+ +	+
Myocardium	+	+ +	+
use as antidysrhythmic drug (p. 283)	0	+	+
side-effects: negative inotropic effect,	+	+ +	±
negative chronotropic effect	0[†]	+	+ +
Vascular smooth muscle			
Arterial more than venous dilation	+ +	+	+
use in hypertension (p. 256)	+ +	+	±
side-effects: flushing, headache,			
swollen ankles	+ +	+	+
Use in angina pectoris (p. 270)	+	+	+

*Structure–activity relationship has some significance for the dihydropyridines but is nebulous for the other classes.
[†]Can cause reflex tachycardia on rapid administration.
+ +, marked; +, present; ±, slight; 0, not used or not present.

with special caution in combination with β-adrenoceptor blocking agents (p. 85), e.g. in the treatment of angina pectoris (10.10) or hypertension (p. 256). *Nifedipine* produces less negative inotropy and is preferred as a vasodilator though this action can give side-effects such as flushing and headache. Recently a few cases of gingival hyperplasia (similar to that caused by phenytoin—Table 7.1—which is stated also to inhibit calcium ion entry into cells) have been observed during nifedipine therapy. *Diltiazem* only shows slight negative inotropy but slows the heart rate significantly: so, again, care is needed in combination with β-blockers.

4.12   Calmodulins

Troponin C is homologous with this group. They are related proteins isolated from calcium-dependent protein phosphokinases (Figs 4.8 and 4.9). These enzymes are found to consist of an enzymatically acting part and a calcium-binding unit (a calmodulin), i.e. calmodulins are intracellular receptors for Ca^{2+} ions. Accordingly, their presence has been reported in association with many of the calcium ion activities shown in Table 4.7, as well as in some other microtubular functions (*see* 4.13). Other important enzymes activated via a Ca^{2+}-calmodulin link include calcium-activated ATPases (p. 114), phosphodiesterase (Fig. 4.6), guanylate cyclase (Fig. 4.8) and phospholipase A_2 (Figs 4.8 and 4.9). Calmodulins have four calcium binding sites, all of which have to be filled for, e.g., microtubular depolymerisation, whereas only one need be occupied for complete phosphodiesterase activation. A commonly-used competitive calmodulin inhibitor is *trifluoperazine* (a piperazinyl phenothiazine, like fluphenazine, Table 7.7); a more potent, but non-competitive inhibitor is calmidazolium.

4.13 Microtubules

These are cytoskeletal systems present in various forms in all eukaryotic (nucleated) cells. The basic unit is a dimer composed of two closely related globular proteins (α- and β-tubulin) which first associate into sheets and then curve to form tubules. These structures may persist by aggregating—to form, for example, cilia, flagellae—but usually differ from microfilaments (such as actin) in their evanescence because, as polymerisation (formation) proceeds at one end of the microtubule, depolymerisation (breakdown) takes place at the opposite pole. Such processes occupy only minutes and therefore can be responsible for quite rapid changes in cellular activity (*see* microtubular theory of general anaesthetic action, 8.7). Microtubules have binding sites for disrupting agents such as colchicine and vincristine (p. 413), which depolymerise cytoplasmic microtubules, or cytochalasin B, which additionally impairs actin gelation and microfilament function.

Microtubular function is usually Ca^{2+}-calmodulin-dependent. In addition to the functions shown in Table 4.7 to be associated definitely with calcium ions, probably with calmodulin and possibly with microtubules, the latter are unequivocally involved with the following:

Changes in cell shape, e.g. amoeboid movements. Rather than having a permanent rigid structure (as with actin) microtubules act as a temporary scaffolding for rapid changes in direction. This property accounts for the phagocytic activity of neutrophil polymorphonuclear leucocytes which may be opposed by the microtubule–disrupting agent, colchicine (*see* treatment of gout, 12.8).

Cell division. Microtubules are essential for the formation of the spindle (so that the chromosomes can correctly orientate), the progression of chromosomes towards respective poles, and elongation of the original cell and its division at the waist into two daughter cells. These processes can be disrupted by the aptly named 'spindle poison', *vincristine* (p. 413).

Axon flow. This is the passage of essential substances which are mainly synthesised in ribosomes near to the nucleus, from the nerve cell body to the periphery. It consists of
- total axoplasmic flow which is slow, e.g. 2 mm day^{-1}
- rapid axonal transport. This is much faster, up to 400 mm day^{-1}, and is prevented by colchicine and vincristine. It carries particular materials including enzymes essential for the synthesis of neurotrans-

mitters (e.g. choline acetyltransferase, 2.2, and enzymes for catecholamine production, 3.2).

See use of specific nerve tract-tracing markers (p. 150).

4.14   Potassium channels

There is a bewildering array of these (many often in the same cell, e.g. patch-clamp recordings on cardiac myocytes have shown at least six) and the difficulties are exacerbated by a relative lack of specificity of the available blocking agents. An attempt is made to classify the presently most important channels in Table 4.9 and to describe them, with identical numeration, below. All channels allow K^+ ions to pass *out* of the cell.

Voltage-operated channels (1)

These pass the current which classically produces repolarisation in excitable tissues, is delayed (compared with the sodium current generated on depolarisation of the cell surface) and activated at about -45 mV. It is blocked by tetraethylammonium (TEA), caesium and barium ions. Its inactivation can have significance in the depolarisation associated with the development of cardiac rhythmicity (pp. 276–8).

It may be preceded by a transient outward current (2), activated over the range -65 to -40 mV, which is preferentially blocked by 4-aminopyridine. *See* phase 1 of the cardiac action potential (p. 274 and

Table 4.9   Characteristics of important potassium channels

Number in text	Type of channel	Activated by	Subtype of channel	Current symbol	Blocking agent(s)*
1	Voltage-operated	Depolarisation to -45 mV	Delayed rectifier†	i_K	TEA‡, Cs^+, Ba^{2+}
2		Depolarisation to -65 mV	Transient outward	i_{to}§	*4-AP*
3		Hyperpolarisation	Inward rectifier†	i_{K_1}	Cs^+, TEA, Ba^{2+}
4	Receptor-operated	Acetylcholine via muscarinic receptors		$i_{ACh(M)}$	Cs^+, Ba^{2+}, 4-AP
5	Calcium-activated	Increase in cytoplasmic Ca^+	High ('big') conductance	$i_{K(Ca)B}$	*TEA*
6		concentration	Low ('small') conductance	$i_{K(Ca)S}$	*Apamin* (p. 126)
7	ATP-regulated	Decreased ATP inside the cell		$i_{K_{ATP}}$	*Tolbutamide* (Fig. 14.4)

*Most blocking agents are not very selective for the different channels: italicised names indicate significant specificity. TEA, tetraethylammonium. 4-AP, 4-aminopyridine.
†This choice of name is unfortunate as most of the potassium currents in *heart* muscle show inward rectification (for definition of this term *see* Fig. 10.15)
‡In squid axon (Table 8.5) only if applied to inner surface
§Usually termed in i_A in tissues other than the heart.

Table 10.6). Channel 3 transmits a background current which is time-independent but voltage-dependent. It is responsible *in heart tissues* for the resting potential, is inactivated on depolarisation and activated on repolarisation — *see* Table 10.6.

Receptor-operated channels (4)

The clearest example here is the effect of stimulation of muscarinic cholinoceptors on cardiac atrial tissues (Table 10.5). As can be seen from Fig. 10.13, combination of an agonist, e.g. methacholine, with the receptor via G proteins not only decreases cAMP formation which lessens Ca^{2+} ion entry but reinforces this effect by opening *potassium* channels, which hyperpolarises the membrane.

Ca^{2+}-activated K^+ channels (5, 6)

An increase in cytoplasmic calcium ion concentration generated (as shown in Fig. 4.8) either via voltage-operated channels and/or receptor activation of phospholipase C, opens potassium channels possibly by combining with calmodulin sites therein. These K^+ channels are separable—by the use of the selective blockers apamin and TEA—into low ('small') conductance (6) and high ('big') conductance (5) types. The latter appear to be generally more important because they are mainly concerned with the repolarisation of excitable membranes and can be visualised as having a negative feedback on calcium entry, i.e. their activation lowers the membrane potential to more negative values than those which trigger voltage-operated calcium (particularly L-) channels to open. Conversely, the application of TEA will depolarise a resting membrane and encourage L-channel activity, e.g. to cause transmitter release at nerve endings (p. 41). *See also* treatment of hypertension by vascular smooth muscle relaxants which act by opening potassium channels and therefore decrease calcium ion entry (p. 259).

ATP-regulated K^+ channels (7)

A rise in the intracellular ATP concentration *in*activates these channels. The resultant depolarisation of, for example, pancreatic β-cells will allow calcium ion entry with subsequent insulin release (Fig. 14.4.): tolbutamide blocks the channels and increases insulin output while diazoxide activates the channels and decreases insulin release.

Summary

Important potassium currents to remember are:

1 i_K—the repolarising current in, for example, nerve (8.2), heart tissues (also involved in the pacemaker potential, Table 10.6).

2 i_{K_1}—a background current mainly important for the resting potential in cardiac cells (Table 10.6).

3 $i_{ACh(M)}$—a receptor-induced current partly mediating the atrial negative inotropic action of acetylcholine.

5 Autacoids

Autacoid has the same middle syllable as pharmacology (derived from Gk: *akos,* a healing substance). Aut- indicates naturally occurring in the body (Gk: *autos, self*). The term is now ascribed to the following groups
- biogenic amines (histamine and 5-hydroxytryptamine, 5-HT)
- peptides and purine compounds
- lipid derivatives.

BIOGENIC AMINES

5.1 Histamine and 5-hydroxytryptamine
Much of the pharmacology of these substances is comparable to that of (nor)adrenaline. The differences are more readily understood when presented in tabular form. Examine Table 5.1 which will now be described in more detail.

Table 5.1 'Pharmacokinetics' of histamine and 5-hydroxytryptamine (5-HT) compared

	Histamine	5-HT
Occurrence	Mast cells Basophil granulocytes Gastric mucosa Central nervous system	Enterochromaffin tissue Platelets Central nervous system
Uptake/synthesis	L-histidine ↓ L-histidine decarboxylase Histamine	L-tryptophan ↓ tryptophan hydroxylase 5-Hydroxy-L-tryptophan ↓ aromatic L-amino acid decarboxylase 5-HT
Storage	Histamine } plus protein Heparin	5-HT } plus protein ATP
Release	*see* text	*See* 5.6 (carcinoid syndrome) and, from platelets, Fig. 17.3
Breakdown (5.4) main sites major products	In most tissues N-methylimidazolylacetic acid Imidazolylacetic acid Imidazolylacetic acid riboside (rat)	Especially liver and lungs; CNS 5-Methoxyindolylacetic acid 5-Methoxytryptophol 5-Hydroxyindolylacetic acid 5-Hydroxytrytophol

Histamine occurs widely in both the animal and the vegetable kingdom. Its main mammalian sites are

- mast cells. These are connective tissue elements which are present in close proximity to blood vessels for which they were originally thought to supply sustenance (mast is acorn mush given to pigs during the winter). They contain granules which are metachromatic (i.e. they do not colour true with a dye: they stain blue-*green* with toluidine blue, due to their additional content of the acidic mucopolysaccharide heparin)
- basophilic leucocytes
- gastric mucosa
- central nervous system. Not yet shown to have functional significance.

5-Hydroxytryptamine (5-HT) also has a wide distribution with a mammalian predominance in

- enterochromaffin cells. These are in the gut (enteron) especially stomach, small intestine and pancreas, and stain yellow with chromium salts (due to the phenolic hydroxyl, and the -NH- group of the pyrrol ring, *see* Fig. 5.2)
- platelets. These cells do *not* synthesise 5-HT but absorb it from the blood plasma
- central nervous system. Here this autacoid has well-authenticated functions (Chapter 6).

There is some overlap, e.g. mast cells of rat and mouse also contain 5-HT (and bradykinin, 5.10); rabbit platelets also contain histamine.

5.2 Uptake, synthesis and storage

Histamine (Fig. 5.1). Uptake of L-histidine is followed by the action of L-histidine decarboxylase (different to aromatic L-amino acid decarboxylase, 3.2) to produce histamine which (as a base) combines with acidic groups in the protein of the granules, the basic groups of the granular protein combining with the accompanying acidic heparin.

5-HT. Enterochromaffin and certain central nervous system cells take up L-tryptophan which is first converted to 5-hydroxy-L-tryptophan (by tryptophan hydroxylase) and then, by aromatic L-amino acid decarboxylase to 5-HT (Fig. 5.2). The autacoid is stored in combination with adenosine triphosphate and protein—similar to catecholamines (Fig. 3.1, d).

5.3 Release

Histamine
- from gastric mucosa (13.5)
- from mast cells. The overall process is represented in Fig. 5.3, for an antigen–antibody reaction of type I (*see* Table 20.1). An active

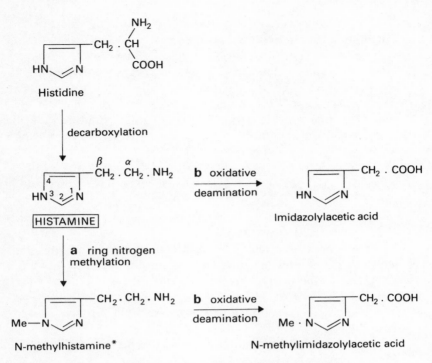

Fig. 5.1 Synthesis and breakdown of histamine. *See* text for enzymes involved. *Nomenclature of N-methylhistamines is complex: the particular compound shown here is *tele*-methylhistamine (N$^\tau$-methylhistamine)—so named because the methyl substituent is on the nitrogen atom furthest away (Gk: *tele*, far) from the side-chain. Note that the 2- and 4-methylhistamines specified as selective agonists in Table 5.2 are substituents upon *carbon* atoms.

extrusion of the granules is produced by a rise in free cytoplasmic Ca^{2+} ions brought about by a membrane phospholipid hydrolysis resulting in an increased passage of calcium into the cell. In the extracellular fluid—stripped of their protective perigranular membrane—the granules liberate their histamine by cation exchange with sodium (and, to a lesser extent, calcium) ions. Two further pathological processes which produce mast cell degranulation are inflammation (via complement factors C3a and C5a) and tissue damage.

Many naturally occurring substances can release histamine from mast cells, e.g. bee venom which contains phospholipase A_2 and three basic peptides, including apamin (Table 4.9).

Non-immunological releasers (e.g. the polymer 48/80, morphine, D-tubocurarine, substance P) act at a site distinct from the IgE receptor and *are less dependent on the presence of extracellular calcium*. Beta-adrenoceptor *agonists* inhibit histamine release (Fig. 11.2).

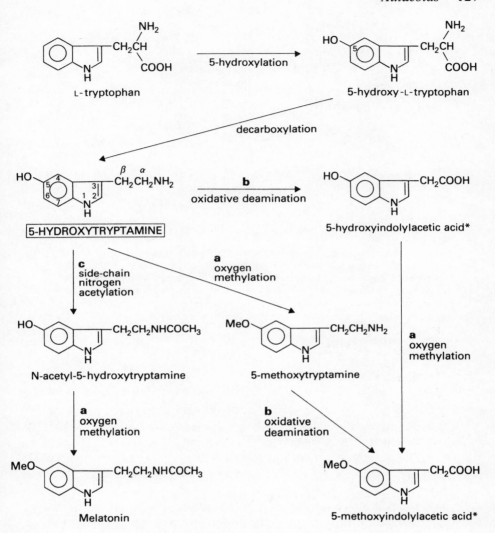

Fig. 5.2 Synthesis and metabolism of 5-HT. *See* text for enzymes involved.
*Or corresponding tryptophol (primary alcohol).

5-HT

- from enterochromaffin (carcinoid) tumours, p. 134
- from platelets (important in clotting mechanisms, Fig. 17.3)

Both histamine and 5-HT are sufficiently ionised to prevent their crossing the blood–brain barrier in significant quantities and, therefore, any central nervous system effects must be produced by these autacoids synthesised and liberated within the neuraxis.

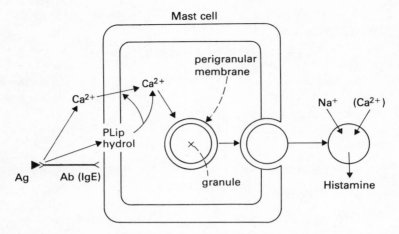

Fig. 5.3 *Immunological* release of histamine from a mast cell (schematic). A type I antigen (Ag)-antibody (Ab-IgE) reaction activates a serine esterase which hydrolyses a membrane phosphatidyl serine (PLip hydrol) with a consequent increase in free cytoplasmic calcium ions. These initiate an energy-dependent process which extrudes the granule from the cell: histamine is then released by cation exchange.
Note: It is important to realise that type I hypersensitivity reactions can release or generate other autacoids in addition to histamine (*see* Fig. 11.2). Heparin (Fig. 17.4) is also released from mast cells.

5.4   Metabolism

Metabolism of both these autacoids results in the formation of less active compounds with the exception of 5-HT conversion to N-acetyl-5-methoxytryptamine (melatonin) in the pineal gland, which may be important in controlling circadian rhythms (p. 162).

The chemical transformations show very marked species variations but are, nevertheless, analogous to those for catecholamines (Fig. 3.2) namely

a   *methylation* of a nitrogen in or oxygen on a heterocyclic nucleus
b   *oxidative deamination* of the amine group on the side-chain
c   *conjugation* of an amino or hydroxyl group.

Histamine (Fig. 5.1). The major pathways, which can take place in most tissues of the body, are

a followed by **b**. Thus, imidazole-N-methyl transferase forms N-methylhistamine (*see* footnote to Fig. 5.1) which is then converted by either monoamine oxidase or diamine oxidase (histaminase) to the corresponding methylimidazolylacetic acid

b   (can be followed by **c**). Here, diamine oxidase (preferential substrate putrescine, NH_2—$(CH_2)_4$—NH_2, or its next higher homologue, cadaverine) converts the autacoid to imidazolylacetic acid which is mainly excreted unchanged, except in the rat where the riboside is formed preferentially.

5-HT is mainly metabolised in the liver and lungs (and also the CNS) by the following processes (Fig. 5.2)

a followed by **b**. 5-hydroxyindole-oxygen-methyltransferase (5-HIOMT) forms 5-methoxytryptamine which is then converted by monoamine oxidase to 5-methoxyindolylacetic acid, or its corresponding primary alcohol, 5-methoxytryptophol

b If followed by **a** this results in the same end-products; if not it produces 5-hydroxyindolylacetic acid or 5-hydroxytryptophol (corresponding primary alcohol)

c followed by **a**. Forms N-acetyl-5-methoxytryptamine (melatonin, p. 162).

5.5 Actions

There is a tremendous overlap between the physiological, pathological and pharmacological effects of both histamine and 5-HT. For CNS effects *see* p. 155 *et seq.* (5-HT) and p. 165 (histamine).

Histamine

On the basis of selective agonists and antagonists (Table 5.2) the receptors can be subdivided into H_1 and H_2. Go down the list in Table 2.3 (smooth muscle, heart tissue and glands—omitting bladder and eye) for the major autonomically innervated tissues affected.

Smooth muscle
- bronchial: constriction (H_1)—*see* Fig. 11.1
- gut: contraction (H_1)
- uterine: contraction (H_1); exception, relaxation (H_2) in rat and mouse
- vascular: species differences become very important here
  Larger vessels (arteries or veins)—isolated—usually contract (H_1).

Intermediate vessels (arterioles and venules) —*in situ*— show overall vasoconstriction in the rat and rabbit but overall vasodilation in cat, dog and human. All these effects are mediated via both H_1 and H_2 receptors, as they require the exhibition of both groups of antagonists to block their actions.

Miscellaneous
- capillaries: There is dilation (H_1 and H_2, red reaction of the triple response) with increased permeability—w(h)eal—mainly mediated via H_1 receptors.

The vascular smooth muscle and capillary effects determine the immediate blood pressure responses in the whole animal, as the direct cardiac effects only occur at high concentrations (*see* below). Thus there is hypertension in the rat and rabbit and hypotension in cat, dog and human (the latter is not very sensitive, except in severe type I allergic reactions, see Tables 5.2 and 20.1). Reflex actions on the heart can secondarily modify the initial responses.

Heart
Direct effects occur when high concentrations are applied to isolated tissues. Again, there are wide species variations but, essentially, a positive chronotropic effect occurs via H_2 receptors: positive and

Table 5.2 Pharmacodynamics of histamine and 5-hydroxytryptamine (5-HT) compared

	Histamine		5-HT	
	H_1	H_2	$5\text{-}HT_2$	?
Agonist	2-Methylhistamine	4-Methylhistamine	α-Methyl-5HT	
Antagonist	Mepyramine (US: pyrilamine)	Cimetidine	Methysergide Ketanserin	
Smooth muscle				
Bronchial	C†		C†	
Gut	C		C* (strong, rat fundic strip)	
Uterine	C (except rat, mouse)	R (rat, mouse)		
Vascular				
artery/vein	C		C	
intermediate vessels	Contraction or relaxation (*see* text)		Contraction or relaxation (*see* text)	
Total peripheral resistance	Overall decrease in human giving hypotension†			
Capillaries‡				
calibre	Relaxation ('red reaction')*			Relaxation
permeability	Increased ('wheal')*			Increased (only rat paw)
Heart, isolated (*see* text)				
force of contraction		+++	+++ (*see*	− − −
rate		+++	+++ text)	− − −
Glands				
Alimentary		+++		
Adrenal medulla	++			++
Mechanism of action	Phosphatidyl inositol hydrolysis	Increasing cAMP	Phosphatidyl inositol hydrolysis	

For smooth muscle: C, contraction R, relaxation; for other functions: + + +, marked stimulation; + +, moderate stimulation; − − −, marked inhibition. ? indicates 5-HT responses which are usually not blocked by methysergide. For CNS actions of 5-HT, *see* 6.3.
Responses to pathological release of the autacoid: * mild, † moderate to severe.
‡ Includes small arterioles and venules.

negative inotropic actions are mediated, usually via H_2 and H_1 receptors respectively. However, in the *guinea-pig* for example, the right auricular positive inotropic effect is predominantly H_2 while the left auricular positive inotropic effect is mainly H_1.

Glands

Histamine causes an increase in all alimentary exocrine secretions from the salivary glands onwards but the major action is to activate acid secretion from the gastric mucosa, which is an H_2-effect. This autacoid also liberates catecholamines from the adrenal medulla either directly (H_1) or in response to a fall in blood pressure (e.g. in cat, dog or human).

5-Hydroxytryptamine

The present classification of 5-HT receptors is unsatisfactory (particularly for the non-CNS actions of the autacoid) due to the lack of sufficiently specific agonists and antagonists for the different subgroups. This will be obvious from a study of Table 5.3 which is an attempt to classify present knowledge. As 5-HT_2 receptors are most important for peripheral actions, these are separated in Table 5.2 and now *all* the effects tabulated there will be discussed.

Go down the list (Table 2.3; smooth muscle, heart muscle, glands) for the major actions.

Smooth muscle

- bronchial: constriction
- gut: contraction (rat fundic strip is very sensitive. Table 5.5)
- uterine: contraction
- vascular: there are significant species and regional differences. One

Table 5.3 A provisional classification of 5-hydroxytryptamine (5-HT) receptors

	$5\text{-HT}_{1A/1B/1C/1D}$	5-HT_2	5-HT_3
Agonist	5-Carboxyamido-tryptamine	α-Methyl-5-HT (also 5-HT_{1C})	2-Methyl-5-HT
Antagonist(s)	Spiperone (also antagonises 5-HT_2, α_1- and D_2-dopamine)	Methysergide (also '5-HT$_1$-like' p.ag.) Ketanserin (also antagonises of α_1, and H_1-histamine)	ICS 205–930 MDL 72222 (not ileum)
Actions			
bronchoconstriction		+++	
gut contraction	+ (rat fundic strip)	+++	++ (ileum)
vasoconstriction	++	+++	
platelet aggregation (Fig. 17.3)		+++	
nervous system — p. 159	CNS +++	CNS+	Peripheral NS +++

Actions: +++, major; ++, moderate; +, minor. P.ag., partial agonist.
* Also *see* Table 6.5 for separation of 5HT_{1A} and 5HT_{1B} receptors in the CNS.

of the original names for 5-HT was serotonin, indicating a substance derived from serum (produced as we now know by platelet aggregation) which gave a pressor response—in the anaesthetised *dog*. Yet, the threshold dose in the *cat* is usually depressor, due to dilator responses in intermediate vessels (these effects appear to be endothelium-dependent and mediated mainly via 5-HT$_1$ receptors, Fig. 10.5). Higher concentrations show a pressor predominance due to vasoconstrictor effects both in large and intermediate vessels and direct positive inotropic and chronotropic effects upon the heart (*see* later). Even higher concentrations of 5-HT cause adrenal medullary secretion of catecholamines and the Bezold–Jarisch reflex (10.1). Direct responses of extra- and intra-cerebral vessels to 5-HT and the involvement of central and peripheral nervous pathways in cardiovascular and pain pathways seem to be significant in migraine (10.6). All sub-groups of 5-HT receptors appear to be involved in migraine remedies: ergotamine is a '5-HT$_1$-like agonist/partial agonist; methysergide and pizotifen (US: pizotyline) are primarily 5-HT$_2$ antagonists; 5-HT$_3$ blockers are undergoing clinical trials (also anti-emetic, p. 317).

Miscellaneous
Capillaries dilate with 5-HT but there is no increased permeability, except in the rat paw. The expansion of the capillaries allied to an overall greater veno- than arterio-constriction results in the skin flushing observed in malignant carcinoid syndrome in man (p. 134).

Heart
The responses of isolated hearts to 5-HT show considerable species variations but, with ascending concentrations, the following successive phases can generally be distinguished
• negative inotropic and chronotropic effects which are blocked by atropine and are therefore mediated via muscarinic receptors
• positive inotropic and chronotropic actions produced either directly (e.g. cat, guinea-pig) via methysergide-sensitive (5-HT$_2$) receptors or indirectly (e.g. rabbit) by noradrenaline release
• negative inotropic and possibly chronotropic effects, due to membrane stabilisation.

Glands
Liberation of catecholamines from the adrenal medulla, usually by a direct action.

5.6   A superfusion (cascade) technique
As shown in Fig. 5.4, this involves an (external) analysis of blood (or other fluid) content by the use of a battery of suitably chosen test tissues. The following determinations can be made:

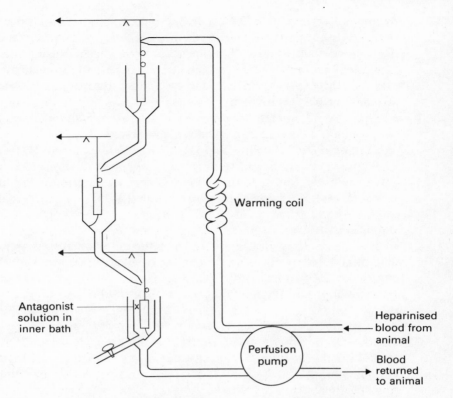

Fig. 5.4 A superfusion technique. Blood is circulated extracorporeally through a series of test tissues to determine the autacoid content. Antagonists can be confined to any particular tissue (as shown in the lower bath).

Qualitative. This requires the selection of appropriate preparations so that specific autacoids can be detected (*see* Table 5.6). The finding(s) can be confirmed by the use of selective antagonists bathing any specific tissue.

Quantitative. Once the actual autacoid has been identified, its content can be estimated by comparison of the responses with those produced by the superfusion of known concentrations of the pure substance.

Release of autacoids. If the blood in the adrenal vein is sampled before and after the injection of 5-HT into the abdominal aorta, any enhanced release of adrenaline (from the adrenal gland) can be determined. Alternatively, using the cascade system alone, with a previously sensitised guinea-pig ileum in the top bath, it can be shown that the addition of the correct antigen results in the liberation of histamine detectable by the use of appropriate tissues in the lower baths.

Destruction of autacoids. Essentially the experiments are the converse of those just used, e.g. if right atrial perfusion of $10 \mu g$ min^{-1} of X results in the same concentration of X in the arterial blood as perfusion into the ascending aorta of $1 \mu g$ min^{-1}, then 90% destruction of X occurs in the lungs. On this basis, autacoids can be divided into two broad groups (excluding CNS metabolism):

i   Those mainly metabolised in the portal and/or pulmonary circulations when liberated physiologically or pathologically—5-HT, prostaglandins, bradykinin, angiotensin I (activated to angiotensin II, *see* 5.9)
ii   Those normally inactivated in the systemic circulation (e.g. in the gut, kidney and limbs)—adrenaline, noradrenaline, histamine, angiotensin II; also 5-HT, prostaglandins and bradykinin, if pharmacologically injected intra-arterially.

Important corollaries are
• if the actions of, for example, adrenaline on blood vessels are to be determined independently of changes in blood pressure producing passive or reflex effects (10.3), the substance should be given intra-arterially (e.g. into the femoral artery) when insufficient will appear in the venous blood to cause systemic changes
• in carcinoid syndrome, a tumour of enterochromaffin tissue produces 5-HT which results in diarrhoea and colic. However, hepatic secondaries of the tumour usually occur later and then the inactivating mechanisms in the liver and lungs are overwhelmed, resulting in bronchoconstriction and skin flushing (p. 132). Note that bradykinin is also released in this condition.

5.7   Antagonists of histamine
This provides a useful classification for antagonistic mechanisms in general.
1   Prevention of release. In the treatment of bronchial asthma (Fig. 11.2) with sodium cromoglycate or adrenal glucocorticoids; a *subsidiary* effect of β-adrenoceptor agonists.
2   Increased destruction. Diamine oxidase preparations have, so far, not been useful therapeutically, probably because this enzyme is not the most important in the removal of the autacoid from its sites of action (5.4).
3   Functional antagonism. This implies that the effects of the agonist are reversed by an agent which, however, does not act upon the same receptors. Thus, as shown in Table 5.4, adrenaline is the best general human functional antagonist for use in emergency situations (e.g. anaphylactoid reactions; angioneurotic oedema with glottic oedema). Salbutamol is valuable in bronchial asthma (11.5).
4   Competitive antagonism. This results in a parallel shift to the right in the agonist log dose-response curve (Fig. 4.2, Ia).

Table 5.4 Actions of histamine and some functional antagonists in humans

| Agent | Bronchioles | Blood pressure | Capillaries* | |
			Calibre	Permeability
Histamine	Constriction	Fall	Dilation	Increased
Noradrenaline	Dilation (weak)	Rise	Constriction	
Adrenaline	Dilation	Rise†	Constriction	Decreased
Isoprenaline	Dilation	Fall	Dilation	
Salbutamol	Dilation	Negligible change†		Decreased

*Includes small arterioles and venules.
†In normal therapeutic dose.

H_1-*receptor blocking agents* (type substance, mepyramine). There are a large number of these with a general chemical structure based upon the—N—C—C—X—configuration (X is nitrogen—most commonly—carbon, oxygen or sulphur). Go down Table 5.2 to obtain their effects. These agents are valuable in some allergic conditions (e.g. urticaria, hay fever) but are not used in bronchial asthma where other mediators are activated along with histamine (Fig. 11.2). As shown in Table 5.5, they may have two other major effects: an antimuscarinic action resulting in characteristic side-effects (e.g. dry mouth and loss of accommodation) and CNS-sedation. The latter may be valuable in a motion sickness remedy (p. 317) but can be disadvantageous in the working patient, e.g. lorry driver, and it also shows an extremely high degree of synergism with ethanol: even *two pints of beer while on anti-H_1 therapy can really be a knock-out* (p. 439). Newer compounds, exemplified by astemizole and terfenadine, cross the blood–brain barrier very slowly and have only slight CNS effects: they also have negligible antimuscarinic actions. Application of anti-(H_1)-histamines to the skin can cause local reactions (18.8).

Table 5.5 Other major actions of anti-(H_1) histamines

Drug	Antimuscarinic effect	CNS sedation*
Promethazine	+ +	+ +
Cyclizine†	+ +	+
Mepyramine (US: pyrilamine)	+	+
Astemizole‡	0	±
Terfenadine	0	±

+, present; + +, marked; ±, slight; 0, negligible.
* Usually manifested as drowsiness. Paradoxically, in children, anti-(H_1) histamine poisoning can initially result in *excitant* CNS effects.
† Liable to abuse—taken with opiates or ethanol.
‡ Poisoning can cause tachycardia and ventricular dysrhythmias.

H_2-receptor antagonists (type substance, cimetidine) are usually thio-derivatives attached to an imidazole ring. The latter is replaced by a furan ring with an aminoalkyl substituent in the newer compound, ranitidine. Pharmacologically, they oppose all the H_2 actions shown in Table 5.2; therapeutically, their major use is in peptic ulcer treatment.

5.8   Antagonists of 5-HT

Like α-adrenoceptor blocking agents, with which they show much overlap, 5-HT antagonists are a heterogenous group chemically and are rarely selective for the different sub-groups. For instance, methysergide—the classical $5\text{-}HT_2$ antagonist—can reduce the diarrhoea and colic of carcinoid syndrome but does not prevent the bronchoconstriction and flushed skin associated with hepatic metastasis of the tumour, probably because of the involvement of other autacoids (e.g. bradykinin). However, $5\text{-}HT_3$ receptors might be important in ileal stimulation and flushed skin, which actions are opposed by ICS 205–930 (Table 5.3). Like many other α-adrenoceptor antagonists (e.g. ergotamine, 15.6), and other 5-HT blockers, methysergide can act as a partial agonist (e.g. on isolated blood vessels, Table 15.5). Any of the above properties could be relevant to its prophylactic use in migraine (10.6): but it is not commonly prescribed now due to the danger of fibrosis in the pleural, pericardial and retroperitoneal spaces if given for more than 3 months. Its replacement is pizotifen (US: pizotyline) *see* 10.6—another $5\text{-}HT_2$ antagonist (p. 132).

PEPTIDES AND PURINE DERIVATIVES

There are an extremely large number of peptides both occurring naturally throughout the animal and vegetable kingdoms, and produced by organic chemists. They have been subdivided in various ways which indicate particular interests (e.g. animal venoms, mammalian hormones, CNS transmitters, e.g. endogenous opioid peptides, p. 167). Here we can give only an inkling of their protean nature, using *bradykinin, angiotensins* and *vasopressin* (in high concentrations), as prime examples. Separation of these from other autacoids by a superfusion technique can be achieved using the tissues shown in Table 5.6.

Table 5.6 Separation of some major autacoid groups

Tissue	5-HT	Bradykinin	Angiotensin II	Vasopressin	Prostaglandin E_2
Rat fundic strip	+ +				+ +
Cat jejunum		+ +			
Rat colon			+ +		+ +
Rabbit rectum				– –	

Contraction: + +, marked. Relaxation: – –, marked.

5.9   Genesis and breakdown

Bradykinin (Fig. 5.5) This is generated from a precursor (itself derived from a plasma α_2-globulin) by the action of kallikrein (activated by tissue damage or bacterial infection which converts Factor XII to its active form Factor XIIa; or by plasmin—*see* Fig. 17.4 for both these substances). The decapeptide—lysyl bradykinin—is converted to bradykinin which is subsequently inactivated, initially by carboxypeptidases which split off one or two terminal amino-acids (kininases I or II, respectively).

Angiotensins (Fig. 5.5). Renin is liberated (from the juxtaglomerular cells)—either directly or reflexly—by a low sodium ion concentration in the macular densa, a fall in blood pressure, diminished extracellular fluid volume, or β-adrenoceptor agonists. Renin converts a precursor (again produced from a plasma α_2-globulin) to the decapeptide, angiotensin I. This is pharmacologically inert until changed, mainly in the lungs, into angiotensin II by the dipeptidyl carboxypeptidase ('converting enzyme') which is very similar to kininase II. Therefore any drug antagonising converting enzyme (e.g. captopril, 10.5) and thus preventing the formation of angiotensin II, will simultaneously *inhibit the breakdown* of bradykinin (? resulting in afferent nerve stimulation

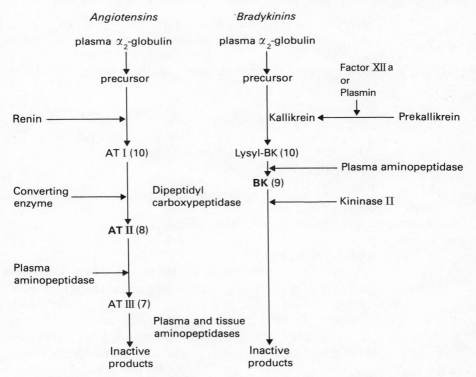

Fig. 5.5 Production and breakdown of angiotensins (AT) and bradykinins (BK). Numbers in brackets indicate amino acid contents.

leading to a persistent cough, p. 256). The removal of another amino acid from angiotensin II produces the heptapeptide, angiotensin III, which may be an active agent especially for aldosterone release (p. 333). Further peptide cleavage results in inactivation.

Vasopressin. This peptide is synthesised mainly in the supraoptic and paraventricular nuclei of the hypothalamus, from whence it passes in the supraopticohypophysial tract for storage in the posterior pituitary gland. Release due to increased plasma tonicity or decreased extracellular fluid volume involves the *same* tract as its major final common path. A dynorphin—*see* p. 167—is also released. Vasopressin is inactivated by a variety of peptidases, which are less effective if the first amino acid in the molecule is deaminated (e.g. desmopressin, 12.7).

5.10   Occurrence and functions

Bradykinin. Its major (pathological) role is in inflammation (5.17) where it directly produces capillary dilation and increased permeability and is potentiated by prostaglandins (which it generates) to cause pain. It is also present in (and can be released from) human carcinoid tumours and rodent mast cells.

Angiotensin II production is particularly involved with the maintenance of blood pressure, blood volume and sodium content of the body which it mainly achieves by direct (and potentiation of sympathetic) vasoconstriction, the release of aldosterone and increased thirst (by a CNS action).

Vasopressin, in physiological concentrations in the blood, exerts the usual effects associated with 'antidiuretic hormone'. In severe haemorrhage, it is released in much larger amounts when it produces significant cardiovascular actions (*see* next section).

5.11   Actions (go down Table 5.7)

Bradykinin has significant bronchoconstrictor action in man (and, for example, guinea-pig) which may contribute to the bronchospasm of bronchial asthma and certainly does to that of malignant carcinoid tumour (5.6). Bradykinin also contracts uterine smooth muscle, especially of the rat; whereas *vasopressin* has only a slight effect on both this tissue and the myoepithelial cells of the mammary gland compared with its structurally related peptide, oxytocin (Chapter 15). The effects on the gut musculature of different species has already been used to separate these compounds (Table 5.6). In parenthesis, the prefix *brady* (Gk: *bradys*, slow) indicates that the compound produces a *slow* contraction of smooth muscle (e.g. guinea-pig ileum); there are *tachy*-kinins (p. 166).

Table 5.7 Pharmacological actions of bradykinin, angiotensin II and vasopressin

Tissue	Bradykinin	Angiotensin II	Vasopressin
Smooth muscle			
Bronchial	+ +		
Gut (*see* Table 5.6)			
Uterine	+ +	+	(+)
Vascular			
resistance	− −	+ + +	+ +
capacitance	+	+ +	+/−
*Capillaries**			
calibre	−	+/−	+ +
permeability	+ +		
Heart			
force of contraction			
(direct)		+	
sinus rate (reflex)	+	−	−

Contraction, increased permeability or quickening of the heart rate: + + +, very marked; + +, marked; +, present; (+), slight. Relaxation or slowing of the heart rate: − −, marked; −, present. Variable response: +/−.
* Includes small arterioles and venules.

Cardiovascular actions

None of these peptides (except angiotensin II) has a marked direct effect upon the heart, but their vascular actions are very interesting.

Bradykinin is a hypotensive substance with dilator effects on resistance vessels (and capillaries) but it contracts the capacitance vessels, thus helping in the production of the skin flush in malignant carcinoid syndrome (5.6). The actions of bradykinin on resistance and capacitance vessels are reported to be mediated by the release of prostaglandins (Table 5.10).

Angiotensin II is the most potent endogenous vasoconstrictor known (about 40 times stronger than noradrenaline) with a proclivity for resistance vessels—acting both directly (major effect) and by potentiation of sympathetic actions (increases synthesis, release and receptor effectiveness of noradrenaline and decreases uptake$_1$). This is important in haemorrhagic shock (10.9), as contraction of the immediate postcapillary resistance vessels (r, Fig. 10.2) results in an increased capillary filtration pressure, causing loss of blood volume (bradykinin release contributes by increasing 'capillary' permeability) while prolonged, intense constriction of the precapillary sphincters produces severe capillary hypoxia.

Vasopressin (as its name indicates) raises blood pressure but it is too dangerous for routine use due to coronary vasoconstriction. A synthetic derivative—felypressin—may be used in place of (nor)adrenaline with local anaesthetics (*see* footnote * to Table 8.2). It especially constricts resistance vessels and capillaries with a potentiating effect upon noradrenaline actions at these sites.

Evidence is accruing that the production of angiotensin II and the release of vasopressin and noradrenaline in haemorrhagic shock results in such a severe capillary hypoxia that (if not relieved within about 2 hours by the transfusion of fluid) the integrity of these vessels is lost and subsequent transfusion is in vain ('irreversible shock').

5.12   Antagonists

Bradykinin (BK) receptors have been subdivided into
- B_1 mediating some smooth muscle actions and antagonised by, for example, leu^8-$desarg^9$-BK
- B_2 involved in effects upon other smooth muscles but, more importantly, in inflammatory phenomena (increased capillary permeability, vasodilation (Fig. 10.5) and pain production—with the associated release of prostaglandins: *see* Table 5.12). A potent antagonist is lys-lys-hyp^3-$(thienyl)ala^{5,8}$-phe^7-BK.

Angiotensin II responses are antagonised competitively by sarcosyl derivatives, one of which, saralasin (a partial agonist), has been shown to diminish the development of haemorrhagic shock in experimental animals. *See also* angiotensin converting enzyme (and renin) inhibitors (p. 256).

Vasopressin receptors have been subdivided into
- V_1 mediating smooth muscle contraction, particularly vasoconstriction: felypressin (*see* above) is an agonist
- V_2 involved in renal water reabsorption (ADH, Fig. 12.1) and selectively activated by desmopressin (p. 310).

Selective antagonists for these receptors have been discovered but commonly vasopressin has been considered to be involved in a response if the latter is absent after section of the supraopticohypophysial tract or in Brattleboro rats (a strain with congenital lack of endogenous vasopressin).

A note on tachykinins/neurokinins

The original member of this group was substance P (an undecapeptide contained in a dried Powder/Preparation originally extracted from the gastrointestinal tract and CNS). Peripherally, it has many actions which are similar to those of bradykinin, e.g. gut contraction (though it produces a more rapid response, hence its description as a *tachy*kinin— Gk: *tachys*, swift); e.g. increased capillary permeability and vasodilation (it has been implicated in the production of the wheal and flare of the triple response; also in the inflammatory response, Table 5.12). In contradistinction to bradykinin, it has significant CNS effects.

Many *neuro*peptides which also act directly on smooth muscle tissues have since been isolated from a variety of sources. Those which show most homology to substance P in the possession of a common pentapeptide(–phe–X–gly–leu–met–NH$_2$) at the C-terminus are the *undeca*peptides eledoisin (from the salivary gland of an octopod) and physalaemin (from skin of a South American frog)—so that originally substance P receptors were subdivided into E and P subtypes; and the *deca*peptides, neurokinins A and B (originally found in *mammalian* CNS extracts) which form the basis of the present classification. Antagonists at these receptors are not very specific and are relatively weak (low pA$_2$ values) so that the subgroups of the *neurokinins*—as they are now termed—are based on the relative strength of agonist actions, *viz.* NK$_1$ (substance P most potent), NK$_2$ (neurokinin A best) and NK$_3$ (neurokinin B most active).

5.13   Purinergic neurotransmission

The effects following stimulation of motor neurones to autonomically innervated organs are not invariably completely prevented by adequate concentrations of the appropriate cholinergic or adrenergic antagonists. The most likely explanation suggests the release of non-adrenergic, non-cholinergic (NANC) transmitters either as *co-transmitters* simultaneously liberated with the primary transmitter or from separate nerve fibres (Fig. 11.1). While any autacoid could be involved there is convincing evidence for purinergic neurotransmission at several sites. Undoubtedly ATP is liberated along with noradrenaline at nerve terminals (Fig. 10.4) and is certainly stored in synaptic vesicles with acetylcholine.

The concept of purinergic nerves which produce effects such as a short-lived relaxation of the gut or contraction of the urinary bladder, receives support by satisfying most of the relevant criteria (Chapter 2), namely *c*ontent, *r*elease and *a*pplication giving a similar response to nerve stimulation. The transitory nature of these effects and the increased amounts of adenosine (rather than ATP) found in tissue perfusates following nerve stimulation suggests that ATP may be rapidly degraded (via ADP and AMP) to adenosine which itself may act as the agonist and then be inactivated by adenosine deaminase or removed by an uptake process (*see* p. 269). Additionally, ATP and adenosine can also act on *pre*synaptic receptors to modify release of the primary transmitters. P$_1$-(subdivided into A$_1$ and A$_2$, which decrease and increase cAMP, respectively) and P$_2$-purinoceptors have been postulated with the differential properties shown in Table 5.8.

LIPID DERIVATIVES

A variety of substances, fatty in provenance, were isolated from many tissues and secretions since the 1930s but only much later were their fundamental natures and some of their functions realised. Fatty acids (of 20 carbon atoms) containing 3–5 double bonds are present in the phospholipids of cell membranes from which they can be liberated by

Table 5.8 One suggested subdivision of purinoceptors

	$P_1(A_1/A_2)$	P_2
Actions	Bronchoconstriction (A_1)	Relaxation of gut
	Bronchodilation (A_2)	
	Negative inotropic effect (A_1, *see* Fig. 10.13)	
	Presynaptic *inhibition* of noradrenaline or acetylcholine release	Presynaptic *facilitation* of noradrenaline release
Agonists	Adenosine > ATP	ATP > adenosine
	2-Chlorodenosine*	
Selective agonist	8-Phenyltheophylline†	
	Theophylline‡	

* Not broken down by adenosine deaminase.
† *c.* 200 times more effective than theophylline as an adenosine antagonist: equipotent as a phosphodiesterase inhibitor.
‡ In concentrations 1–2 orders of magnitude less than those required to produce phosphodiesterase inhibition (Table 4.4; *see also* p. 235 and Fig. 11.1).

phospholipase A_2 (Figs 4.6–4.8)—or related acyl hydrolases—activated by Ca^{2+} ions produced by a large number of physiological, pathological and pharmacological stimuli. To simplify matters, Fig. 5.6 shows the relevant fatty acid containing four double bonds (arachidonic acid: mainly derived from dietary linoleic acid). Following release from the cell membrane some arachidonic acid (AA) becomes available to the cellular microsomal enzymes which convert it into *eicosanoids* (Gk: *eicosi*, twenty) either prostaglandin-type derivatives (upwards in the figure) or leukotrienes (downwards).

5.14 Eicosanoids: genesis and metabolism

Prostaglandins (originally isolated from prostate and seminal vesicles but now recognised as ubiquitous in the body) result from the action of a *cyclo-oxygenase* upon arachidonic acid, to produce the series designated by the subscript *two* (as there are two double bonds in the final product). Derivatives of the corresponding fatty acids containing three or five double bonds result in prostaglandins (PGs) with one or three double bonds, thus producing the corresponding subscript *one* and *three* series, respectively. To continue with the *two* series (Fig. 5.6): arachidonic acid is converted by microsomal cyclo-oxygenase into the unstable endoperoxides (PGG_2 and PGH_2) which, within a few minutes, are enzymatically changed into the products also shown in Table 5.9. Most of these have only brief actions due to the corporeal ubiquity of their inactivating enzymes.

The chemical name of arachidonic acid is 5,8,11,14-*eicosa*tetra*enoic acid so that the 5-*hydro*peroxy derivative which immediately results due to the action of *lipoxygenase* is 5-HPETE. This is converted by a dehydrase to leukotriene A_4 (LTA_4) from which the other LTs are

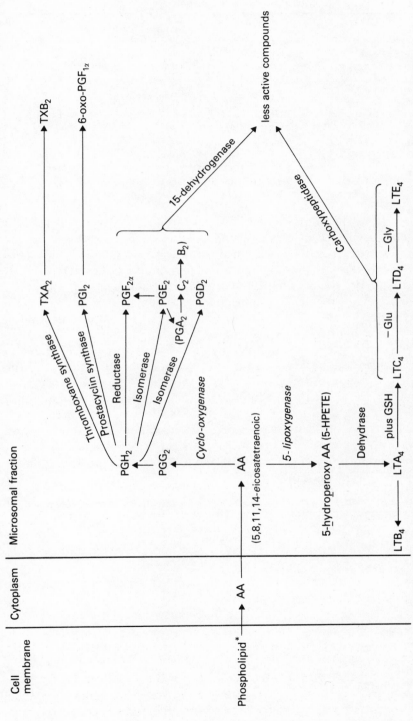

Fig. 5.6 Genesis and breakdown of prostaglandin (PG) and leukotriene (LT) compounds: termed eicosanoids because they are derived from fatty acids containing 20 (Gk: *eicosi*, twenty) carbon atoms, e.g. arachidonic acid (AA). TX, thromboxane; GSH, glutathione (γ-glutamylcysteinylglycine); − Glu, minus glutamic acid; − Gly, minus glycine.
*See action of phospholipase A₂ (PLA₂), Fig. 4.7a.

Table 5.9 Formation and breakdown of major prostaglandin-like substances

| Enzyme for production from PGH_2 | Active product(s)* | Inactivation (main route) | |
		Enzyme involved	Product
Reductase	$PGF_{2\alpha}$†	15-Dehydrogenase	
Isomerase	PGE_2, PGD_2	15-Dehydrogenase	
Prostacyclin synthetase	PGI_2 (prostacyclin)		6-oxo-$PGF_{1\alpha}$†
Thromboxane (TX) synthase	TXA_2		TXB_2

* More stable derivatives have been synthesised: they are termed prostanoids.
† Subscript α in the F series indicates the steric position of the 9-hydroxyl group.

obtained as shown in Fig. 5.6. The terminology is derived as follows: *leuko*, because they were originally obtained from white blood cell extracts; *triene*, as they contain three *alternating* double bonds; subscript four because they have a *total of four* double bonds. LTC_4, LTD_4 and LTB_4 are the commonest naturally occurring agents of this group (the original 'slow reacting substances of anaphylaxis'—SRSAs—were mixtures of these): their main catabolic enzyme is a carboxypeptidase.

Agents modifying eicosanoid content are shown in Table 5.10. Bradykinin effects mediated via prostaglandins (*see* p. 139) are due to an increase in deacetylation resulting in enhanced release of the lipid precursor. Adrenal glucocorticoids, via intracellular receptors (Fig. 4.5, 2) induce the synthesis of proteins (lipocortins) which inhibit phospholipase A_2 activity: they also increase prostaglandin breakdown. As there are negligible stores of *active* eicosanoids, formation and inactivation control effective tissue concentrations—hence the therapeutic importance of the aspirin-like and adrenal glucocorticoid drugs (*see* specific effects on p. 147).

Table 5.10 Substances affecting the genesis and/or breakdown of eicosanoids

| Stage(s) affected | Resultant effect on effective eicosanoid content | |
	Increased	Decreased
Release of arachidonic acid		
increased	Bradykinin	
decreased		Adrenal glucocorticoids
Cyclo-oxygenase inhibition		Aspirin-like drugs*
Cyclo-*and* 5-lipoxygenase inhibition		BW 755C
Thromboxane synthase inhibition		l-benzylimidazole
Breakdown by prostaglandin 15-dehydrogenase		
increased		Adrenal glucocorticoids

* Aspirin *acetylates* the enzyme irreversibly: other members of this group act differently.

5.15 Actions of eicosanoids

Many physiological, pathological and pharmacological processes are modulated by prostaglandins whose involvement can be inferred by the usual criteria (*see* Chapter 2, Introduction).

Content. Presence of enzymes for synthesis and breakdown. Ubiquitous.

Release, e.g. of metabolites, found in the local tissues, blood or CSF draining the relevant area or in the urine.

Application (of, for example, arachidonic acid or a relevant prostanoid) results in a similar response to that occurring naturally.

Modification. Antagonism (e.g. by prevention of synthesis—aspirin-like drugs—or by receptor blockade) or potentiation (e.g. by inhibition of prostaglandin dehydrogenase) affects both natural release and application of the putative agent similarly.

However, the situation is extremely complex because in many instances the release produces a mixture of prostaglandins or prostaglandin-like substances which can have opposing actions. Thus the overall *qualitative* effect depends upon which prostaglandin is predominately formed and which receptors specific to a particular prostaglandin are present in the tissue concerned; the *quantitative* action is dependent upon the total amount and persistence of the specific prostaglandin released and the number of specific receptors available in the tissue. In the following sections an attempt will be made to indicate areas where pharmacological actions of eicosanoids or their inhibition are presently important in relation to therapeutic uses and/or side-effects of drugs.

Table 5.11 Actions of representative prostaglandins (and thromboxane A_2)

Tissue	Inhibition	Excitation
Smooth muscle		
Bronchial (Figs 11.1, 11.2)	E_2	$F_{2\alpha} < D_2$, TXA_2/B_2
Gut (excluding sphincters)		E_2, $F_{2\alpha}$
Uterine (human)		
body		
non-pregnant	E_2	$F_{2\alpha}$
pregnant	I_2	E_2, $F_{2\alpha}$
fallopian tube	E_2	$F_{2\alpha}$
Vascular	$C_2 > A_2 > E_2$, $F_{2\alpha}$, I_2	TXA_2
Heart muscle		
force of contraction		(weak direct, mainly reflex) E_2, $F_{2\alpha}$
Glandular		
Alimentary (Fig. 13.2)		
gastric oxyntic	E_2, $F_{2\alpha}$	
mucous		E_2, $F_{2\alpha}$

Prostaglandin actions

There are marked species variations but the most common effects upon autonomically innervated tissues or organs are shown for the prostaglandin *two* series of compounds in Table 5.11—go down the list as in Table 2.3 (smooth muscle, heart muscle, glands).

For discussions of the significance of prostaglandin actions in particular areas, *see* bronchial muscle, Fig. 11.1; gut, p. 321; and female genital system, 15.3. The vascular effects are included with clotting mechanisms (17.2). A further major role is in the intermediation of pyrogen-induced fever (7.8). Finally, these substances are intimately involved in the processes of inflammatory response (*see* Table 5.12) and pain (7.9).

Prostaglandins can be liberated as co-transmitters but the resultant effects vary with the tissue and eicosanoid involved, e.g. sympathetic nerves to the *rabbit* heart simultaneously release noradrenaline and prostaglandin E_2, which decreases the release of noradrenaline and opposes its action on the heart—yet on other tissues prostaglandins can potentiate sympathetic effects. Also, hormones or transmitters which increase cyclic AMP can activate prostaglandins which oppose their actions (*see* Fig. 13.2).

Leukotriene actions

In the production of the inflammatory response, LTB_4 is chemotactic for polymorphs, and LTC_4 and LTD_4 increase 'capillary' permeability (Table 5.12). The latter two compounds additionally produce bronchoconstriction in bronchial asthma (Fig. 11.2).

5.16   Platelet activating factor (PAF, PAF-acether)

This is formed by the action of phospholipase A_2—activated by Ca^{2+} ions—on a cell membrane (choline-containing) phospholipid, which

Table 5.12 Autacoids and their contribution to the acute inflammatory response

Autacoid	Local vasodilation	Increased vascular permeability	Pain
Histamine*	+	+	
Bradykinin	+	+	+
PGE$_2$/PGD$_2$	+	p	p
LTC$_4$/LTD$_4$		+	
PAF†	+	+	

+, present; p, potentiates response(s) to other agent(s); PG, prostaglandin; LT, leukotriene; PAF, platelet activating factor.
* Not significant in all types of inflammation.
† *See* text for mechanisms of action; also liberates LTB_4 (which is chemotactic for inflammatory cells) and arachidonic acid (eicosanoid precursor)—*see* Fig. 4.7,b.

generates PAF and arachidonic acid (Fig. 4.7b). As its name implies, it is important in platelet clotting mechanisms (Fig. 17.3) but it has much wider significance in connection with inflammation and allergic conditions. It is produced by sensitised macrophages, eosinophils and platelets and liberates chemotactic substances, e.g. leukotriene B_4, and other eicosanoids which mediate vasodilation and bronchoconstriction (Table 5.12 and Fig. 11.1). It appears to mediate increased 'capillary' permeability by a direct action on post-capillary venules.

5.17 Pharmacology of inflammation

Acute inflammation is associated with the liberation or generation of the autacoids shown in Table 5.12.

Treatment of inflammation
Useful agents are:

Steroidal anti-inflammatory drugs (SAIDs), i.e. adrenal glucocorticoids. They have several actions (via specific *intra*cellular receptors)
• formation of lipocortins which depress phospholipase A_2 activity and, so, lessen the production of eicosanoids and PAF
• decreased activation of plasmin, hence less production of bradykinin and eicosanoids
• blockade of uptake$_2$ with consequent prolongation of (nor)adrenaline functional antagonism of autacoid-induced vascular dilation
• increased prostaglandin breakdown
• decreased production of complement fragments C3a and C5a so that there is less mast cell degranulation.

Non-steroidal anti-inflammatory drugs (NSAIDs). The type substance is aspirin (7.9). These primarily *inhibit cyclo-oxygenase* (thereby preventing prostaglandin and thromboxane synthesis) but they can also depress the formation of plasmin (leading to less bradykinin and eicosanoid production) and some (e.g. fenamates) may even (weakly) block bradykinin receptors.

Additional drugs used in resistant cases of rheumatoid arthritis (which is essentially an immune reaction with a superimposed inflammatory response) are shown in Table 5.13.

Interleukin-1 is an additional factor which assumes importance here. This is a general term for a series of related proteins which are secreted by macrophages during *acute inflammation*: it is chemotactic, liberates eicosanoids and is an endogenous pyrogen (Fig. 7.4). In *chronic inflammation* it increases fibroblast activity but also causes joint tissue (bone and cartilage) breakdown: *immunologically*, it increases the responses of T- and B- lymphocytes to antigens.

Table 5.13   Drugs which may be used in rheumatoid arthritis

Drug	Mechanism of action	Side-effects	Reference
Gold salt (sodium aurothiomalate)	Inhibition of lysosomal enzyme activity (?) Modification of connective tissue metabolism	Skin rashes Kidney albuminuria* nephrotic syndrome Red bone marrow depression* granulocytopenia thrombocytopenia aplastic anaemia	18.8 12.9 17.3
Penicillamine	Chelation of immune complexes	Similar to gold but thrombocytopenia more common* Pyridoxine deficiency*	16.5
Sulphasalazine	Suppression of T lymphocytes	Headache Nausea Skin rashes Granulocytopenia*	p. 325
Chloroquine	Lysosomal stabilisation Decreased interleukin-1 production	Ocular* Nausea Skin rashes	19.8
Azathioprine	Destruction of lymphocytes	Antimitotic (Table 19.2, most commonly gastrointestinal)	Fig. 19.7

(?), possible mode of action.
* Side effects uncommon if urinary, haematological, ocular and nervous system checks are made regularly during treatment .

Note on itch

This symptom which commonly occurs in association with cutaneous inflammation is often produced by similar substances, particularly histamine, bradykinin and eicosanoids. But other autacoids may be implicated (e.g. substance P, p. 166). The afferent fibres involved are those associated with pain.

6 CNS Transmitters

Unlike the peripheral nervous system which conveys simple messages to and from the executive organs, the CNS has to coordinate and constantly modify motor function according to sensory input, hormonal and other blood-borne signals. Thus, many more transmitters are required to provide the necessary integrative processes with sufficient flexibility. These exist within a three-dimensional meshwork of neuronal 'hard-wiring' which is extremely intricate, rendering analysis difficult. Progress has been made by initial study of relatively simple situations such as the Renshaw cell loop (*see* Fig. 6.1), and retinal and cerebellar layers; with subsequent disentanglement of the labyrinthine connections present in areas such as the brainstem. Here, the classical neurophysiological procedure of punctate excitation followed by the detection of any resultant electrical changes at distant sites and traditional anatomical lesion-degeneration experiments have been reinforced with pharmacological and neurochemical techniques to compile 'maps' of specific transmitter pathways. Before describing particular methods in greater detail, however, an important caveat is necessary: the anatomy of the CNS in experimental animals (rat, rabbit) can be markedly different to that of humans, especially in brainstem connections to the cerebral cortex or the neocerebellum. Finally, the use of isolated parts of the neuraxis, e.g. slices of cerebral cortex or of spinal cord, e.g. synaptosomes (nerve terminals from homogenised brain which seal to form spheroids) or single (including cultured) neurones can provide fundamental clues to molecular mechanisms of transmitter (or drug) action. However, such techniques are artificial because in the whole animal there are important modulating influences on simple transmitter functions, e.g. other locally present transmitters, hormonal and ionic contents of bathing fluids, glial activity.

6.1 Elucidation of CNS transmitters

Go through the criteria stated in Chapter 2, Introduction.

Content

In different areas of the neuraxis this was originally determined by extraction and bioassay (physicochemical methods, e.g. high performance liquid chromatography, are now used). But remember that some central transmitters (e.g. glycine, 6.4) are almost universal cellular constituents, and therefore only *enhanced* amounts are significant. Histochemical (including immunoreactive) staining and autoradiographic methods are available to pinpoint many agents, e.g. catecholamines (6.3), relevant anabolic or catabolic enzymes (such as choline acetyltransferase, *see* 6.2), uptake sites and, even, specific receptors (*see* below).

Pathways can be delineated at suitable times after nerve lesions when accumulation (of, for example, transmitters, precursors, anabolic enzymes, or vesicles) proximal to the cut will accompany distal loss, or by the use of specific tract-tracing markers (e.g. horseradish peroxidase or a tritiated amino acid). Also, neurotoxins are available for the selective destruction of, for example, catecholaminergic and/or 5-hydroxytryptaminergic neurones (p. 156). However, neurotoxins are seldom *wholly* selective and, further, adaptive changes in surviving pre- and postsynaptic receptors or in other associated transmitter systems may complicate the interpretation of the results, particularly of protracted experiments.

Caveat. While for most of the 'classical' transmitters, e.g. acetylcholine, noradrenaline (which are mainly resynthesised in or re-uptaken into the pre-synaptic terminal) the presynaptic content and specific receptor density are in close proximity), for other neurotransmitters (particularly peptides—which, like proteins, are synthesised in the ribosomes of the nerve cell body or which act diffusely as neuromodulation) the main transmitter content may be remote from the release and receptor sites (as localised by the techniques described next).

Autoradiographic and immunohistochemical techniques have been used to localise *receptors* for visualisation by light or electron microscopy. The use of a selective ligand containing a radioactive isotope which emits a positron on decaying, allows visualisation of the relevant receptors by a non-invasive method (positron emission tomography, PET) *in vivo* and is applicable to humans. Quantitative determinations of receptor numbers are also possible, particularly with autoradiography or PET. Finally, specific receptor isolation (p. 104) and determination of the mechanism(s) of receptor–response linking (4.8) provide sound bases for the qualitative separation of receptor types and subtypes.

Release

Even a fine micropipette introduced within the brain tissue samples the effluent from several cells (which are not necessarily homogenous). Further difficulties are rapid inactivation (e.g. of acetylcholine by its specific esterase; overcome by eserine in the perfusing fluid) or re-uptake (e.g. uptake$_1$ for catecholamines, requiring inhibition with desmethylimipramine $=$ desipramine). If release is sufficiently close to an external or internal surface of the neuraxis, strategically placed cups (cerebral cortex) or micropipettes (into cerebrospinal fluid pathways) may allow collection of a transmitter or a breakdown product (e.g. homovanillic acid from dopamine, 6.3). More commonly perfusion of tissue slices or whole brains via implanted semipermeable fibres (fibre dialysis)—combined with the prior administration of a radiolabelled transmitter (or precursor) plus a high affinity uptake carrier (if available)—enables the effects of nerve stimulation or drug application on transmitter release to be examined.

Application
This is achieved most directly via a micropipette which is multi-barrelled (to allow simultaneous electrical current or voltage application and/or measurement, and the application of modifying agents). From the pipette, placed using a stereotaxic manipulator, the ionised drug solution is ejected by iontophoresis at a rate dependent upon the polarity and strength of current applied. Direct monitoring of the resultant effect by intracellular electrode (if possible) avoids secondary changes in experimental conditions, either drug-induced or otherwise. In place of the possible transmitter, *more potent and/or more selective* agonists may similarly be employed. Drugs which act *pre*synaptically will affect release (*see* previous section).

Of course, drugs used in medical practice (except when given intrathecally such as local anaesthetics, *see* Table 8.2) can only affect CNS structures if they cross the blood–brain barrier in sufficient concentration. This obstacle can be circumvented experimentally by systemic injection into newly born animals in which the barrier is incompletely developed (e.g. chickens up to 10 days old) or by drug introduction at a preselected point into the cerebral ventricles (intracerebroventricular injection, icv), or the subarachnoid spaces of the brain or spinal cord.

Modifications
To eliminate access problems and non-specific effects, the potentiating or antagonising agent must be applied directly by microiontophoresis. It should alter *similarly* the identical responses obtained both following natural activation and local administration of the putative transmitter.

6.2   Acetylcholine

General evidence

Content
Content is shown in Table 6.1 and is paralleled by choline acetyltransferase (visualised by immunohistochemical labelling). Acetylcholinesterase has a wider distribution but is not so specific a marker for

Table 6.1 Contents of acetylcholine, dopamine, noradrenaline and 5-hydroxytryptamine in specific areas of the neuraxis

	Acetylcholine	Dopamine	Noradrenaline	5-Hydroxytryptamine
Cerebral cortex neopallial/limbic	+	+	+	+
Basal ganglia caudate nucleus lentiform nucleus globus pallidus	+++	+++		+
Thalamus			+	+
Hypothalamus	+	+	+++	++
Brainstem	+	+	++	++
Cerebellum			+	+
Spinal cord anterior horn lateral horn posterior horn	+		+ +	+

Concentration: +++, high; ++, moderate; +, significant.

cholinergic neurones. Ethylcholine mustard aziridium ion acts as a neurotoxin at low concentrations but does not destroy *all* cholinergic neurones. Choline uptake sites have been mapped autoradiographically using tritiated hemicholinium.

Release
Has been shown most convincingly into cerebral cortical cups containing eserinised saline.

Application
Acetylcholine is not the ideal agent due both to its rapid hydrolysis and its relative non-selectivity between muscarinic and nicotinic cholinoceptive sites. Any of the selective agonists shown in Table 2.4 may be iontophoresed directly but the fully charged members, e.g. methacholine, will not cross the blood–brain barrier. Drugs which produce significant central effects when give systemically are shown in Table 6.2.

Table 6.2 Agents which can cross the blood–brain barrier and affect central cholinoceptors

Subtype of receptor	Agonist	Antagonist(s)
Muscarinic	Oxotremorine	Hyoscine, atropine, benzhexol (US: trihexyphenidyl), orphenadrine
Nicotinic	Nicotine	Dihydro-β-erythroidine

Modifications

Potentiation. Eserine is extremely effective in enhancing both the strength and duration of acetylcholine responses but does not distinguish between muscarinic and nicotinic receptor sites.

Antagonism. In general, using selective drugs, it is possible to classify most synapses as predominantly muscarinic or nicotinic, although there is some overlap in a few areas (compare autonomic ganglia peripherally, 2.8).

Summary

Except for the Renshaw cell loop—where practically all of the transmitter criteria have been satisified—most progress has been made by the use of histochemical methods confirmed by microiontophoretic experiments. Separation into muscarinic and nicotinic receptors (both of which can be visualised by autoradiography) is fairly satisfactory but not invariably clear-cut.

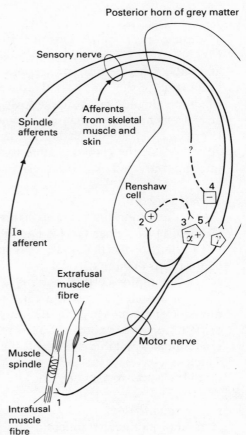

Fig. 6.1 Hemisection of grey matter of the spinal cord to show spinal control of skeletal muscle activity by the following transmitters: 1, 2, acetylcholine; 3, glycine; 4, γ-aminobutyric acid (GABA: presynaptic inhibition); 5, L-glutamate(?)—*see* p. 165. Continuous lines indicate excitatory and interrupted lines inhibitory neurones. ?, connection unclear. α and γ indicate corresponding motor neurones. +, excitatory and −, inhibitory postsynaptic potentials; ▱, presynaptic inhibition.

Specific sites

Renshaw cell circuit
As shown in Fig. 6.1, the anterior horn neurone (*a*) is controlled on its motor side by a negative feed-back loop arising from an efferent nerve collateral which releases acetylcholine to activate the Renshaw cell. The latter, in turn, produces an inhibitory postsynaptic potential (IPSP) by the intermediation of glycine (6.4). This mechanism allows the alternation of motor units essential to avoid prolonged passive constriction of small blood vessels by the surrounding, contracting muscle fibres. The receptors on the Renshaw cell body are primarily of the nicotinic type since dihydro-β-erythroidine antagonises the responses elicited either by antidromic stimulation of the motor nerve or by the application of acetylcholine—neither of which are significantly modified by the local use of atropine. However, as at autonomic ganglia, muscarinic receptors are present, which produce excitation of the Renshaw cell on iontophoretic injection of methacholine (antagonised by atropine), though they are not the normal route of transmission across this synapse.

Recticular activating system (RAS)
The anatomical connections of this arousal mechanism are shown in Figs 8.7 and 9.1. Cholinergic synapses are present throughout the RAS and, also, the cortical projections liberate acetylcholine in direct proportion to the state of wakefulness—most when awake, much less when asleep and least when heavily anaesthetised (e.g. with barbiturates). Conversely, acetylcholine can induce rapid eye movement (REM) sleep (Fig. 9.1), but the physiological significance of this is uncertain. At all these sites the cholinoceptors involved are predominantly muscarinic, e.g. activated by oxotremorine and blocked by atropine.

Corpus striatum
The caudate nucleus contains a high concentration of acetylcholine (Table 6.1) partly derived from neurones originating in the anteroventral nucleus of the thalamus. This is an important way-station of the dento-rubro-thalamocortical tract which is essential for cerebellar control of motor cortical activity and coordination. Any imbalance between this cholinergic (muscarinic) system and the opposing dopaminergic one results in a manifest motor disorder, such as parkinsonism or Huntington's chorea (7.2). Tremor occurs when acetylcholine predominates and this is probably the mechanism whereby tremorine— which is converted to the active agent oxotremorine in the liver— produces its most characteristic effect.

Hypothalamus
Here the cholinergic innervation has been shown most clearly in neurones which activate the supraoptic and paraventricular nuclei,

resulting in the liberation of vasopressin (5.9) and oxytocin (15.3), from the neurohypophysis. The receptors involved are nicotinic in type.

Temperature regulation (see p. 189)

Memory (7.7). There is evidence that acetylcholine is involved in the initial, short-term cataloguing process ('storage') of information by activation of Papez's circuit (hippocampus–fornix–mammillary body). This could explain the retrograde amnesia produced by hyoscine (2.7).

Emesis. It is likely that there are muscarinic cholinergic links either in the vomiting centre and/or in one of its connections (p. 317). This could account for the effectiveness of hyoscine in motion sickness.

Envoi
We are still some way from understanding all the interactions of cholinergic synapses within the neuraxis. For example, nicotine block-ade of spinal cord reflexes is readily explained by stimulation of the Renshaw cells, but when this substance is injected systemically into experimental animals it usually causes centrally mediated convulsions: these could be due to a depolarising block at the Renshaw cells or action(s) elsewhere in the neuraxis. The latter could also be the mechanism whereby anticholinesterases which enter the CNS readily (e.g. eserine, DFP, 2.6) engender fits. However, toxic doses of atropine can also exert initial excitant and convulsive effects centrally. Thus, increases in motor activity produced via cholinergic receptors must be multifactorial in origin. Further, the peripheral subdivision of cholino-ceptive cells into muscarinic and nicotinic types may not be equally satisfactory centrally.

6.3 Dopamine (DA), noradrenaline (NA), 5-hydroxytryptamine (5-HT)

General evidence

Content
The main sites for DA, NA and 5-HT are shown in Table 6.1, and the appropriate synthetic and catabolic enzymes are also present within these areas. The nerve pathways involved have been elucidated by the use of two main techniques.
1 *Histochemical.* Treatment of nervous tissue with formaldehyde results in compound which fluoresce in ultraviolet light: green with the catecholamines, yellow with 5-HT. Differentiation of the dopaminergic from the noradrenergic neurones is achieved by immunofluorescent staining of dopamine-β-hydroxylase, and the use of neurotoxins (*see* next subsection).

The relevant synthetic pathways are collated in Table 6.3. Enzyme blockade (by the agent shown below in brackets) results in loss of the corresponding transmitter(s), namely
• tyrosine hydroxylase (by α-methyl(para)tyrosine) diminishes DA and NA
• tryptophan hydroxylase (by parachlorophenylalanine) decreases 5-HT
• aromatic L-amino acid decarboxylase (by α-methyl(meta)tyrosine) causes exhaustion of DA, NA and 5-HT
• dopamine-β-hydroxylase (by disulfiram) prevents NA formation.

The administration of radiolabelled transmitters confirms that they pass into the expected sites, although some exogenous NA is taken up by dopaminergic neurones and 5-HT can enter catecholaminergic (NA and DA) terminals.

2 *Neurotoxins* are usually applied via a syringe fixed to a stereotaxic manipulator which, by the use of a particular set of coordinates, ensures their introduction into a preselected area of the neuraxis.

6-hydroxydopamine is taken up by catecholaminergic neurones and converted into quinone derivatives which destroy the nerves. *5,6-and 5,7-dihydroxytryptamine* exert a similar influence upon neurones containing 5-HT and/or NA—the latter are unaffected if uptake$_1$ is blocked by pretreatment with - desmethylimipramine (DMI, desipramine): dopaminergic neurones are not depleted by this toxin (*see also* MPTP, p. 174). *Note caveats re neurotoxin use* (6.1).

Release

Direct measurement. NA (especially in the presence of DMI) and 5-HT have been found in the effluent from a transected spinal cord following descending-fibre activation. Stimulation of the substantia nigra results in an increase of 3-methoxy-4-hydroxyphenylacetic (homovanillic) acid, which is a major metabolite of DA, in a perfusate of the anterior horn of the lateral cerebral ventricle.

Indirect measurement. Decrease in content is usually masked by rapid restitution of stores. Attempts to prevent the latter by the combined use of a synthesis inhibitor and an U$_1$ blocker have sometimes been successful, for example in showing a fall in limbic NA after stimulation of the medial forebrain bundle.

Turnover. The concentration of icv-administered ^{3}H-NA in the hypothalamus declines with time but this could indicate release from non-neuronal tissues. Even if it is certain that the radiolabelled compound has entered nerve terminals (e.g. give ^{3}H-DA and measure ^{3}H-NA), this does not necessarily imply transmitter function.

Table 6.3 Properties of dopamine (DA), noradrenaline (NA) and 5-hydroxytryptamine (5-HT) useful in the determination of CNS presence

	DA	NA	5-HT
Colour of fluorescent compound formed with formaldehyde	Green	Green	Yellow
Synthesis Precursor	tyrosine	tyrosine	L-tryptophan
Enzyme and product tyrosine hydroxylase tryptophan hydroxylase	→ dopa →	→ dopa →	→ 5-hydroxy-L-tryptophan →
aromatic L-amino acid decarboxylase	DA	DA	5-HT
dopamine-β-hydroxylase		NA	
Breakdown (major products only) Enzyme(s) and product(s) COMT/MAO	3-Methoxy-4-hydroxyphenyl-acetic acid* (homovanillic acid)	3-Methoxy-4-hydroxy-mandelic acid* (vanillyl mandelic acid)	
MAO	3,4-Dihydroxyphenylacetic acid* (DOPAC)	3,4-Hydroxymandelic acid*	5-Hydroxy-indolylacetic acid* (Table 5.1)
Selective blocker of re-uptake	Nomifensine Amphetamine Amantadine	Des(methylim)-ipramine	Paroxetine Fluoxetine

(The precursors L-tryptophan → 5-hydroxy-L-tryptophan → 5-HT cross the blood–brain barrier.)

COMT, catechol-oxygen-methyltransferase; MAO, monoamine oxidase.
* Also, some of the corresponding primary alcohol (*see* Figs 3.2 and 5.2).

Application

This must be by micropipette iontophoresis as these transmitters do not significantly cross the blood–brain barrier (Table 6.3). Under these circumstances NA and 5-HT, for example, depress *spinal* neurones and DA is inhibitory to caudate nucleus cells. Attempts to classify central adrenoceptors using the selective agonists shown for the peripheral system in Table 3.1 have been moderately successful in separating α- and β-effects; much less so in subtyping them. At some sites, adrenaline (A) rather than NA may be the transmitter (*see* 10.4). Agonists for D_1 and D_2 dopamine receptors are shown in Table 6.4. The best characterised CNS receptors for 5-HT are the subsets 5-HT_{1A} and 5-HT_{1B}: sites and agonists for these are shown in Table 6.5.

Modifications

Potentiation. This can generally be achieved by inhibition of reuptake (Table 6.3). Desmethylimipramine at low concentrations prevents U_1 of NA but slightly interferes with the return of DA and 5-HT into their respective neurones. More selective inhibitors for DA are nomifensine, amphetamine and amantadine; these block U_1 in higher concentrations. Paroxetine is a more selective inhibitor for 5-HT. Potentiation may also be obtained by inhibition of MAO which decreases breakdown of NA, DA and 5-HT (7.5).

Antagonism of NA actions by selective drugs as used in the peripheral nervous system (α, 3.4; β, 3.5) is not always satisfactory in classifying CNS receptor subgroups. *For DA*, CNS receptor antagonists are shown in Table 6.4. While many effects appear fairly straightforward through a

Table 6.4 Subdivision of dopamine receptors in the central nervous system

	D_1	D_2
Adenylate cyclase	Stimulated	Inhibited or unaffected
Agonists		
most selective	SKF 38393	Quinpirole
dopamine	+++	++
apomorphine	+++	++
bromocriptine	++	+++
Antagonists		
most selective	SCH 23390	Sulpiride
α-flupenthixol	+++	++
haloperidol	++	+++
chlorpromazine	+	++
domperidone		+++

Activity: +++, strong; ++, moderate; +, weak.

single type of receptor (e.g. prolactin release-inhibiting hormone, Fig. 15.1, via D_2), others (e.g. midbrain pathways) appear to contain a multiplicity of dopamine receptor types, both pre-and postsynaptic (*see* Fig. 7.1, caveat). *5-HT* antagonists for subsets 1A and 1B are shown in Table 6.5.

Summary

For NA, DA and 5-HT the main breakthrough was achieved using histochemical techniques and confirmatory evidence is being provided using neurotoxin, iontophoretic and receptor mapping studies.

Specific sites

Brainstem

The most clearly defined pathways are illustrated diagrammatically in Fig. 6.2 for *rat* brain.

NA neurones arise from cell groups (named A1–A7, not all shown) in the medulla and pons. They project *rostrally* (via medial forebrain bundle) to the limbic system, also to thalamus and hypothalamus; *dorsally* to the cerebellum; *caudally* to the spinal cord, particularly the lateral horn of grey matter at the sympathetic outflow (thoracic and upper lumbar segments) but also to the posterior horn. Locus caeruleus (A6) cells* occupy a pivotal position in this system (e.g. in sleep, Fig. 9.1).

5-HT neurones have a rather similar distribution. Their main origin is in the raphe nuclei (cell groups B1–B9) in the medulla and pons, from

Table 6.5 Important 5-hydroxytryptamine receptor groups in the CNS

Subset	1A	1B
Agonist(s)	5-Carboxyamidotryptamine	
	8-Hydroxy-DPAT	RU-24969
Partial agonist	Buspirone	
Antagonist	Spiperone* (also antagonises 5-HT$_2$, α_1 and D$_2$-dopamine receptors)	Iodo-cyanopindolol
Main site(s)	Limbic system	Globus pallidus
	Raphe nuclei	

DPAT, 2(*di*-n-*propylamino)tetralin; RU-24969, 5-methoxy-3-(1, 2, 3, 6-tetrahydropyridin-4-yl)-1-*H*-indole.
* Has also been used as a ligand for D$_2$-receptors.

*Cells in this area have a blue colour (L: *cæruleus*; uncommon variant *cœruleus*). American usage should avoid this pitfall by simplification of the diphthong to ceruleus in either case.

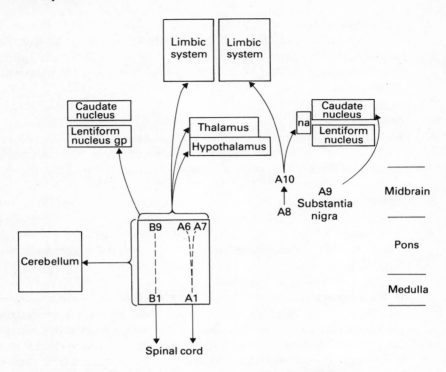

Fig. 6.2 Major connections of neuraxial areas containing significant concentrations of (right) DA, (left) 5-HT and NA; common lines do not necessarily indicate identical pathways: gp, globus pallidus; na, nucleus accumbens. For details, *see* text.

which they project rostrally and dorsally like NA neurones (and additionally to the globus pallidus) and also caudally, mainly to the posterior horn.

DA neurones project rostrally from cell groups A8–A10 in the midbrain, via two major pathways

• *nigrostriatal*—from the pars compacta of the substantia nigra (particularly A9) to the caudate nucleus (*see* Fig. 7.1)

• *mesolimbic*—from the ventral tegmentum (A10) to the nucleus accumbens (on the ventral surface of the fused rostral ends of the caudate and lentiform nuclei) and to the limbic system.

All three transmitters can affect the limbic system which is particularly important when considering psychotropic agents (Chapter 7). Evidence is also accruing that some or all of them are involved in brainstem cardiovascular (*see* migraine, 10.6) and respiratory control. DA receptors are present in the chemoreceptor trigger zone (which activates the vomiting centre, Fig. 13.1). Their activation accounts for the emetic actions of substances such as apomorphine, ergotamine and ergometrine; their antagonism accounts for the uses of chlorpromazine, metoclopramide or domperidone against vomiting (p. 317).

Hypothalamus and pituitary gland
Temperature regulation (p. 189) and feeding (9.5) may involve any or all of these transmitters. Posterior pituitary vasopressin and oxytocin release via the supraoptic and paraventricular nuclei, produced by parasympathetic stimulation, is prevented by sympathetic activation or noradrenaline iontophoresis—indicating 'classic' autonomic control of these processes.

Anterior pituitary hormone release. There is evidence that all the transmitters under discussion can modify the output of adenohypophysial hormones. The clearest example is dopamine released from the median eminence which (via a D_2-dopamine receptor) activates the prolactin release-inhibiting hormone; thus, bromocriptine (Table 6.4) can be used to inhibit lactation (15.1) and galactorrhoea may be a side-effect of chlorpromazine (Table 7.6).

Spinal cord
NA neurones descending from the brainstem nuclei are intimately involved with sympathetic outflow (lateral horn) but also possibly with afferent sensory neurones (as next). 5-HT neurones pass caudally from the raphe nuclei and impinge mainly on afferents and interneurones in the posterior horn where they have important interconnections with peptidergic fibres (6.5 and pain, 7.10).

Memory. There is some evidence that all three transmitters can modify the early stages of sensory registration (7.7).

Sense organs. Dopamine appears to be important locally, in the chemoreceptors of the carotid and aortic bodies, the olfactory bulbs and (together with 5-HT) in the amacrine cells of the retina.

Adrenaline as a CNS transmitter
This is much less common than the other catecholamines (noradrenaline, dopamine). Methods for detection centre essentially on the enzyme necessary for the conversion of noradrenaline to adrenaline (which is also present in the adrenal medulla and other chromaffin tissues), namely *p*hen(yl)ethanolamine-*N*(itrogen)-*m*ethyl*t*ransferase (PNMT). This can be specifically detected by immunofluorescent staining and inhibited by, for example, dichloro-α-methylbenzylamine.

Cell groups C1–C3 have been defined in the lower brainstem with C1 particularly important in the control of blood pressure (p. 249).

Envoi
The monoamines discussed above have well-defined motor and sensory roles involving the mind (psyche) and central homeostatic mechanisms; these can often be exploited therapeutically.

Circadian rhythms. 5-HT metabolism (Fig. 5.2) by acetylation on the side-chain nitrogen atom followed by 5-oxygen-methylation results in the formation of melatonin. This is particularly to be noted in the *mammalian* pineal gland, where the necessary enzymes are inhibited by light striking the eye, so that melatonin decreases during the day and increases at night. Many diurnal rhythms occur in mammals but melatonin formation may well be one controlling factor. A good example is in seasonal breeders where melatonin secreted during the night decreases the releasing hormones for gonadotrophins, particularly in winter. Note that in the *frog*, melatonin is *produced* under light conditions to aid in camouflage (18.5).

The suprachiasmatic nucleus in the anterior hypothalamus also appears to be involved in the control of circadian rhythms. Putative transmitters in this area are GABA and acetylcholine.

6.4   Amino acids

The major substances implicated are
- inhibitory. Glycine, γ-aminobutyric acid (GABA)
- excitatory. L-glutamic acid, L-aspartic acid.

Inhibitory amino acids

General evidence

Content. Because of the ubiquity of amino acids, possible transmitter sites must contain them in enhanced amounts compared with other

Table 6.6 Contents (above basic cellular levels) of four amino acids in specific areas of the neuraxis

	Glycine	GABA	L-glutamic acid	L-aspartic acid
Cerebral cortex				
neopallial		+	+	
Basal ganglia				
caudate nucleus		+	+	
lentiform nucleus				
globus pallidus		+++		
Thalamus		+		
Hypothalamus		++		
Brainstem	+	+++*	+	
Cerebellum		+	+	+
Spinal cord				
anterior horn	+++	+		
posterior horn		+	+	++
posterior columns			+	

Concentration: +++, high; ++, moderate; +, significant.
* Particularly substantia nigra (pars reticularis)

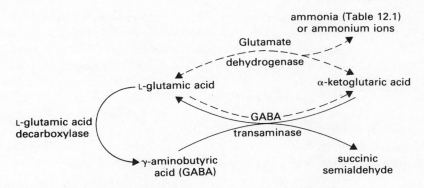

Fig. 6.3 Main pathways of GABA synthesis and breakdown. Interrupted lines indicate other interconversions between α-ketoglutaric acid and L-glutamic acid: the latter can, however, be formed or degraded via other routes.

tissues. The relative distributions, shown in Table 6.6, indicate fairly localised functions for all these agents, with the exception of GABA. Other amino acids (e.g. taurine) are concentrated in certain areas of the CNS, where they could possibly act as transmitters. Compared with glycine, glutamic acid and aspartic acid, which are involved in many different biochemical pathways, the formation and breakdown of GABA is relatively restricted so that the simple scheme portrayed in Fig. 6.3 is valid. Distributions of the necessary enzymes, namely L-glutamic acid decarboxylase (L-GAD) and GABA transaminase (GABA-T) respectively, in the CNS agree well with those of GABA. Inhibition of L-GAD with 3-mercaptopropionic acid decreases GABA content. Both GABA and glycine receptors have been mapped using autoradiographic techniques.

Release. Amino acid transmitters are rapidly removed from the synaptic cleft by specific uptake mechanisms—not only into central neurones but also into glial cells, which can provide a subsidiary source of transmitter on subsequent depolarisation (e.g. by locally available extracellular K^+ ions). Nipecotic acid specifically inhibits re-uptake of GABA into neuronal (but less into glial) sites. Much work has been performed on brain or spinal cord slices pre-incubated with the radiolabelled putative agent, which has then been shown to be increasingly released on application of an appropriate stimulus.

Table 6.7 A subdivision of GABA receptors

	$GABA_A$*	$GABA_B$
Selective agonist	Muscimol	Baclofen
Selective antagonist	Bicuculline	(Bicuculline-insensitive)
Ionic characteristic	Cl^--dependent	Cl^--independent

* *See* Fig. 7.2.

Application. Both glycine and GABA (a conformationally restricted form is muscimol, Table 6.7) produce hyperpolarisation, associated with an increased Cl^- ion conductance, Fig. 7.2. Glutamic acid depolarises many neurones in the CNS and is sometimes used to produce a non-specific activation. Aspartic acid also causes excitation when applied electrophoretically.

Modifications
• *Potentiation* of GABA effects can be achieved by blocking GABA transaminase with amino-oxyacetic acid, γ-vinyl GABA (vigabatrin) or sodium valproate (p. 172 and Fig. 7.2).

• *Antagonism.* Presynaptic prevention of release of either glycine or GABA can be produced with tetanus toxin. Postsynaptic blockade of glycine is achieved by strychnine; and of GABA by bicuculline (which appears to be a competitive inhibitor) or picrotoxin (? post-receptor block of GABA $\rightarrow$ Cl^- channel opening)—*see* Fig. 7.2.

Summary. That the Renshaw cell liberates glycine can be proved by most of the necessary criteria. For GABA-ergic synapses, $GABA_A$ and $GABA_B$ subtypes (Table 6.7) are present in the brain and spinal cord (*see* baclofen, 7.3). The $GABA_A$ receptor, which acts as an ion channel for Cl^- ions has been characterised. It is commonly (but not invariably) intimately associated with benzodiazepine receptors which are present on the $GABA_A$-chloride ion channel complex (*see* Fig. 7.2).

Specific sites

Glycine. This is unequivocally the transmitter released by the Renshaw cell. Antidromic stimulation of a somatic motor nerve results in an IPSP on the anterior horn cell (Fig. 6.1) which can not only be duplicated by the iontophoretic application of glycine but also *shows the same reversal potential.* Tetanus toxin blocks only the antidromic nerve stimulation (indicating a presynaptic action) while strychnine additionally prevents the effect of applied glycine and displaces its dose–response curve of inhibition to the right in a parallel fashion (indicating postsynaptic, competitive antagonism). Thus, tetanus toxin and strychnine are both spinal convulsants (9.7).

GABA-ergic synapses
• *Spinal cord.* Afferents, both from the skin and skeletal muscle, inhibit motor neurone activity by presynaptic inhibition—mediated by GABA—at site(s) along the CNS section of the reflex arc (Fig. 6.1). This GABA release is prevented by tetanus toxin and its receptor action by both bicuculline and picrotoxin.

- *Basal ganglia.* GABA-ergic neurones pass from the globus pallidus to the pars reticularis of the substantia nigra (*see* Fig. 7.1). These sites are of significance in motor disorders especially Huntington's chorea (p. 174).
- *Cerebral and cerebellar cortices* contain modest excesses of GABA which assume importance with regard to antiepileptic drugs (7.1), minor tranquillisers (7.4), hypnotics (9.1), and penicillin toxicity (19.3). GABA is released from the occipital cortex after stimulation of the lateral geniculate body and into the fourth ventricle by activation of cerebellar Purkinje fibres.
- *Others.* There have been recent suggestions that GABA is involved in memory (7.7), cardiovascular control (p. 249), circadian rhythms and functioning of the horizontal cells of the retina.

Excitatory amino acids

The distributions of L-glutamate and L-aspartate within the CNS are shown in Table 6.6. Release is difficult to prove due to high-affinity (re)uptake. Most work has involved the iontophoretic application of synthetic compounds which act more selectively as agonists. On this basis excitatory (acidic) amino acid receptors have been divided into *NMDA* (N-methyl-D-aspartate), *quisqualate* (AMPA* *is a more selective agonist) and kainate*—*see* below—subtypes. The NMDA receptors are blocked *competitively* by 2-amino-5-phosphonopentanoate (AP5) and *at their associated ion channel* by ketamine and phencyclidine (p. 220) and σ-opiates (p. 197). There are no selective antagonists for the other two subtypes but kynurenic acid (a tryptophan metabolite) blocks at all three sites. AP5 prevents penicillin fits (p. 404).

Excitatory glutaminergic pathways have been postulated at the terminations of Ia afferents on motor neurones (Fig. 6.1, blocked by kynurenic acid but not by AP5), and passing from the cerebral cortex to the caudate nucleus (Fig. 7.1, caption). *See also* cardiovascular control (p. 249).

Kainic acid, a stable heterocyclic analogue of glutamic acid, produces (via kainate receptors—*see* above) initial excitation of many types of CNS cell (e.g. cholinergic, adrenergic, GABAergic) followed by destruction of the cell body with subsequent degeneration of the rest of the neurone.†

6.5 Autacoids (except 5-HT)

Biogenic amines

Histamine, together with its anabolic (p. 125) and catabolic (p. 128) enzymes, occurs in significant amounts within certain areas of the CNS

---

* α-amino-3-hydroxy-5-methylisoxazole-4-propionic acid.
† Substances which first stimulate and later destroy neurones are termed '*excitoxins*'.

and binding studies have revealed specific receptive sites; but, so far, a transmitter function has not definitely been ascribed to this autacoid.

Anti-(H_1) histamines which cross the blood–brain barrier have an anti-emetic action (p. 317) and produce sedation (Table 5.5): the degree of drowsiness induced by different members of the imipramine group of antidepressants (p. 182) has been correlated with their relative abilities to block histamine receptors.

Peptides and purines

Hypothalamo-pituitary axis (14.1)
The presence of peptidergic neurones is firmly established here, namely to the:
- neurohypophysis: vasopressin, oxytocin
- adenohypophysis: releasing or release-inhibiting factors. Some of these, e.g. somatostatin (which primarily prevents growth hormone release; also does the same for thyrotrophin centrally and for insulin, glucagon and gastrin, peripherally), probably have wider functions within the CNS (*see* below).

Tachykinins/neurokinins
High CNS concentrations occur in the substantia nigra (Fig. 7.1, caption) where there is extensive NK_2 and NK_3 (but not NK_1) receptor binding—*see* Caveat, 6.1. In the spinal cord area, the posterior horn and roots contain significant amounts of substance P which appears to mediate some C fibre pain activity (p. 207). Capsaicin—an irritant principle of some red pepper plants (*Capsicum* species) specifically affects unmyelinated primary sensory peptidergic neurones. It first releases their transmitters (e.g. substance P, somatostatin) resulting in depletion and then destroys them by a neurotoxic action.

Endogenous opioid peptides
Extracts of hypothalamus and the pituitary gland contain—among other peptides—opiocorticotropin, the content of which is illustrated in Table 6.8. The 'opio' part of the names arises because the peptide includes sequences (e.g. β-endorphin) which produce marked, maintained analgesia (similar to that occurring with morphine, Table 7.13—the classical opiate agonist) after introduction into the third ventricles of cats.

Extraction analysis of areas of the neuraxis known to contain high concentrations of opiate receptors (by the use of specific binding ligands, Table 4.3) led to the separation of two pentapeptides, differing by only one amino acid and, accordingly, termed [met](methionine) and [leu](leucine) enkephalin. Although the peptide sequence of [met]enkephalin is present in β-endorphin, *the latter does not appear to*

Table 6.8 Opiocorticotropin and its subdivision into important peptides

Amino acid number*	Subdivisions		Analgesia† Duration	Potency
1 13 24 39 41 58	} tetracosactrin } } ACTH	} −α-MSH } −β-MSH		
61 65 91/2	} (methionine) enkephalin β-endorphins N-methyl (methionine) enkephalin amide		+ + + } + + +	+ + + + + +

ACTH, corticotrophin: MSH, melanocyte-stimulating hormone.
Duration: +, short; + +, moderate; + + +, long. Potency: +, weak;
+ +, moderate; + + +, strong (slightly greater than morphine).
* Guide list only: varies widely with species and part of hypothalamo-pituitary area extracted.
† Analgesia (following introduction into the third ventricles of cats).

be the natural precursor of the former. The enkephalins are rapidly (within seconds) and β-endorphin (rather more slowly) inactivated by tissue peptidases, which makes release difficult to prove. Application of the more stable amide derivatives (e.g. of [met]enkephalin) into the feline third ventricle results in analgesia slightly greater in potency and duration than that obtained with morphine. This is perhaps less unexpected if you realise that morphine can be synthesised from two molecules of tyrosine (Fig. 6.4).

Endogenous opioid peptides can be subdivided into:
• *β-endorphin family.* These occur mainly in relation to endocrine function in the hypothalamo-pituitary axis
• *enkephalin family.* Widespread in nervous tissue, e.g. amygdala, periaqueductal grey matter and the spinal cord (particularly posterior horn): the implications for pain mechanisms and their relief are considered in 7.10. Enkephalins are also present in the myenteric plexuses of the gut and are released along with catecholamines from chromaffin tissue (p. 64)
• *dynorphin family.* A group found in submucous gut plexuses, with [leu]enkephalin in nervous tissue and with vasopressin in the posterior pituitary gland. All contain [leu]enkephalin at one terminus.

Purinergic mechanisms
Adenosine and related nucleotides, together with enzymes for their synthesis and breakdown, are widespread within the neuraxis and can

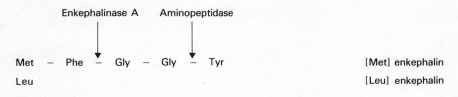

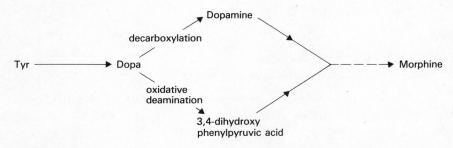

Fig. 6.4 Structural analogy between enkephalins (catabolising enzymes, arrowed above) naturally occurring in the CNS and the synthesis of morphine. Interrupted line indicates multi-stage reaction.

be released from a number of areas on the appropriate nerve stimulation. Applications of relevant agonists elicit similar responses which may *either be potentiated* by block or re-uptake (e.g. of adenosine by dipyridamole) or prevention of inactivation (e.g. by inhibitors of adenosine deaminase) *or be antagonised* by methylxanthines (e.g. theophylline); however, these latter have other actions (*see* Table 5.8 and p. 235).

At the moment central purinergic neurones have not been postulated. CNS adenosine receptors (P_1, Table 5.8) are subdivided into A_1 (which *de*crease cAMP) and A_2 (which *in*crease cAMP) subtypes—both found pre- and postsynaptically—and considered to play a neuromodulatory rather than a primary neurotransmitter role (*see* co-transmitters, p. 141).

Lipid derivatives
Eicosanoid production within the CNS has important functions with respect to
- pyrexias due to infections (7.8)
- pain mechanisms, which possibly may be partly central in origin (7.9).

7 CNS Transmitters and Drug Action

Many drugs when given experimentally, either by intracerebroventricular injection or in high concentrations (by other routes), produce CNS actions which are normally not manifest under therapeutic conditions; such effects are only considered here if they have possible toxicological significance in humans. Otherwise only major, or important subsidiary, responses to drugs will be discussed.

Broadly, agents modifying CNS function may be classified as

1 *Non-selective.* This implies that they affect the neuraxis in the reverse order to that of phylogenesis (i.e. the more recently developed faculties are disturbed before the more primitive ones). General anaesthetics (8.6) and ethanol (9.2) fall into this category: thus the highest centres (involving, for example, intellectual discrimination) are dulled first, followed by loss of coordination at the motor and sensory level, with the vital centres (controlling the respiratory and cardiovascular systems) being most resistant to drug action.

2 *Selective.* These agents produce an effect upon one (or more) CNS function(s) at doses which have negligible actions on other neuraxial responses. For example, anti-epileptic drugs, which depress motor cortical activity preferentially without producing much drowsiness; antidepressants, which enhance mood but do not cause excitement or convulsions.

DRUGS AFFECTING MOTOR ACTIVITY

7.1 Epilepsy
The commonest disability is *grand mal* (originating in the cerebral motor cortex); this can be symptomatic but is usually idiopathic. Termination of the fit—which begins with a tonic phase and then progresses to clonic movements (Table 9.3)—and prevention of its recurrence are the major considerations in therapy. Effective agents include hydantoins (e.g. phenytoin, US: diphenylhydantoin), barbiturates with a phenyl group (e.g. phenobarbitone, Table 1.3), a dibenzazepine (carbamazepine, *see* Fig. 7.3, *note* in legend), sodium valproate and benzodiazepines (e.g. diazepam).

Possible mechanisms of drug action

1 *An increase in forebrain GABA* (or increased efficiency of GABA-ergic synapses, 7.4) which produces a raised Cl^- ion conductance and hyperpolarisation. It has been suggested that cerebral endogenous anticonvulsant peptides are present, together with 'phenytoin' receptors which respond to anticonvulsant hydantoins and barbiturates and interact in a complex manner with both GABA- and benzodiazepine-receptor systems, *see* Fig. 7.2.

2 *A decrease in excitatory amino acid function* (p. 165). Phenobarbitone blocks quisqualate receptors : lamotrigine, a new anticonvulsant, prevents glutamate release.

3 *Prevention of post-tetanic potentiation* (of the type mentioned on p. 71, when increased activity of a junction results in enhanced presynaptic release of transmitter). This could account for the successful use of phenytoin in trigeminal neuralgia—which is associated with a high frequency of impulses in the fifth cranial nerve—and in cardiac dysrhythmias. Similar rapid neuronal firing may be present in cerebral 'circus movements' maintaining epileptogenic activity. Carbamazepine also possesses this action.

4 *Membrane stabilisation* (Chapter 8). This could also account for the suppressive effects of phenytoin in certain cardiac dysrhythmias (10.13).

5 *Modulation of the Na^+, K^+-activated ATPase* (vital to maintain transmembrane ionic gradients). This might be a relevant consideration for phenytoin which stimulates the enzyme.

Drugs used in the treatment of grand mal epilepsy are usually given prophylactically for prolonged periods—3 years after the last attack—sometimes in fairly high doses. Therefore, in addition to acute side-effects, longer-term disadvantages assume significance (Table 7.1). *Phenytoin* is a very useful drug in this connection, which indicates that the side-effects shown are uncommon but they illustrate a number of important principles. For example, as mentioned in Chapter 1, the simplest way to make a benzene ring more water-soluble is to (para)-hydroxylate it (*see* Table 1.7, phenytoin, phenobarbitone). This reaction requires folic acid as a co-factor which may become exhausted during prolonged therapy resulting in a folate-deficiency megaloblastic anaemia (p. 378). Interference with vitamin D hydroxylation (p. 370) results in a low plasma 25-hydroxycholecalciferol—probably due to induced hydroxylation to compounds which are less active than the 1,25-dihydroxycholecalciferol (1,25-DHCC) normally produced and essential for gut absorption of calcium. Nevertheless there is sufficient precursor to maintain 1,25-DHCC plasma levels but these must be *less* effective in phenytoin-induced osteomalacia.

Table 7.1 Possible side-effects of the most important anti-epileptic drugs

	Phenobarbitone	Phenytoin (US: diphenyl-hydantoin)	Carbamazepine	Sodium valproate	Ethosuximide
Drowsiness	+++*	+	+	+	++
Cerebellar ataxia	++	++	+		+
Visual					
nystagmus	+	+			
diplopia		+	+		
photophobia					+
Hypersensitivity (p. 435)				‡	
(more common) rash	+	++	+		+
(less common) blood dyscrasia					
leucopenia†		+			+
aplastic anaemia		±	+		+
Blood dyscrasias					
folate-deficiency anaemia	++	++	++		
leucopenia (non-allergic)					++
Osteomalacia	++	++	+		
Nausea and vomiting		+	+	+	+
Liver function depression		(Table 20.4, 3)		+	
Gingival hyperplasia		++ especially in the young			
Lymphadenopathy		+			
Hirsuties		+			
Teratogenicity: increased incidence of hare-lip and cleft palate in offspring		+ +		+ (rats)	
Porphyria (in susceptible individuals)	+	+			

Incidence/severity: +++, common/marked; ++, less common/moderate; +, occasional/mild; ±, uncommon.
* Also, irritability (children); confusion (elderly). Therefore not much used.
† Type II hypersensitivity reaction, Table 20.1.
‡ Rarely can produce Reye's-like syndromes (*see* p. 193).

Phenytoin has further interesting pharmacokinetic properties

- plasma protein binding is normally about 90%
- microsomal metabolism may change from first- to zero-order kinetics around the therapeutic concentration (p. 20)
- it induces microsomal enzymes: *can nullify 'the pill'.*

Thus phenytoin has interactions with many drugs (including other anti-epileptics) and for this reason single drug therapy is recommended.

In other forms of epilepsy (and status epilepticus) the same drugs are used except that, in *petit mal*, ethosuximide (mechanism unknown, toxicology shown in Table 7.1) and sodium valproate are the first-line agents.

Valproate antagonises GABA transaminase but this is not considered to be its (sole) mechanism of the anti-epileptic effect which it can exert at lower doses than those required for GABA transaminase block (*see* Fig. 7.2).

7.2   Basal ganglia defects

Conditions which are not due to a specific loss in transmitter function, e.g. Wilson's disease (where the copper-carrying plasma protein, caeruloplasmin, is abnormal or deficient and the metal is accordingly deposited in the liver and lentiform nucleus) are treated with an appropriate therapy, namely chelation of the copper ions with penicillamine (20.9) in this uncommon condition.

Parkinsonism

Parkinsonism is the most common defect and can arise in a number of ways; iatrogenic, degenerative, infective (post-encephalitic) or toxicological see *Note* on MPTP at end of this section. Whatever the cause, there is an overall deficiency in dopamine function compared to acetylcholine (muscarinic) activity in the caudate nucleus (Fig. 7.1), this is manifested as hypokinesia, rigidity and tremor (lessened during voluntary movement). However, the situation is not so simple since, depending on the aetiology, the symptoms are relieved to differing

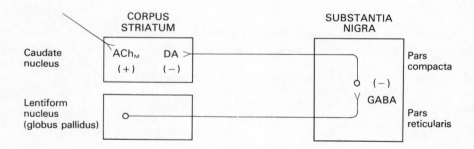

Fig. 7.1 Major pathways (diagrammatic) necessary for correct motor function between the substantia nigra and the caudate nucleus (which requires a balance of dopaminergic and cholinergic inputs). Transmitters: ACh_M, acetylcholine, muscarinic—excitatory (+); DA, dopamine—inhibitory (−); GABA, γ-aminobutyric acid exerting a negative feed-back on DA neurone. *Caveat.* This view of locomotor control in the nigrostriatal circuit is simplistic because: ACh may activate the GABA neurone; presynaptic DA receptors have been reported on many of these fibres; and other putative transmitters occur, e.g. excitatory corticostriatal glutaminergic fibres (p. 165), e.g. neurokinin receptors in the substantia nigra (p. 166).

extents by the two major forms of therapy which are thus preferentially indicated (Table 7.2). Pharmacologically, the options are, simply:

1 To block acetylcholine (muscarinic) receptors. This major therapy necessitates agents which cross the blood–brain barrier (e.g. benzhexol, orphenadrine, see Table 6.2). Additionally, these drugs may increase dopamine release by a presynaptic action. Their immediate side-effects are similar to those of atropine (*see* Table 2.7) and may be beneficial (e.g. less salivation, *see* Table 20.2); but, centrally, the necessary chronic administration may induce a confusional state which has to be distinguished from a recrudescence of the parkinsonism.

2 To increase activation of the dopamine receptors

a by more transmitter passage

• raise presynaptic content, i.e. levodopa (*see* later)

• facilitate release and/or decrease re-uptake of dopamine, e.g. amantadine (an antiviral drug, 19.9); a minor, but often initial, form of treatment

b by direct receptor stimulation, e.g. with bromocriptine (*see* later).

Levodopa is the L-isomer of DOPA (the D-isomer is toxic). Dopamine is inactive when given systemically because it does not cross the blood–brain barrier (Table 6.3). The effectiveness of levodopa implies that sufficient dopa decarboxylase activity remains within the surviving neurones for adequate dopamine formation and/or that denervated receptors acquire increased sensitivity. This therapy often fails within

Table 7.2 Use of the two major treatments in parkinsonism

	Antimuscarinic drug (e.g. orphenadrine)	Production of dopamine (i.e. levodopa)
Symptoms relieved		
hypokinesia	0	+ +
rigidity	+	+ +
tremor	+	±
Preferred for which type	Iatrogenic	Others
Side-effects		
peripheral	Dry mouth*	Hypotension†
	Cycloplegia	Cardiac dysrhythmias
central	Confusion	Nausea and vomiting
		Dyskinesias—especially choreoathetoid facial movements
		Psychological disturbances

Symptomatic relief: + +, marked; +, some; ±, slight; 0, negligible.
* *See* Table 20.2.
† Central component also involved.
Note: For iatrogenic parkinsonism *see* p. 178.

3–5 years as manifested by 'on-off effects' (i.e. abrupt reversions to parkinsonian symptoms—'*off* effects'—occurring many times during each dosage period) and 'end of dose deterioration'. The addition of a direct dopamine agonist, e.g. bromocriptine (Table 6.4) is then indicated. This is not very effective *alone* because it only acts on *low affinity* D$_2$ receptors which require *some* dopamine to be present if they are to produce an adequate response.

Nevertheless, levodopa is still widely used. Its side-effects are shown in Table 7.2 but the peripheral actions can be eliminated by the simultaneous administration of domperidone (an anti-emetic, peripheral dopamine antagonist, *see* p. 317) and/or a dopa decarboxylase inhibitor which does not cross the blood–brain barrier (type substance, carbidopa, Fig. 3.3). The latter also increases the effectiveness of the treatment by allowing more of the transmitter precursor to pass into the CNS. Further potentiation can be obtained by the addition of selegiline (deprenyl) a monoamine oxidase-B inhibitor which prevents dopamine breakdown and rarely causes hypertension, p. 184 (although selegiline can be metabolised to amphetamine; however, remember that excessive dopamine can result in dyskinesias (Table 7.2).

Note. MPTP(1-*m*ethyl-4-*p*henyl-1,2,3,6-*t*etrahydro*p*yridine)—an illicitly manufactured pethidine derivative—produces parkinsonism in addicts. After crossing the blood–brain barrier it is converted by MAO-B to the 1-*m*ethyl-4-*p*henyl*p*yridium ion (MPP$^+$) which enters dopaminergic neurones and is neurotoxic. It has been suggested that idiopathic parkinsonism might be caused by a similar 'naturally occurring' toxin.

Huntington's chorea

Huntington's chorea is an uncommon, familial condition of progressive mental and physical deterioration. Choreiform movements are produced which can be ascribed to changes in nigrostriatal function that are the opposite of those seen in parkinsonism, i.e. excessive dopamine function compared to cholinergic (muscarinic) stimulation. These are possibly due to deficiency of glutamic acid decarboxylase (*see* Fig. 6.3), resulting in less GABA synthesis and inhibitory feedback (Fig. 7.1). The treatment of choice at the moment is depletion of CNS dopaminergic neurones with tetrabenazine (which acts in a reserpine-like manner, 3.2). Alternative strategies include dopamine receptor blockade—haloperidol is preferable to chlorpromazine here, as it also increases GABA release (*see* Table 7.7)—and muscarinic (cholinergic) activation; eserine (2.6) will cross the blood–brain barrier and is the most suitable agent. Unfortunately, the progressive mental impairment is unaffected by drugs.

7.3 **Spasticity**

The final common path for skeletal muscle tone is the α-motor neurone which is controlled most immmediately by spindle afferent activity (Fig. 6.1) but also by many supraspinal (particularly extrapyramidal) centres. The major mechanisms of drugs used in the treatment of spasticity are shown in Table 7.3. *Diazepam* decreases presynaptic inhibition in the spinal cord (Fig. 6.1) but has the disadvantage of drowsiness (Table 7.5). *Baclofen* is a derivative of GABA which more readily crosses the blood–brain barrier, where it exerts depressant actions mainly at the spinal cord level. $GABA_B$ receptors are defined as baclofen-sensitive and bicuculline-resistant (*see* Table 6.7). *Dantrolene* acts primarily on excitation–contraction coupling in skeletal muscle.

DRUGS AFFECTING THE PSYCHE

Many drugs act upon the mind (Gk: *psyche*) but in this section first consideration will be given to those agents which *selectively* modify mental function. These may conveniently be divided into

● *psychotherapeutic substances* which are used in the treatment of psychiatric disorders

● *psychotomimetic substances* which can be employed experimentally, to induce psychotic states for pharmacological analysis. Clinically some are important as drugs of dependence.

A grossly simplified classification of psychological abnormalities is shown in Table 7.4. *Neuroses* may be regarded as relatively mild upsets involving an exaggeration of normal behaviour of which the patient is aware (i.e. has insight). They are often precipitated by an obvious cause (as indicated by the adjective 'reactive' for the depressed condition). *Psychoses* are much more severe bouts of *ab*normality, during which insight is lacking. They usually appear without apparent reason.

The groups of drugs used in these conditions are also shown in Table 7.4. It must be realised that intermediate or mixed situations exist, e.g. anxiety neuroses with depressive phases, e.g. manic-depressive psychosis: the treatment of these is more complicated.

Table 7.3 Major mechanisms of antispastic agents

Drug	Main effect	Main site
Diazepam	Increase in efficiency of $GABA_A$ergic synapses (Fig. 7.2)	Central nervous system
Baclofen	$GABA_B$ agonism	Spinal cord
Dantrolene	Decreased intracellular release or increased sequestration of calcium ions (4.10)	Skeletal muscle*

* Also used in malignant hyperthermia (p. 442).

Table 7.4 Psychiatric conditions and their treatment

Condition	Excited state	Indicated drug	Inhibited state	Indicated drug
Neurosis	Anxiety neurosis	Anxiolytic (minor tranquilliser)	Reactive depression	Antidepressant
Psychosis	Schizophrenia	Antischizophrenic (major tranquilliser)	Endogenous depression	

7.4 Tranquillisers

Anxiolytics (minor tranquillisers)

Those used clinically are mostly benzodiazepines—type substance, diazepam—with the actions shown in Table 7.5.

These effects are mediated via specific benzodiazepine receptors which increase the efficiency of transmission at $GABA_A$ synapses.

The GABA receptor is a tetramer consisting of two α and two β subunits. The latter contain the GABA recognition site (Fig. 7.2). Drug combination with one benzodiazepine recognition site on an α subunit results in allosteric modulation of the $GABA_A$ mediated Cl^- ion channel opening, but is *ineffective in the absence of GABA*.

Positive modulators, such as diazepam, increase the probability of channel opening by GABA or, if the latter is already present on the β subunit, prolong the channel open time (? by binding to the 'open' form of the channel). *Negative modulators* ('inverse agonists'), e.g. DMCM*, stabilise the channel in its inactivated ('closed') state and/or shorten channel open time: they therefore produce the opposite actions to those of diazepam, namely convulsions, anxiety and insomnia. The benzodia-

Table 7.5 Actions of diazepam

Effect	Major site(s) of action	Reference
Anticonvulsant (grand mal)	Motor cortex	7.1
Amnesia	?	7.7 and p. 193
Anxiety relief (minor tranquilliser)	Limbic system	7.4
Hypnotic action (sleep)	Sleep/awake centres	9.1
Muscle spasm alleviation	Spinal cord ? Higher centres controlling muscle tone	7.3

* 6, 7-*di*methyl-4-ethyl-β-*c*arboline-3-carboxylic acid *m*ethyl ester.

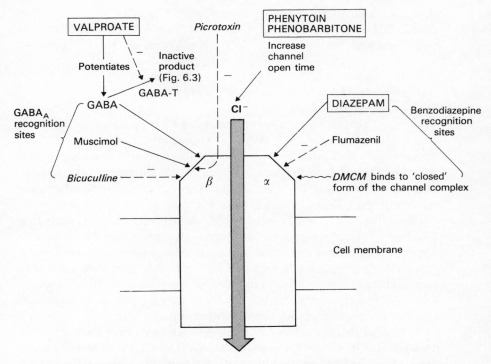

Fig. 7.2 The benzodiazepine-GABA$_A$-chloride ion (Cl$^-$) channel complex in relation to drug effects. Interrupted lines show inhibitory ($-$) actions. Activation of *one* of the GABA$_A$ recognition sites on the β subunit by GABA or muscimol (Table 6.7) opens the Cl$^-$ ion channel which hyperpolarises the cell membrane. This effect is opposed by *either* bicuculline (competitively) *or* picrotoxin (which non-competitively prevents GABA activation opening the channel). Drug combination with the benzodiazepine recognition sites on the α subunits can result in (*see* text): positive modulation, e.g. diazepam; negative modulation, e.g. DMCM; or antagonism of positive or negative modulation, e.g. flumazenil. Possible sites of action of other *anti-epileptics* (names in rectangles) are indicated. GABA-T, GABA transaminase. Names of *convulsants* are italicised.

zepine antagonist, flumazenil, blocks the binding of both positive *and* negative modulators.

Ideally, minor tranquillisers should relieve anxiety and tension without producing unconsciousness (difference from general anaesthetics) or sleep (difference from hypnotics). However, they may induce confusion in the elderly, and drowsiness is a common side-effect; in higher dosage they are used as hypnotics (9.1). As anti-anxiety agents, benzodiazepines are preferable to their predecessors, the barbiturates, because they produce less drowsiness, less respiratory depression in overdose (and specific antagonist available, flumazenil) and less induction of hepatic microsomal enzymes (for their metabolism *see* p. 229). Diazepam is very heavily bound (*c.* 99%) to α_1-acid glycoproteins in the plasma (p. 15).

Realisation of the physical dependence produced by these drugs (Table 7.9) has exerted a great brake on their prescription and they are only indicated for short-term (2–4 weeks) relief of severe, disabling anxiety.

Antischizophrenics (also termed major tranquillisers, antipsychotics, neuroleptics)

The type substance is chlorpromazine. Its trade name, Largactil®, conveniently indicates that it has a large number of actions. This is because the phenothiazine molecule with its dimethylaminopropyl side-chain (Fig.7.3) forms a multifaceted whole which can interact with many different types of receptor site. The major resultant effects are summarised in Table 7.6. This does not exhaust the possibilities. For example on some isolated preparations, chlorpromazine can antagonise 5-hydroxytryptamine and also, histamine (H_1) responses; however, it is obvious in this latter case, that it has one carbon atom too many in the side-chain to be generally effective (*see* 5.7). Further, it has a strong local anaesthetic action but is too painful when injected to be of use in this way; and it potentiates the effects of many centrally acting drugs (e.g. morphine p. 203). *See also* hypothermic effect, p. 189.

It is unusual for such a relatively non-selective drug to be so often prescribed. Tolerance develops within weeks to some side-effects, e.g. drowsiness, and others are relatively uncommon or treatable (but *see* tardive dyskinesia later), even when the medicament is taken over a number of years, as is necessary in schizophrenia (*acute* types with positive symptoms, e.g. delusions, hallucinations—p. 186—respond better to these drugs than *chronic* types with negative symptoms, e.g. loss of drive and emotional responsiveness).

The side-effect most commonly observed is *iatrogenic* parkinsonism but other extrapyramidal syndromes (e.g. akathisia, dystonic reactions) can occur. From Table 7.6, it can be seen that the incidence of

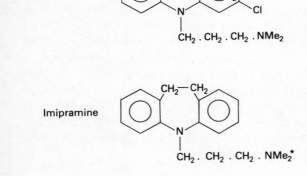

Chlorpromazine

Imipramine

Fig. 7.3 (*Above*) chlorpromazine—a (2-chloro substituted) phenothiazine ring with a dimethylaminopropyl side-chain. (*Below*) imipramine—a dibenzazepine. *Replacement of one methyl group by a hydrogen atom produces desmethylimipramine (desipramine). *Note*: carbamazepine (anti-epileptic) is a dibenzazepine derivative.

Table 7.6 Major actions of chlorpromazine

Receptor effect	Site	Action	Use	Possible side-effects
Dopamine blockade	Mesolimbic system	Antischizophrenic	Schizophrenia	
	Chemoreceptor trigger zone	Anti-emetic (except in motion sickness)	Vomiting (except in motion sickness)	
	Corpus striatum	*See* text	Huntington's chorea (7.2)	Parkinsonism Akathisia Tardive dyskinesia (*see* text)
	Hypothalamo-pituitary axis	Block of prolactin release inhibiting hormone		Galactorrhoea
		Block of gonadotrophin releasing hormone (*see* Fig. 14.7)		Menstrual irregularities
Acetylcholine (muscarinic) blockade				
central	Corpus striatum	Anti-parkinsonism		
peripheral	Autonomic nervous system			Dilated pupil Loss of accommodation Dry mouth
Noradrenaline				
central α-facilitation	Brainstem			Hypotension
peripheral α-blockade	Sympathetic nervous system			Hypotension
Other				Drowsiness Allergic cholestatic jaundice (13.9) Allergic rashes (18.8) Leucopenia (17.5) Cataract (18.4) Photosensitisation (Table 18.3)

parkinsonism depends upon the relative blockade by the major tranquilliser of dopamine and muscarinic receptors. In this connection Table 7.7 is illustrative. It shows the side-effects of different chemical groups of major tranquillisers. Those which have most antimuscarinic action produce least extrapyramidal (parkinsonism) symptoms and vice versa. Interactions of chlorpromazine with *noradrenergic* synapses are complicated. On the peripheral autonomic nervous system, it is clearly an α-blocker as it can produce adrenaline reversal (10.2). However, centrally, noradrenaline synaptic α-facilitation is another possible mechanism for the observed hypotension (10.4, Fig. 10.7).

Tardive dyskinesia consists of involuntary movements of the facial, tongue or limb muscles appearing tardily, i.e. after prolonged drug treatment. Stopping the major tranquilliser worsens the condition which seems to be an imbalance of the Huntington's chorea type, i.e. a *relative* dopamine hyperactivity in the corpus striatum (7.2). A simple explanation implicates receptor hypersensitivity in response to the postsynaptic block, but this is usually a short-term phenomenon and increased dopamine release (by a presynaptic mechanism) or increased receptor number may be involved in the longer term (*see* p. 93).

This introduces a further point. The antischizophrenic potency of, for example, the phenothiazines (but not a series of butyrophenones) correlates well with their ability to antagonise dopamine activation of brain adenylate cyclase, i.e. they can act by blocking D_1-dopamine (postsynaptic) receptors (*see* Table 6.4). However, all the major tranquillisers shown in Table 7.7 (except cis(α)-flupenthixol) show a good parallelism between antipsychotic effect and displacement of ^{3}H-haloperidol in brain homogenates. This indicates involvement of D_2-dopamine receptors—probably presynaptic but, possibly, those postsynaptic ones not linked to cyclic AMP. The exact sites of all these receptors are still speculative.

In addition to their use against psychoses, major tranquillisers are also employed in a number of other situations including the treatment of vomiting (13.4) and Huntington's chorea (7.2), and with morphine in terminal cancer cases (p. 203). For hypothermic action *see* p. 189.

7.5   Antidepressants (antidepressives)

Drugs which relieve depressive symptoms without inducing mental excitement or delirium (difference from psychotomimetic agents, 7.6), or fits (difference from convulsants, Table 9.3) are called antidepressants.

The original antidepressives—monoamine uptake blockers and MAO inhibitors—primarily (acutely) increase synaptic monoamine levels in the CNS (Table 7.8). This led to the hypothesis that depressive states were due to monoamine deficiencies. Such a view is now considered too facile for the following reasons:

Table 7.7 Major tranquillisers: relative incidence of common side-effects

Chemical class	Subgroup	Type substance	Side-effects			
			Antimuscarinic	Extrapyramidal	Hypotension	Drowsiness
Dibenzodiazepine		Clozapine	+++	+		
Diphenylbutylpiperidine		Pimozide	+++	+		±
Phenothiazine	Piperidinyl	Thioridazine	+++	+	++	++
	Dimethylaminopropyl	Chlorpromazine	++	++	++	+++
	Piperazinyl	Fluphenazine	+	+++	+	++
Butyrophenone		Haloperidol*	+	+++	+	+
Thioxanthene		Cis(α)-flupenthixol	+	+++		+

+++, above average; ++, average; +, below average; ±, slight.
* Also increases GABA release (important in the treatment of Huntington's chorea, 7.2)

Antidepressant drug actions
- in general correlate with the ability to increase synaptic noradrenaline and/or 5-HT *but not dopamine*
- take 2–4 weeks to commence whereas uptake block or MAO inhibition are rapid in onset
- *chronically* produce down regulation of β_1-adrenoceptors and/or 5-HT$_2$ receptors. Up regulation of α_2-(presynaptic) adrenoceptors and GABA$_B$ receptors have also been reported *inter alia*
- for the additional effect of sedation have been stated to be due to anti-histamine activity (particularly for the impramine-like group).

So, the antidepressive effect is probably related to *chronic* rather than acute changes. Therefore, therapeutically
- treat agitated patients with the more sedative drugs and withdrawn patients with the less sedative ones.
- encourage all to persist with treatment and ignore the immediate effects, e.g. antimuscarinic actions such as dry mouth, loss of accomodation and hesitancy of micturition, particularly with imipramine and amitriptyline
- consider electroconvulsive therapy in severe cases.

Imipramine
This drug (as shown in Fig. 7.3) is closely related to chlorpromazine chemically and in some animals can in fact act as a tranquilliser. When given to humans, its antidepressant effect usually takes 2–4 weeks to appear. During this period antimuscarinic block is often prominent (Table 7.8) which the patient must be encouraged to bear in the interest of subsequent antidepressive relief. Other side-effects are drowsiness and hypotension (the latter possibly centrally mediated by increased synaptic noradrenaline, *compare* chlorpromazine). An allergic cholestatic jaundice can occur. Combinations with monoamine oxidase inhibitors can result in mutual potentiation and are dangerous.

Poisoning is not uncommon and the lethal manifestations are
- CNS antimuscarinic effects (like atropine poisoning, p. 57): treat with eserine plus diazepam if there are associated convulsions
- cardiac dysrhythmias (due to peripheral potentiation of noradrenaline by prevention of uptake$_1$): give appropriate antidysrhythmic therapy.

The imipramine group are often designated 'tricyclic' antidepressants (i.e. having a structure possessing three rings). This is a poor term as many drugs have such structures, including anthracene purgatives (13.6) and chlorpromazine (Fig. 7.3). Even among antidepressants (Table 7.8) some 'bicyclics' (properly, '*di*cyclics') act mainly as uptake blockers (e.g. viloxazine); and some 'tetracyclics' mainly increase noradrenaline release (e.g. mianserin, possibly by presynaptic α_2-block,

Table 7.8 Potential antidepressives: primary effects on brain monoamine and acetylcholine (muscarinic) receptors, and sedative actions

	Release of			Uptake of			Breakdown of			Antimuscarinic side-effects	Sedative (hypnotic) action
	DA	NA	5-HT	DA	NA	5-HT	DA	NA	5-HT		
Amphetamine*	+++	+++		--	-		--	--	--		
Mianserin		++†								+	+++
Viloxazine					-					+	+
Imipramine					--	-				++	+
Desmethylimipramine					--	-				++	
Amitriptyline				-	--	-				+++	+++
Monoamine oxidase inhibitors											
phenelzine		+					--	--	--		
tranylcypromine		++					--	--	--		

DA, dopamine; NA, noradrenaline; 5-HT, 5-hydroxytryptamine.
Increases: +++, marked; ++, moderate; +, some. Decreases: ---, marked; --, moderate; -, some; 0, negligible.
* Not used because of its psychotic tendency (Table 7.9).
† Produces α-adrenoceptor block, presynaptically.

3.6). Other drugs overlapping such simple chemical and pharmacological classifications will doubtless be discovered in the future. This is further exemplified by the wide range of these effects possessed by amphetamine—which has *one* ring, Table 3.2.

Monoamine oxidase inhibitors

Monoamine oxidase (MAO) consists of at least two mitochondrial isoenzymes: MAO-A, selectively antagonised by clorgyline; and MAO-B, selectively inhibited by selegiline (p. 174). MAO-A is mainly concerned in the antidepressive action of MAO inhibitors. This is an interesting pharmacological group, though of limited significance therapeutically (*see* later). They are subdivisible into

1 *Reversible competitive antagonists* (e.g. amphetamine, ephedrine). They are sympathomimetic agents which can cross the blood–brain barrier and are not catabolised by MAO (Table 3.2). Nevertheless, they prevent its action and, together with the release of catecholamines (Table 7.8), this probably accounts for most of their (marked) central nervous system actions (*see* 9.4 for amphetamine).

2 *Irreversible antagonists.* This is the group usually referred to by the term 'monoamine oxidase inhibitors'. The type substance is phenelzine but (as can be seen from Table 7.8) it is also an indirectly acting sympathomimetic drug.

MAO inhibitors can cause the following adverse effects.

Blood pressure changes. There is a variety of these under different conditions, namely

1 *Hypotension* (a common side-effect; probably multifactorial in origin) possibly, like imipramine, by increased synaptic noradrenaline concentration centrally: peripheral hypotheses also exist, e.g. the formation of octopamine (Table 3.2) which acts as a false transmitter with only a weak agonist action.

2 *Hypertension*

a In the presence of uptake$_1$ blockers, e.g. imipramine.

b Due to an indirect sympathomimetic action (i.e. noradrenaline release) by

- the MAO inhibitor itself, e.g. tranylcypromine, (uncommon) phenelzine
- a food item which is normally destroyed by MAO in the gut wall and liver, e.g. tyramine in certain cheeses: uncommon with MAO-B inhibitors
- a storage blocker, e.g. reserpine, which usually results in increased presynaptic cytoplasmic noradrenaline which is rapidly inactivated by mitochondrial MAO (Fig. 3.1,e) but, in the presence of the MAO inhibitor, releases the transmitter.

Decreased liver function
- this may result in lessened metabolism and, therefore, greater systemic toxicity of, for example, pethidine which is normally partly N-demethylated by hepatic enzymes (Table 1.7)
- allergic hepatocellular jaundice can occur (13.9)

Additional side-effects on the central nervous system (particularly) and the gastrointestinal tract have resulted in MAO inhibition being used progressively less and less in the treatment of depressive states.

Finally, note that the actions of phenelzine can be increased in 'slow' acetylators (Table 20.3,2).

Lithium
This agent (used as the carbonate) is difficult to classify *simply*, because it is used both to calm manic patients and, prophylactically, as a mood-stabiliser in manic-depressive illnesses. The mechanism of action is unknown, but is likely to be related to the interruption of phosphatidyl inositol recycling shown in Fig. 4.8.

Like sodium, it is actively absorbed from the gut and passes into the extracellular fluid; it gradually enters the cells but, unlike sodium, it is not easily extruded so that, after about a week, it is distributed throughout the total body water. Plasma levels are then monitored as they are critical both for therapeutic effectiveness and to avoid central nervous system toxicity, which varies from tremor, muscular twitching and drowsiness in mild cases to convulsions or coma in frank overdose. At acceptable plasma concentrations nausea and diarrhoea are the commonest early side-effects. Nephrogenic diabetes insipidus due to inhibition of the specific adenylate cyclase necessary for antidiuretic hormone action (p. 310) can occur—presenting with polyuria and thirst; goitre (mainly due to decreased thyroid hormone synthesis, Fig. 14.2) is rare. Lithium ions can be teratogenic.

Lithium is eliminated via the kidney: it is reabsorbed mainly in the proximal tubule (like sodium) but not in the distal convoluted tubule (unlike sodium). Diuretics acting primarily on the distal tubules, e.g. thiazides, can cause compensatory increases in the proximal tubular reabsorption of sodium (and lithium) resulting in toxic effects. Conversely, in acute lithium poisoning give an i.v. NaCl infusion.

7.6   Psychotomimetic drugs: dependence
Amphetamine. This can induce a psychosis on repeated usage (Table 7.9); as also can cocaine and LSD (*see* below).

Lysergic acid (Ger:* *S*äure, acid) *Diethylamide* —*LSD. As with all psychotomimetic drugs*, the response varies with the individual and the

* Ger, German.

Table 7.9 Types of drug dependence

Type substance	Emotional dependence	Physical dependence	Tolerance (to central nervous system effects)	Cross-tolerance to	Reference(s)
Morphine	+ + +	+ + +	+ + +*	Other opioids	7.10
Barbiturate	+ + +	+ + + +	+ + +	Ethanol and other central depressants	
Ethanol	+ + +	+ +	+ +	Barbiturates and other central depressants (including general anaesthetics)	9.1
Diazepam	+ +	+ +	+†		Table 7.5, 9.1
Amphetamine	+ +	+‡,§	+		9.4
Cocaine	+ +	+‡,§	±		Table 8.2 (footnote)
Tobacco	+	±‡	+		2.5
Cannabis	+	±‡	+		7.6
Lysergic acid diethylamide	+	0§	+ + +		7.6

+ + + +, very strong; + + +, strong; + +, moderate; +, present; ±, slight; 0, absent.
* Except miosis (in human).
† Tolerance to the hypnotic and anticonvulsant actions develops more rapidly than tolerance to the anxiolytic effect.
‡ No characteristic withdrawal symptoms.
§ Psychoses can develop *during* chronic usage.

surroundings, but common psychological manifestations are
• hyperaesthesia (enhanced sensory perceptions)
• synaesthesia (transpositions of sensory perceptions, e.g. colours heard, sounds tasted)
• distortions of time or space
• illusions (incorrect interpretations of sensory data)
• delusions, hallucinations (mental images unrelated to external events)
• depersonalisation (sense of withdrawal, i.e. loss of personal participation in events which are being perceived)
• increased lability of mood (euphoric generally exceed depressive phases).

The majority of these effects appear to be related to diminished 5-hydroxytryptamine transmission brought about either by inhibition of release or by antagonism at receptor sites (LSD is closely related chemically to methysergide, which blocks $5HT_2$ receptors, Table 5.3).

However, other central transmitters may be involved. In addition there may be somatic manifestations, especially of skeletal muscle activity (incoordination, increased tone, weakness) and sympathetic activation (mydriasis, tachycardia, hypertension).

Cannabis (hashish, marijuana). The psychological effects can include similar changes to those occurring with LSD but there is a predilection for sedation ('dream-like states') rather than euphoria. Further, this mixture of compounds (of which tetrahydrocannabinol is the most psychoactive constituent) can produce a deficit in the stage of consolidation and transfer to long-term storage in mental processing (memory, 7.7). Present evidence implicates both 5-hydroxytryptaminergic and catecholaminergic mechanisms in these responses. Somatic effects include tachycardia, hypertension and a decrease in intraocular pressure. *See also* anti-emetic effect of nabilone (p. 317).

Unfortunately neither LSD nor tetrahydrocannabinol produces a reasonable model of a human psychosis but pharmacological analysis of their actions is providing some insight into psychoactive drug mechanisms.

Opium (morphine). Smoking of opium—as once practised extensively by the Chinese—results in very similar phenomena to those experienced with LSD, probably with an overall sedative element. Modern users of morphine or diamorphine by the intravenous route tend to obtain more of the euphoriant aspects of these drugs, thus accounting for their popularity as drugs of physical dependence. (For other actions *see* 7.11.)

Drug dependence

This may be defined as a state harmful to the individual, and (usually) also to society, resulting from the compulsive chronic intake of a drug. It can involve any combination of

- *emotional dependence*—if the agent is not taken psychological distress ensues
- *physical dependence*—abstinence produces somatic symptoms (termed a withdrawal syndrome)
- *tolerance* (*see also* p. 93)—lessened response to the same (repeated) dose necessitating greater and/or more frequent administration to produce the same (therapeutic) effect. It may be associated with either emotional or physical dependence but is not by itself an indicator of drug dependence, as it can be manifested in the absence of the latter (e.g. drowsiness with chlorpromazine, p. 178). It usually also applies to chemically related compounds but such cross-tolerance can be more widespread, as indicated in Table 7.9. Tolerance may be of two types (often mixed):

1   *Pharmacokinetic.* Here the effective concentration of the drug at the active site is decreased. For instance barbiturates, by inducing microsomal enzymes, can be metabolised faster; but excretion might be expedited in the tolerant individual (e.g. with cannabis).

2   *Pharmacodynamic.* Here the action is lessened. For example, chronic alcoholics do not metabolise ethanol *much* more rapidly than naïve subjects (9.2) yet they are capable of imbibing much greater quantities of alcoholic drinks before appearing inebriated.

Different spectra of these three phenomena are exemplified by the type substances shown in Table 7.9, which also indicates the reference section for each particular agent. Theories underlying dependence and pharmacodynamic tolerance are gradually emerging and are discussed in the relevant sections. *See also* Misuse of Drugs Regulations (21.6).

7.7   A note on memory

This involves a series of overlapping processes including initial sensory registration, cataloguing and placement in a short-term store, later consolidation by rehearsal and passage into a long-term store, and subsequent retrieval. These complicated procedures appear to be mediated via existent 'hard wiring' (e.g. sensory fibres, Papez's circuit: hippocampus–fornix–mammillary body), *de novo* 'soft wiring' producing new synaptic connections, and new formation of protein. The latter (under RNA control) is not only necessary for 'soft wiring' but also, within the neurones, for coded storage of information: it is prevented by inhibitors of protein synthesis.

Cholinergic transmission is considered necessary for early storage processes (6.2). Hyoscine produces retrograde amnesia (2.7) and atropine inhibits activation of Papez's circuit. A corollary has been attempts to enhance cholinergic functions (e.g. with anticholinesterases) in the treatment of Alzheimer's disease (a presenile dementia), so far without much success.

The catecholamines (particularly noradrenaline but possibly dopamine) and, probably, 5-hydroxytryptamine—via their brainstem connections—mainly affect attention and information analysis during the initial stages of sensory registration and short-term storage. They do not seem to be necessary for long-term memory. Benzodiazepines can produce amnesia (pre-operative medication, 8.6; use as hypnotics, 9.1). β-endorphins, vasopressin and GABA are currently being intensively investigated as endogenous substances involved in memory processing.

DRUGS AFFECTING BODY TEMPERATURE

In the warm-blooded animal there is a balance between heat production and heat elimination. Blood temperature and activation of hot or cold receptors in the skin are monitored by centres in the hypothalamus (anterior, particularly preoptic area, heat loss; posterior-lateral, heat gain). Through a series of interneurones (employing, as transmitters, catecholamines, 5-hydroxytryptamine and acetylcholine—probably varying with the species, and termed 'thermogenic amines' in this connection), these centres reciprocally engender the appropriate *acute* thermoregulatory mechanisms as follows. For heat loss, cutaneous vasodilation, sweating, panting; for heat gain, vasoconstriction in the skin, shivering, adrenal medullary secretion. More *chronic* temperature changes also induce longer-term metabolic effects mainly modulated via adrenal medullary (including heat production from brown adipose tissue) and thyroid hormones.

Some important drug effects and medical conditions associated with these categories are shown in Table 7.10. A *hypothermic* agent (e.g. chlorpromazine, by hypothalamic blockade of 'thermogenic amines' and/or vasodilation) renders the subject poikilothermic, i.e. it adopts the temperature of its surroundings. However, in the case of humans (particularly), this effect can only be achieved if compensatory mechanisms (such as sympathetic activation, shivering) are simultaneously blocked. Thus patients taking chlorpromazine are not normally affected. An *antipyretic* agent (e.g. aspirin), will only lower a pathologically raised temperature (*see* next section).

7.8   Antipyretic agents

Some ways by which endogenous pyrogens, e.g. interleukin-1 (p. 147) are generated and produce fever are shown in Fig. 7.4. However, a number of points are still tentative. For example, by what mechanisms do endogenous pyrogens (or substances released by them, e.g. interferon-γ, Table 19.7) produce prostaglandin-like autacoids, which of these latter are involved, and how do they interact with the 'thermogenic amines'? The fine details are irrelevant when considering the antipyretic properties of the non-steroidal anti-inflammatory agents which, by their blockade of cyclo-oxygenase would prevent the formation of *all* prostaglandins and thromboxanes.

The type substance of the non-steroidal anti-inflammatory drugs is acetylsalicylic acid (aspirin). Its properties relative to those of other similarly acting agents are shown in Table 7.11. It will be seen that there is a reasonable parallelism between prostaglandin cyclo-oxygenase inhibition and anti-inflammatory potency, but this does not extend to the antipyretic and analgesic actions. As the temperature-lowering effects are confined to pathologically induced fevers (exercise-produced pyrexias are not reduced), prostaglandin-like substances are probably mainly involved (Fig. 7.4) and one suggestion is that the stronger antipyretic agents—paracetamol, aspirin, mefenamic acid (Table 7.11)—produce this action by blocking the isoenzyme of prostaglandin cyclo-oxygenase *occurring in nervous tissue*. As these drugs are also the most useful general analgesics within this group, they might have a (?

Table 7.10 Clinical situations which produce changes in body temperature

Factor involved	Site involved	Increased temperature		Decreased temperature	
		Mechanism	Clinical situation(s)	Mechanism	Clinical situation(s)
Heat production	Peripheral	Stimulation of metabolism	Thyroxine overdose (14.3); aspirin poisoning (7.9)	Inhibition of metabolism	Myxoedematous coma (14.3)
		Increased muscular movement	Amphetamine overdose* (9.4); malignant hyperthermia (20.6)		
Heat balance	Central	Pyrogen production	Microbial infection	Prevention of pyrogen-producing prostaglandins Inhibition of central control	Antipyretic agent† (e.g. aspirin) Hypothermic agent*† (e.g. chlorpromazine)
Heat loss	Peripheral	Decreased sweating	Atropine poisoning‡ (Table 2.7)	Increased cutaneous vasodilation Increased sweating	Barbiturate overdose Acute ethanol poisoning (9.2) Morphine in febrile patient (p. 203)*

* Other factors may be involved.
† For distinction between antipyretic and hypothermic agents, *see* text.
‡ In this case, the decreased sweating has more effect than the concomitant peripheral vasodilation.

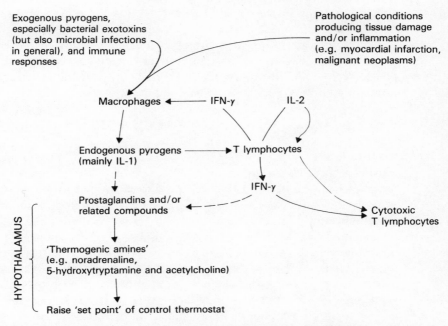

Fig. 7.4 The genesis of pyrogen-induced fever. Interrupted lines indicate actions produced *either* outside the blood–brain barrier (BBB) *or* by crossing into the brain at sites where the BBB is deficient. IL, interleukin. IFN-*γ*, interferon-*γ*, which has three actions on this diagram: it increases the release of IL-1 from macrophages, has a pyrogenic effect itself and activates cytotoxic T lymphocytes. *Lymphokines* are substances released from lymphocytes, e.g. interleukins, interferons: as they are often also released by other cells, a preferable, more general term is *cytokines*.

Table 7.11 Aspirin-like drugs: comparison of properties

	Relative potency as inhibitor of prostaglandin E_2 synthesis *in vitro*[*]	Action		
Type substance		Anti-inflammatory	Antipyretic	Analgesic[†]
Paracetamol (US: acetaminophen)	±	0	+	+
Aspirin	+	+	+	+
Mefenamic acid	+	+	+	+
Ibuprofen[‡]	+ +	+	±	±
Indomethacin	+ + +	+ +	±	±

+ + +, Very strong; + +, strong; +, moderate (satisfactory); ±, weak; 0, negligible.
* Using an isoenzyme prepared from a prostate gland extract.
† For definition of 'aspirin-like' analgesic action, *see* text.
‡ Type substance of the 'propionic acid derivatives'.

central) nervous system *pain-relieving* action in addition to their peripheral analgesic effect (*see* next section).

Antipyretic drugs, as such, are obsolete. The modern method is to attack the cause of the pyrexia; if this is infective, give chemotherapeutic agents. Should the temperature demand immediate reduction, physical measures, e.g. fans, ice-bags are used.

DRUGS AFFECTING PAIN MECHANISMS

7.9   'Aspirin-like' analgesia

Pain is a cardinal symptom in the practice of medicine, alerting the patient to seek advice and a valuable aid to the doctor in diagnosis. As soon as the latter has been achieved, the production of analgesia is paramount and can be brought about by one or more of the various means shown in Table 7.12. The salient differences between aspirin and morphine when used as analgesic drugs are shown in Table 7.13. To reiterate, when aspirin-like substances are used as anti-inflammatory agents, they relieve pain by their local inhibition of prostaglandin synthesis. However, when they act as general analgesics (e.g. in headache, migraine, neuralgia), an additional nervous system action—possibly central—appears to be involved. Their particular niche (as indicated in Table 7.13) is in mild-to-moderate pain without much psychological distress.

Toxicity

For distinction between side-effects and overdose, *see* 20.1.

Aspirin

In recommended analgesic dosage (see current British National Formulary).

1   *Gastric irritation.* This is multifactorial in origin due, in part, to ion-trapping (*see* Fig. 1.3) combined with inhibition of prostaglandin synthesis. Any bleeding is intensified by diminished platelet aggregation (17.3). The so-called 'soluble' aspirins are certainly solutions at about neutral pH, i.e. when dissolved in water by the patient, but precipitate a considerable proportion of the drug (albeit in a finer form) in the acid milieu of the stomach. Buffering, at its simplest by taking the tablets with milk, reduces ion-trapping by lessening gastric absorption.

2   *Hypersensitivity reactions* (p. 435) often consist of inoffensive responses (e.g. watering of the eyes and nose, mild rashes) but sometimes may be life-threatening, e.g. bronchoconstriction in the asthmatic. Many of these cases are not allergic. An intriguing suggestion is that (in such patients) blockade by aspirin of cyclo-oxygenase may encourage lipoxygenase activity resulting in leukotriene formation (Fig. 5.6) with consequent bronchoconstriction (Fig. 11.1). An interesting

Table 7.12 Methods available for the relief of pain (excluding hypnosis)

Method	Surgical example	Medical examples
Remove cause	Excision of diseased organ (e.g. appendix)	Glyceryl trinitrate in angina pectoris (10.10) Ergotamine in migraine (10.6)
Prevent perception of pain occurring naturally	Cut afferent nerves or tracts	'Aspirin-like' analgesics (7.9) 'Morphine-like' analgesics* (7.10–7.13) Local anaesthetics (8.1)
during operation or manipulation		Local anaesthetics (8.1) General anaesthetics (8.6)

* For acupuncture, *see* Fig. 7.5.

recent finding is that aspirin-like drugs can release oxygen free radicals (p. 29) from the platelets of sensitive individuals.

3 *Reye's syndrome*, an acute encephalopathy associated with changes in hepatic fatty acid oxidation, is *rare* but can occur in feverish children given aspirin. For this reason it is recommended that aspirin should not be given to the 'under twelves' unless there is a very special indication.

Table 7.13 Comparison between aspirin and morphine as analgesic agents

	Aspirin	Morphine
Analgesic action		
Site(s)	Peripheral tissue and nervous system (? central)	Central nervous system
Associated effects	Anti-inflammatory	Mental detachment Relief of anxiety Euphoria Drowsiness

Suitability	Pain
	  mild/moderate
	  superficial
	  discontinuous
		Pain
		  severe
		  deep
		  continuous
		  with
		  psychological
		  overlay

Disadvantages		
Physical dependence	Negligible	Marked
Tolerance	Negligible	Marked
Respiratory centre	Stimulation (only in toxic concentrations)	Depression
Nausea and vomiting	Only in high therapeutic dosage (salicylism)	Marked (*see* p. 202)
Constipation	Absent	Marked
Others	*See* 7.9	*See* Table 7.15

In high therapeutic dosage (e.g. anti-inflammatory use). The syndrome here is referred to as *salicylism* and consists of headache, nausea and vomiting, tinnitus—a useful diagnostic symptom—and hypopro-thrombinaemia (during prolonged therapy).

In overdose. This causes gross acid–base imbalances in which alkalosis usually precedes acidosis.

1 *Alkalosis* is due to activation of respiratory centres either directly, reflexly via arterial chemoreceptors or indirectly. In the latter case, *uncoupling of oxidative phosphorylation* by high concentrations of salicylates produces a deficiency of high-energy phosphate bonds. In an attempt to overcome this, there is increased metabolism with a consequent rise in plasma PCO_2 which stimulates respiration. Associated phenomena include precipitation of alkalotic tetany (16.4), hyperpyrexia (Table 7.10), and excretion of an alkaline urine. The latter is particularly unfortunate in view of the subsequent acidosis (usually significant after an hour or two).

2 *Acidosis.* High drug concentrations cause this by
• depression of the respiratory centres (respiratory acidosis)
• *block of the tricarboxylic acid cycle* (particularly malic and isocitric dehydrogenases) resulting in a ketosis and dehydration like that encountered in diabetic ketoacidosis (metabolic acidosis)
• excessive salicylic acid (the major metabolite of aspirin) in the blood.

Subsequent phenomena include coma and cardiovascular failure which further exacerbate the situation. As there is no specific antagonist to these multifarious actions of aspirin, treatment is largely symptomatic, empirical and *extremely difficult*. Don't forget to produce an alkaline diuresis (pp. 12, 313).

Aspirin-like drugs
These can cause gastric irritation and intestinal upsets if they significantly inhibit prostaglandin cyclo-oxygenase in the alimentary tract; they are least common with paracetamol. All can produce hypersensitivity reactions, particularly rashes. To particularise:

Indomethacin is indicated in rheumatic illnesses and gout (p. 311). It can cause headache and dizziness along with gastrointestinal upsets and hypersensitivity reactions but has a very low incidence of blood dyscrasias. It is excreted in the milk (15.5).

Ibuprofen has similar side-effects. Used in milder rheumatic conditions. The chemically related *naproxen* (both are propionic acid derivatives) is rather more potent.

Paracetamol is often used as a mild-to-moderate analgesic in place of aspirin. It has the advantage of less gastric irritation but can still cause hypersensitivity reactions. In overdose the effects are completely different to those of aspirin and centre round the hepatic metabolism of the drug (*see* p. 26).

Mefenamic acid has not replaced paracetamol as the main analgesic alternative to aspirin. Its most serious side-effects, demanding cessation of treatment, are diarrhoea or haemolytic anaemia. In overdose it can produce epileptiform fits.

Analgesic nephropathy is a renal papillary necrosis occurring in patients who have been steadily consuming mild-to-moderate analgesics over many years—often legitimately, but sometimes due to a psychological dependence. Most commonly, a preparation containing a *mixture* of such substances has been involved so that it is extremely difficult to pin-point the causative agent. Animal experiments have implicated many of the common analgesics but must be accepted with reserve because of the high doses of drug used. The lesson is that such analgesics must not be given to patients for prolonged periods without repeated checks of renal function.

Aspirin—final notes

Pharmacokinetics (oral administration)

Absorption is mainly as the intact drug in the small intestine (1.1).

Plasma content is chiefly in the form of sodium salicylate (due to deacetylation *either* by acetylation of prostaglandin cyclo-oxygenase—*see* footnote to Table 5.10—*or* by hydrolysis in the blood and liver). Sodium salicylate is usually heavily (*c.* 85%) protein bound but this value can fall to 50% with high concentrations.

Excretion (human). Normally, 75% salicyluric acid (produced by conjugation of salicylic acid with glycine), 15% salicylglucuronic acid, either on the phenol or .COOH group, and 10% free salicylate. In poisoning, alkalinisation of the urine expedites removal mainly as free salicylate (Fig. 1.5).

Pharmacodynamics

Uses
- analgesic—moderate dose
- anti-aggregatory (antithrombotic)—low dose
- anti-inflammatory—high dose.

Contraindications
- peptic ulcer
- hypersensitive patients: particular care with asthmatics
- gout: high concentrations of aspirin have a uricosuric action (*see* Fig. 12.6) and were once used, but they are now interdicted because they interfere with the effects of modern uricosuric agents
- patients on warfarin therapy (*see* Table 17.2).

7.10   'Morphine-like' analgesia
The physiological background is depicted in Fig. 7.5 where the classical trineuronal pain pathway is shown, namely
1   Peripheral receptors—via Aδ and C fibres, p. 207—to substantia gelatinosa in the posterior horn of the spinal cord.
2   Passage to the opposite side and ascent via the lateral spinothalamic tract and medial lemniscus to the ventroposterolateral nucleus of the thalamus.
3   From the thalamus to sensorimotor and frontal cortices.

The pathway can be inhibited by intermediate neurones in the spinal cord (possibly liberating enkephalins) which, by a presynaptic action, prevent the release of the primary neurone transmitters. These intermediate neurones can be *activated* by either
a   increased general sensory input (*see* substance P, 6.5) or
b   (from the periaqueductal grey matter and nucleus reticularis paragigantocellularis) generated impulses in monoaminergic neurones (originating in the nucleus raphe magnus, liberating 5-HT and, possibly, from the locus caeruleus releasing noradrenaline) which descend from the raphe nuclei.

Morphine is considered to:
- relieve pain directly
I   by acting as an enkephalin agonist (p. 167) presynaptically on the primary nociceptive neurones
II   by increasing descending antinociceptive mechanisms. This effect is achieved
a   at the periaqueductal grey matter via μ-opiate receptors;
b   at the nucleus reticularis paragigantocellularis
- Produce euphoria
III   by acting on μ-opiate receptors in the amygdala. This and associated areas in the limbic system are probably involved in the mental detachment/anxiety relief characteristic of morphine (Table 7.15).

Opiate receptors
Opium has a long history as an analgesic and euphoriant. These effects are almostly entirely due to its morphine content and the specific receptors involved are legitimately termed 'opiate'. Nowadays, the term has been broadened to include a variety of sites at which other congeners of morphine may act more selectively. Four types of opiate

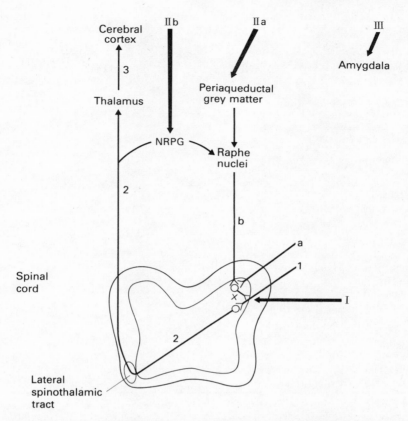

Fig. 7.5 Sites of analgesia and euphoria produced by morphine (schematic). 1, 2, 3, main nociceptive pathway; a, b, main inhibitory pathways; X, inhibitory (?enkephalinergic) neurone; I, IIa, IIb, III major sites of morphine action. NRPG, *n*ucleus *r*eticularis *p*aragigantocellularis. Acupuncture may be analgesic by stimulation of a or b pathways, either directly or by the release of endogenous opioids.

receptor were originally defined (*see* footnote to Table 4.3). Sigma-opiates act particularly on the NMDA receptor ion channel (p. 165).

A comparison of the properties of μ, δ and κ receptors is given in Table 7.14. To summarise (in alphabetical order)

δ These bind enkephalins *selectively* but also endorphins.

κ These bind dynorphins *selectively*. They produce a central analgesia by a different receptor to that for morphine (*see* Table 7.15): the type substance for this particular effect is pentazocine.

μ These bind endorphins better than dynorphins or enkephalins. It is the *typical morphine receptor* specifically producing central analgesia and euphoria (Fig. 7.5).

Drugs which interact with opiate receptors are termed 'opioids' and are divisible into agonists, mixed agonists/antagonists (partial agonists), and antagonists (*see* 7.12).

Table 7.14 A comparison of μ, δ and κ-opioid receptors

	μ	δ	κ
Selective agonist*	DAGO†	DSLET‡	U 50488
Selective antagonist*	Naloxone	ICI 174864	Norbinaltorphimine
Presence in peripheral organs			
guinea-pig ileum	$+++$	0	$+$
mouse vas deferens	$+$	$+++$	0
rabbit vas deferens	0	0	$+++$
Mechanism of action			
peripherally	Decreased transmitter release		
ion channels affected§	K^+	K^+/Ca^{2+}	Ca^{2+}
coupling mechanism	All via G-proteins (not via PtdIP$_2$ hydrolysis)		
inhibition of			
adenylate			
cyclase (Fig. 4.6)	$+$	$+++$	
Responses to			
naturally occurring compounds			
β-endorphins	$+++$	$+++$	$+$
enkephalins (met/leu)	$+$	$+++$(leu)	0
dynorphins	$++$	$+$	$+++$
drugs			
morphine	$+++$	$+$	0
pethidine	$+++$	$+$	0
etorphine	$- +++$	$++$	$\pm$
pentazocine	¶	¶	$+++$
naloxone	$---$	$--$	$--$

Presence, mechanism and responses (major ones italicised): (positive) $+++$, major; $++$, intermediate; $+$, minor; $\pm$, slight; (negative) $---$, major inhibitory; $--$, less inhibitory; ? possible.
* Guide–list only: even more specific ligands are constantly being discovered.
† [D-ala^2-methyl-phe^4-glyol^5] enkephalin.
‡ D-ser-(leu)enkephalin-threonine^6.
¶ Partial agonist at μ- and δ-receptors.
§ Major ionic conductance changes: increase in gK$^+$ pre-and postsynaptically; decrease in gCa^{+2}.

Morphine tolerance and withdrawal syndrome

There have been several unitary hypotheses to explain these pheno-mena, e.g. the effect on noradrenaline release described in the first edition of this textbook (this does explain the use of clonidine to lessen withdrawal symptoms). However, it appears unlikely that a single process is involved: rather there are a series of adaptive events (affecting transmitter release, action on receptor(s) and coupling mechanisms) which diminish the response during tolerance and manifest themselves as exaggerated effects when morphine is withdrawn.

7.11 Pharmacology of morphine

Pharmacokinetics

Absorption from the gut is relatively slow (possibly due to drug-induced gastroduodenal stasis) but adequate for maintenance dosage in the terminal cancer patient. For a rapid effect the drug is administered s.c. or i.m., except in peripheral circulatory failure, where i.v. injection is indicated (1.1).

Plasma concentrations are not very high due to rapid passage into the tissues. Less than half is protein bound (mainly to globulins). Only relatively small amounts cross the blood–brain barrier but they produce very significant central nervous system actions.

Excretion. Mainly as glycuronides or ethereal sulphates on the phenolic (3-position) or alcoholic (6-position) hydroxyl groups: less in the N-demethylated form and/or as the free drug.

Pharmacodynamics
The actions of morphine are collated in Table 7.15; together with their respective uses and disadvantages. Tolerance probably occurs to all effects, to varying degrees—least to miosis and constipation which are prominent in the addict.

Central nervous system actions
1 *Analgesia* with its associated phenomena of mental detachment and euphoria is cardinal, hence its employment in
• severe pain of short duration, e.g. road traffic accident
• severe pain of longer duration in the terminal cancer patient: here physical dependence is not a limiting factor and tolerance is much less than in the addict *provided that pain is never allowed to recur* (this is achieved by regular, adequate dosage)
• relief of anxiety, e.g. haematemesis, myocardial infarction (in addition to analgesia; also, depression of sympathetic activity decreases cardiac work), e.g. preoperatively (formerly, *see* 8.6).
Conversely, euphoria results in the dependence liability. Uncommonly dysphoria occurs.
2 *Sleep* (or at least drowsiness) is a noteworthy concomitant of morphine administration: it can be advantageous (e.g. postoperatively) but may be a nuisance if the cooperation of the patient is desirable.
3 *Respiratory depression*—particularly a decreased response to PCO_2 in the arterial blood—occurs with even the lowest analgesic doses of morphine. This demands care in situations of breathing insufficiency but, paradoxically, has an adjuvant beneficial effect in left ventricular failure (paroxysmal nocturnal dyspnoea) where the respiratory centres are overreacting to the afferent impulses from the congested alveoli.
4 *Antitussive.* Suppression of a cough is valuable if there is not much phlegm to be expectorated, i.e. the cough is unproductive and is merely keeping the patient awake by its annoyance, as in bronchial carcinoma. Fortunately, this action—unlike others—is not only produced by L-morphine but also by its D-isomer, so that specific cough suppressants

Table 7.15 The actions in humans of morphine (with pros and cons) compared with those of pethidine and pentazocine

Site and effect	Morphine	Uses	Disadvantages	Pethidine (US: meperidine; Europe: Demerol®)	Pentazocine
Central nervous system					
Brain					
Psyche					
mental detachment/anxiety relief	++++	Haematemesis		+++	+
hallucinations		Heart failure			+
Amygdala					
euphoria	+++ (μ)	Treatment of severe pain (*see text*)	Physical dependence	+++ (μ)	+
Periaqueductal grey matter and NRPG* (Fig. 7.5): analgesia	++++ (μ)			+++ (μ)	++ (κ)
Oculomotor nucleus pupil constriction	++	Recognition of addict	Loss of localising sign in head injury	0; (−, dilation, in overdose)	
Sleep/awake mechanisms (9.1) drowsiness	+++	Postoperative medication	(*See text*)	+	+
Respiratory centres	− − −	Left ventricular failure	Care in, for example, bronchial asthma, chronic bronchitis	− −	− −
Cough centre†	− −	Suppression of unproductive cough	Postanaesthetic precipitation of pneumonias	0	
Chemoreceptor trigger zone of vomiting centre	+++		Postoperative rupture of stitches: fluid and electrolyte imbalances	+++	++
Vasomotor centre (high doses only)	− −			− −	

		Treatment of severe pain (*see* text)				
Spinal cord analgesia	++++			+++	++	++
Smooth muscle						
Gut motility: constipation peristalsis	––	Antidiarrhoeal	In myocardial infarction (straining at stool)	±		
contraction (including sphincters)	++					
Sphincter of Oddi contraction	++		Biliary (spasm intensified)	+		
Bladder contraction (including sphincter vesicae)	+			0		
Uterus				*See* text		
Bronchioles	+		Care in bronchial asthma	0		
Vascular	–	Heart failure	In head injury—vasodilation can give increased bleeding. In myocardial infarction hypotension intensified (use diamorphine, p. 204)	–		
Other						
Histamine release	++			++ but also antihistamine		
Sweating	++					

Excitation or action: ++++, very marked; +++, marked; ++, present; +, slight; ±, variable; 0, negligible.
Depression: – – –, marked; – –, present; –, slight.
μ, κ indicate opiate receptors (*see* 7.10).
* Nucleus reticularis paragigantocellularis.
† *See Note* in text.

without the disadvantageous central nervous system effects of morphine (e.g. *dextro*methorphan) are available. However, morphine given postoperatively may inhibit coughing, which is necessary in the bedridden patient to clear the airways and prevent hypostatic pneumonia.

Note. Inhalation of a nebulised solution of citric acid by unanaesthetised guinea-pigs induces coughing which can be prevented by pretreatment not only with morphine or codeine but also with a polar enkephalin analogue which does not cross the blood–brain barrier. Conversely, all these preventive effects can be antagonised by the quaternary compound, N-methylnalorphine. These observations suggest a peripheral site of antitussive action in this experimental situation.

5 *Nausea and vomiting* are common after morphine. The vomiting centre is activated via the chemoreceptor trigger zone, *see* p. 315. Although tolerance rapidly (within a week) develops to this effect, in terminal cancer patients an anti-emetic (e.g. chlorpromazine), is often added initially.

Smooth muscle effects

1 *Gastrointestinal* (*see* enkephalins, dynorphins, p. 167). Prevention of acetylcholine release inhibits peristalsis but morphine also increases tone in gut wall and sphincters so that, paradoxically, its stimulant action results in constipation. Other factors are involved—slower passage of gut contents allowing greater water absorption so that faeces become scybalous which, allied to anal sphincter spasm and disregard of the 'call to defaecation', lessens bowel motions. It is possible to achieve a lowering of gut propulsion without significant central effects, for example with codeine which is accordingly useful in the treatment of diarrhoea.

2 *Sphincter of Oddi* contraction raises intrabiliary pressure and may even precipitate colic.

3 *Urinary bladder.* Spasm of the detrusor muscle produces a desire to pass water, but sphincter closure and inattention to the 'call to micturate' usually result in retention of urine.

4 *Bronchial tree.* Although high concentrations of morphine can induce constriction in animal preparations, in asthmatic patients the main respiratory dangers of the drug are due to its central respiratory depression and possible peripheral release of histamine.

Other actions

1 *Histamine release* may account for the fact that itch (often mediated via histamine, p. 148) is the one type of pain/irritation which is not invariably relieved by morphine. It may also manifest itself as a triple response around the site of drug injection. More serious sequelae are bronchoconstriction (*see* above) and hypotension (*see* below).

2 *Cardiovascular actions.* Generally these are not prominent but they may become important under particular circumstances. Essentially there is vasodilation—which is inadvisable in conditions of cerebral bleeding such as head injury—brought about by a combination of direct peripheral effect, histamine release and central vasomotor depression. This effect may be valuable in heart failure, where the venodilation relieves the preload (and therefore work) of the heart.

3 *Body temperature.* Morphine has an antipyretic action due to peripheral sweating (? plus vasodilation) and (possibly) central adjustment of the hypothalamic thermostat.

Species differences
In many animals morphine produces excitement (usually accompanied by mydriasis instead of miosis) rather than drowsiness. Thus, in domestic creatures, e.g. cats, horses, cattle, sheep, pigs and goats, morphine is often not a suitable strong analgesic agent and veterinarians prefer etorphine (*see* later). Marked tolerance to the gastrointestinal effects of morphine has been reported in animal tissues (other than human).

7.12 Opioids
A major aim has been to separate the unique analgesic (or other useful) actions from the disadvantages, as stated in Tables 7.13 and 7.15. Possibilities include

• simultaneous administration of non-opioids, e.g. chlorpromazine, in terminal cancer patients. The rationale is to potentiate the analgesia (usually would increase the opioid dose nowadays) and to prevent nausea and vomiting (rarely a problem after the first week anyway): use declining

• simultaneous use of opioid antagonists. This has not been successful so far because the analgesic action has also been antagonised

• administration of enkephalins or endorphins: not yet applied. However, an inhibitor of enkephalinase A (a dipeptidylcarboxypeptidase which breaks down enkephalins, Fig. 6.4) namely thiorphan, has been shown to produce analgesia in animals

• the use of other opioid compounds. All these can be modelled in a form similar to that of the 'backbone' of the morphine molecule. The drugs to be discussed are shown in Table 7.16.

Agonists
Diamorphine (US: diacetylmorphine; heroin). The present view regards this as a pro-drug of morphine. In the body, heroin is converted (within minutes) to monoacetylmorphine, MAM, and then (more slowly) to morphine. Its major advantage is that protection of the two hydroxyl groups of the parent compound by acetylation allows more rapid

Table 7.16   Representative opioids

Subgroup	Agonists		Mixed agonists/ antagonists	Antagonists
	strong	moderate		
Morphine variants	Diamorphine	Codeine	Nalorphine	Naloxone
Oripavine series	Etorphine		Buprenorphine	Diprenorphine
Benzomorphan			Pentazocine	
Pethidine (US: meperidine) series	Pethidine Fentanyl*			
Methadone series	Methadone	Dextropropoxyphene (US: propoxyphene)		

* Used in neuroleptanalgesia, *see* 8.6.

penetration into the CNS, accompanied by lessened 'peripheral' side-effects, e.g. nausea and vomiting, constipation, vasodilation. Clinically, heroin is used parenterally in the treatment of severe pain short-term, e.g. in myocardial infarction, and in the terminal cancer patient. Among i.v. users the progression is often from morphine to heroin because the latter gives a more rapid 'high' with less constipation.

Codeine. This differs from morphine only in that the phenolic (3-) hydroxyl group is methylated. This confers two advantages: lessened dependence liability and decreased hepatic inactivation. Therefore, the drug is effective orally as a valuable antitussive and antidiarrhoeal agent. It has, however, one major disadvantage, namely, less affinity for opiate receptors. It is thus an analgesic in the aspirin range (suitable in mild-to-moderate pain). In humans, 10% is reported to be converted to morphine and it is considered to have 10% of the analgesic potency of the latter—might this be the key to its analgesic effect?

Etorphine (Immobilon®) is an extremely potent opioid which appears to have no significant advantages over the parent drug for *human* use. It is employed extensively—as its trade name suggests—to immobilise animals where, compared to morphine, it does not produce excitant actions in, for example, cats and horses, and where it is 10^3–10^4 times more potent. The antidote is diprenorphine (Revivon®).

Pethidine (Europe: Demerol®; US: meperidine). This has many similar effects to morphine (Table 7.15), along with some antimuscarinic (e.g. dilation of pupil in overdose) and anti-(H_1) histamine actions (especially in isolated tissue preparations). These two latter actions indicate an antispasmodic element which would be valuable in intestinal, biliary or renal colic and in bronchial asthma. As seen from Table 7.15, this may be justified in the urinary and bronchial tracts. However, the main use of pethidine is as an analgesic with little hypnotic effect. In this connection it is used in childbirth but care must be taken on two counts:

1 If given too early (before 6 cm dilation), it tends to relax the cervix uteri and delay labour.

2 Like morphine, it crosses the placental barrier and depresses the fetal respiratory centres; this is readily reversible with naloxone.

Pharmacokinetically, pethidine is interesting in that:

1 Most is N-demethylated in the liver. Thus, its actions and toxicity, e.g. respiratory depression and (unexpectedly) convulsions, are potentiated by hepatic depressants such as monoamine oxidase inhibitors.

2 a smaller amount is excreted unchanged and, as this drug is a base, elimination is aided by acidification of the urine (1.1).

Methadone is roughly equianalgesic with morphine but produces less euphoria and drowsiness. However, it has a much longer half-life (average, 18–24 hours compared with 3 hours) so that withdrawal symptoms are slower in development and more protracted, *but less severe*. For this reason a daily *oral* (reducing dependence also on the syringe and needle) dose can be used to 'cover' morphine or diamorphine withdrawal. Related drugs are

• *Dextropropoxyphene*, a weaker analgesic often combined with paracetamol (e.g. in Co-Proxamol)

• *Dipipanone*, now the most common opioid drug of physical dependence after morphine/heroin.

Mixed agonists/antagonists
These produce different effects on different opiate receptors.

Nalorphine. Conversion of the N-methyl group of morphine to N-allyl produced this compound. Animal tests showed that it was an antagonist of morphine but, given by itself, acted as a weak agonist. Yet, when administered to dying patients with pain it was a reasonably effective analgesic. This is a classic example of a drug acting differently in the clinical compared with the experimental situation (21.2). Unfortunately it produced psychotomimetic effects, particularly hallucinations, and is never used as an analgesic.

Pentazocine. Although pure morphine was isolated in the early 1800s, its synthesis was only achieved about 150 years later. Round this time, chemists produced many intermediate compounds—pentazocine (a benzomorphan) was a derivative of one of these. Initially, it appeared that the separation of potent analgesic action from physical dependence liability had at last been achieved. The drug is effective orally and this, together with the facts that s.c. or i.m. injection is irritant and that it can produce withdrawal symptoms in morphine addicts (it is a partial agonist at μ-receptors, Table 7.14), lessened the inclination to explore its possibilities illegally. Its properties are shown in Table 7.15. Overall it is less potent than morphine as an analgesic (acts via κ-receptors) and can sometimes produce visual and auditory hallucinations. It is used (commonly orally) for moderate-to-severe pain, when sedation is not required. Physical dependence can be produced by repeated parenteral use, albeit much less commonly and much less severely than with morphine. In humans, unlike morphine, it produces hypertension: avoid in myocardial infarction.

Buprenorphine is unusual because its mixed action is exerted on the *same* receptors. It has an analgesic action via μ-receptors, which becomes less at higher concentrations as the antagonist properties predominate, so that then it can precipitate withdrawal symptoms in morphine addicts. Due to tight binding to the μ-receptors, its effects are only partially reversible with naloxone. It is given sublingually or parenterally, is largely metabolised in the liver and is longer-lasting than morphine.

Antagonists
Naloxone has negligible agonist activity. It is a much more potent antagonist at the μ-compared with the κ- or δ- opiate receptors. Major uses are in opioid poisoning and in the determination of endorphin and opioid effects experimentally. However, it can antagonise certain central actions of some non-opioid drugs and transmitters, which either raises doubts as to its selective usage or indicates that some opioid drugs act via other transmitters. *Naltrexone* is similar.

Diprenorphine is used to antagonise etorphine effects in veterinary practice.

7.13 Uses of opioids
- *analgesia*: the primary indication (*see* Table 7.15)
- *anxiety relief*: an important use, e.g. in haematemesis
- *left ventricular failure* (paroxysmal nocturnal dyspnoea): morphine has three beneficial effects: relief of anxiety, lessened cardiac work due to venodilation, and decreased respiratory centre response to alveolar congestion
- *antitussive* in unproductive cough (p. 294)
- *antidiarrhoeal* (codeine is often used, 13.7).

8 Membrane Stabilisers and Labilisers

It is important to appreciate that the terms stabilisation and labilisation refer to changes in *electrical* (ionic) movements across the membrane. As an analogy, consider a slice of Gruyère cheese with the holes going right through and representing ionic channels; melting it to make a Welsh rarebit would result in closure of ion channels, i.e. electrical stabilisation, even though the 'membrane' had been made more fluid, i.e. mechanically labilised. This, however, would be an irreversible change. Representative substances which have major, usually reversible, actions in this connection are shown in Table 8.1. The most important medical agents in this chapter are local and general anaesthetics; their particular indications as analgesics can be seen in Table 7.12. Additionally, some local anaesthetics are employed in antidysrhythmic therapy (10.13).

8.1 Local anaesthetic drugs

These are used clinically by the routes indicated in Table 8.2 (one suitable experimental test for each type is given). They produce their analgesic effect either
- by depression of pain-sensitive nerve terminals (surface and infiltration types) or
- by blockade of primary afferent algesic neurones (other types). *The site of action is the axon membrane.* Conduction in the C fibres (along their whole length as they are non-myelinated) and in the A-δ fibres (at

Table 8.1 Membrane stabilisers and labilisers

Membrane stabilisers	Membrane labilisers
Local anaesthetics Tetrodotoxin*†, saxitoxin*†	*Veratrum* alkaloids* Batrachotoxin*† α-Scorpion (and sea anemone) toxins*†
Increase in external concentration of calcium ions* General anaesthetics (8.6)	Decrease in external concentration of calcium ions*

* Only useful experimentally († including sodium channel isolation and characterisation).

Table 8.2 Common types of local anaesthesia

Route and site of administration	Type of local anaesthesia produced	Pharmacological test		Numeration (see Table 8.3)	Dangers
		Drug application	Test applied		
Topical application to external or mucous surface	Surface	Into conjunctival sac	Corneal reflex	1	Contact dermatitis (18.8)
Subcutaneous injection round nerve terminals	Infiltration*	As intradermal wheal	Painful stimulus (e.g. pin-prick)	2	Entry into blood vessel with systemic toxicity (see under lignocaine, p. 280)
Deeper injection round nerve trunk	Conduction*	To fluid bathing frog sciatic nerve preparation	Transmission of nerve impulse	3	
Via lumbar puncture into the cerebrospinal fluid in the subarachnoid space (intrathecal)	Spinal	Into lumbar cerebrospinal fluid	Flexor reflex (leg)	4	Cauda equina damage; hypotension†; respiratory depression†
Via a sacral foramen into the epidural space	Caudal	Into sacral epidural space	Flexor reflex (leg)	5	Puncture of blood vessel in epidural space

* Usually with a vasoconstrictor (e.g. adrenaline, 1:80 000–1:200 000) to localise (see text): use felypressin (p. 139) if adrenaline contraindicated, e.g. in patients taking imipramine-like antidepressants.

† Given to patient sitting up. Too forceful injection or patient subsequently lying down can result in progressive ascending block of efferent nerves as they cross the subarachnoid space: sympathetic, preganglionic lumbothoracic leading to hypotension; somatic, resulting in loss of respiration as follows—thoracic (chest wall), cervical 3, 4 and 5 (diaphragmatic).

A note on cocaine. This is sometimes applied topically, e.g. to the eye (18.2). It is an atypical local anaesthetic because of the dependence liability (Table 7.9) and the sympathomimetic effects (due to uptake, block) which produce vasoconstriction and overall cardiac excitation rather than an antidysrhythmic action. It can produce hypersensitivity reactions—which have been fatal.

Table 8.3 Local anaesthetic structures and ionisation

Drug	Use (from Table 8.2)	Hydrophobic end pK_a*	Connecting chain ester; or amide (italicised)	Hydrophilic end pK_a*	Status at body pH (7.4)
Procaine	†	H_2N— ⬡ — 2.5	$CO.O.CH_2CH_2$—N(Ethyl)(Ethyl) 9.0		Charged≫uncharged
Benzocaine (US: ethyl aminobenzoate)	1	H_2N— ⬡ — 2.5	$CO.O.CH_2CH_3$		Uncharged (*see* text)
Lignocaine (US: lidocaine)	1–5	⬡(CH₃)(CH₃)	*NH.CO*—CH_2—N(Ethyl)(Ethyl)	8.0	Charged>uncharged
Prilocaine	2–5	⬡(CH₃)(CH₃)	*NH.CO*—CH(CH₃)—N(H)(Propyl)	8.0	Charged>uncharged
Bupivacaine	5‡	⬡(CH₃)(CH₃)	*NH.CO*—(piperidine, N—Butyl)	7.5	Charged just> uncharged

* pK_a values to nearest 0.5 unit.
† Rarely used clinically.
‡ Long duration but slow onset.

their nodes of Ranvier), which subserve slow and fast pain, respectively, are particularly involved. This is obvious to anyone who has had a dental extraction and *felt* (A-β touch fibres unaffected) the forceps grasp the tooth painlessly.

At high concentrations most drugs which are sufficiently hydrophobic to dissolve in the membrane will exert local anaesthetic effects; but, the changes are often irreversible, rendering them unsuitable for medical use. Thus, clinically acceptable local anaesthetics may be defined as 'substances which produce short- to moderate-lasting, *reversible* blockade of pain impulses peripherally at concentrations of the drug which do not damage either the nerve or surrounding tissues'.

The chemical structures of five representative local anaesthetics are depicted in Table 8.3. The type substance—effective by any route—is lignocaine (US: lidocaine).

The *intermediate chain* of each molecule is a major determinant of duration of effect. The *esters* are relatively rapidly hydrolysed by butyryl (plasma) and acetylcholinesterases; the *amides* are more slowly inactivated by hepatic microsomal enzymes which first N-dealkylate and then hydrolyse the amide group. Metabolism (excluding antidysrhythmic use) is only significant in infiltration and conduction anaesthesia, and is minimised in these cases by the addition of a *low* concentration of a vasosonstrictor (*see* footnote*, Table 8.2) which maintains the drug concentration locally and lessens systemic toxicity. However, in anatomical extremities (e.g. ring block of a digit) the vasoconstrictor is omitted as it may compromise the local circulation.

The *hydrophobic end* is negligibly ionised in body fluids even if it contains an amine group. The latter, which a pK_a of 2.5, is about five pH units lower than body pH at which benzocaine, for example, has roughly 10^5 times uncharged compared with charged molecules.

The *hydrophilic end* is usually a secondary or tertiary amine with a pK_a in the range 7.5–9.0, within which experimental manipulation of the ambient pH can significantly alter the ratio of ionised to unionised molecules, e.g. for lignocaine (pK_a, 8.0) at pH 7 *c*.90% is ionised and vice versa at pH 9. It must be stressed that such pH variations are only employed in the laboratory to investigate possible cellular mechanisms of action. In clinical practice, the local anaesthetics are applied at tissue pH (usually 7.4) and then the effects of ionisable drugs depend upon the relative numbers of charged and uncharged molecules present.

Experimental work on the squid axon—where it is easy to apply drugs internally or externally—using membrane stabilisers of widely varying ionisability, elicits the results shown in Table 8.4. These indicate that

- the *uncharged* drug acts equally well from either side
- *charged* forms are effective when applied internally (with the important exception of tetrodotoxin where the converse is true)

Table 8.4 Sites of action of local anaesthetics: squid axon

| Drug | Status at pH 7.4 | Effectiveness when applied | |
		Externally	Internally
Benzocaine	Uncharged	+	+
Lignocaine	Charged>uncharged	+	++*
Quaternary ammonium derivative of lignocaine†	Charged	0	+
Tetrodotoxin	Charged	++	0

++, very effective; +, effective; 0, ineffective.
* pH-dependent: more effective at lower pHs, i.e. when more ionised molecules present.
† Made by the addition of a third ethyl group to the tertiary nitrogen atom; short name, QX-314.

- pH change only significantly affects lignocaine.

These findings will be explained in the next section.

8.2 Ionic mechanisms of local anaesthetic action

In nerves, depolarisation produces a rapid inward movement of Na^+ ions (which generates the action potential) and a slower outward K^+ ion current which repolarises the axon membrane so that it is ready to respond to the next stimulus. Local anaesthetics can be shown by voltage-clamp experiments to block conduction in excitable tissues by diminished entry of Na^+ ions during the generation of the action potential (Table 8.5). As the concentration of the drug is increased, this results (Fig. 8.1, upper) in

- a progressive fall in the rate of the rising phase of the spike (ab_1, ab_2, ab_3) causing a corresponding slowing of conduction velocity. This is

Table 8.5 Ionic mechanisms of local anaesthetic action

| Drug | Ionic movement of | | Local anaesthetic effect |
	Sodium ions inward	Potassium ions outward	
Tetrodotoxin	−	0	+
Lignocaine	−	(−)	+
Tetraethylammonium (Table 4.9)	0	−	0

Ionic movement: −, depressed; (−), slightly depressed at high drug concentrations; 0, no change.
Local anaesthetic effect: +, present; 0, absent.

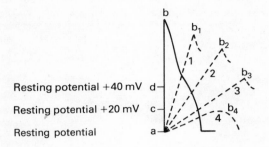

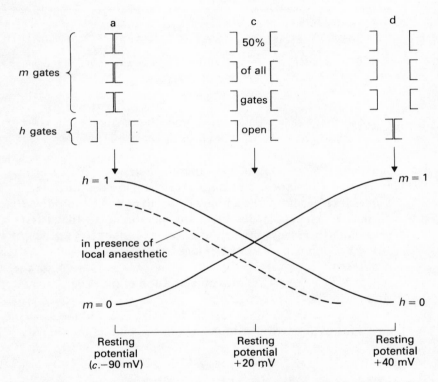

Fig. 8.1 (*Upper*) Progressive effects of increasing concentrations (1–4) of a clinically useful local anaesthetic (e.g. lignocaine) on the generation of an action potential in a nerve; b, maximum depolarisation. (*Middle*) Schematic representation of m ('activating') and h ('inactivating') sodium gate positions at the resting potential (a) and *in the steady state* after depolarising voltage clamps of 20 mV (c) and 40 mV (d) from that potential (*see* text). (*Lower*) Voltage-dependence of m and h gate positions over the range, resting potential to resting potential plus 40 mV. Ordinate: 1, all gates open; 0, all gates closed. Interrupted h curve indicates effect produced by *one concentration* of a local anaesthetic. *Caveat.* This diagram is schematic. In fact, complete recovery from inactivation usually necessitates hyperpolarisation to about -120 mV and at -90 mV, $h = c.$ 0.9, normally.

because the less intense the depolarisation at any point, the shorter the range of local circuits induced

• finally (ab$_4$), inability of the local depolarisation to reach the threshold potential, resulting in conduction block.

Although lignocaine in higher concentrations can decrease exit of K$^+$ ions this is irrelevant to its local anaesthetic action which can occur without any change in resting potential (which is mainly dependent upon outward movement of K$^+$ ions, p. 108): *see also* Table 10.5, possibly decreased *calcium* current at high lignocaine dosage contributing to the negative inotropic effect.

The current (I) of any ion across an excitable membrane can be determined by the application of Ohm's Law:

$$I = \frac{E}{R} = E \times g \text{ (conductance)} \qquad (1)$$

For example, for sodium ions:

I_{NA} (or i_{Na})	$= (E_m - E_{Na})$	$\times \bar{g}_{Na}$	$\times m^3 h$	(2)
current	ionic transfer function	maximum conductance	gating function	

Representing

current flow	the difference between the membrane potential (E_m) and the equilibrium potential (E_{Na}) of the Na$^+$ ion determined using the Nernst equation	conductance when all gates open	the possibility of three m and one h gates being open simultaneously (these numbers of gates were found to give the best fit to the original equations derived experimentally)

Control

	Voltage-dependent		Voltage-dependent (Fig. 8.1, lower)
			Time-dependent *The m gates open faster than the h gates close*

This last fact (shown in Fig. 8.2 and discussed in the next paragraph) is the key to the production of the action potential because it allows the gating situation shown in c, Fig. 8.1 (middle) to arise, i.e. 50% (or more) of the *m* gates to be open while most of the *h* gates are still open (due to slower closure) and to persist sufficiently long to ensure generation of the spike potential.

On *depolarisation* of the axon membrane from the resting state, the time-dependent sodium gate movements involve (*see* Fig. 8.2)

• opening of the *m* gates ('*activation*'): rapid with a time constant* (τ_m) in the range of tenths of a millisecond

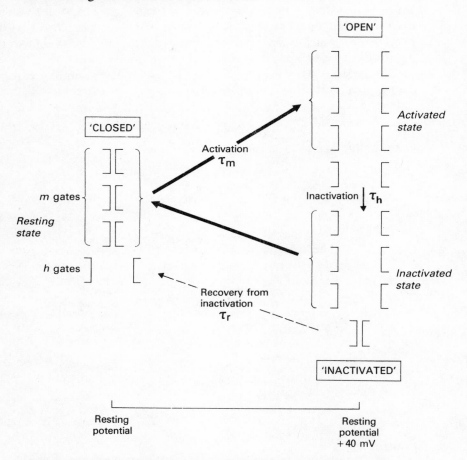

Fig. 8.2 Modification of the voltage-dependent openings and closures of the *m* and *h* gates of the sodium channel (illustrated in Fig. 8.1, lower) by *time*-dependent movements of these gates. *On depolarisation* the *m* gates open rapidly, allowing passage of the sodium current: then inactivation of the *h* gates occurs so that the channels are closed. *On repolarisation*, while the *m* gates rapidly close, the *h* gates only open very slowly so that recovery to the (normal) resting state is delayed. Arrows indicate relative speeds of processes: thick arrows, fast; thin arrow, moderate; interrupted arrow, slow. *See* text for approximate values of time constants.

*The time constant (τ) of an exponential process is the time required for $1-(1/e)$ (approximately two-thirds) of the change to occur.

- closure of the h gates ('*inactivation*'): approximately ten times slower i.e. time constant (τ_h) is several milliseconds (3–15 times τ_m).

These gating movements are shown in Fig. 8.2 over the potential range where voltage-dependent changes are important.

On *repolarisation*, the sodium gate movements are

- closure of the m gates: rapid
- opening of the h gates ('*recovery from inactivation*'): much slower than the movements previously described. The time constant for this process (τ_r) is tens of milliseconds (30–150 times τ_m) so that there is a significant time delay before the next action potential can be propagated.

Local anaesthetics in increasing concentrations do not modify the m-gate voltage curve but progressively depress the maximum of the h-gate curve and displace it to the left (e.g. interrupted line in Fig. 8.1, lower) so that fewer and fewer h gates are open at any given potential. Finally their number falls below the minimum necessary for depolarisation to the threshold potential and block ensues.

8.3 Modification of local anaesthetic actions by calcium ions

Calcium ion changes *within* cell membranes can affect charge distributions (p. 5). The intracellular fluid concentration of calcium ions is much less than the extracellular fluid concentration (Fig. 4.10). When the latter is decreased, membrane labilisation occurs with the production of tetany in excitable tissues (*see* Fig. 8.6).

When the *external* calcium ion concentration is raised (e.g. from 2 mM to 20 mM)

- alone, there is a local anaesthetic effect
- in the presence of an unionised anaesthetic (e.g. benzocaine) there is an increased (additional) effect, i.e. the two mechanisms are different (*see* 8.4)
- in the presence of an ionised local anaesthetic, there is a decreased effect, i.e. the two mechanisms appear to be competing with each other.

The first and last of these experimental findings are explicable (Fig. 8.3) if we now redraw Fig. 8.1 (lower) and add the gating effects of increased external calcium ion concentration. It will be seen that

- alone, this moves the m-gate curve to the right, thus procuring membrane stabilisation over the vital depolarising range (-90 to -50 mV). The dextral movement of the h-gate curve is irrelevant in this connection (as h-gate movements are slower) but it assumes a prime importance (*see* next)
- in the presence of the *ionised* local anaesthetic when it opposes the sinistral displacement of the latter's h-gate curve and thus diminishes its effect.

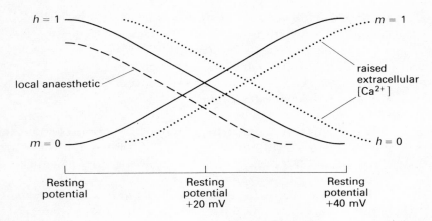

Fig. 8.3 Repetition of Fig. 8.1 (*lower*), with the addition (dotted lines) of the effects of increased (e.g. ten times normal) extracellular calcium ion concentration on the *m* and *h* gate voltage-dependence curves. *See* caveat to Fig. 8.1 (*lower*).

8.4   Cellular mechanisms of membrane stabilisation

Figure 8.4 summarises present views on sites of action.

Tetrodotoxin contains a charged base (guanidine) which combines with acidic groups on the outer part of the sodium channel. There are 'plug' and 'lid' theories. Binding of tritiated tetrodotoxin is diminished by saxitoxin (which contains two guanidino groups) but is unaffected by the charged form of, for example, lignocaine which, therefore, must be acting at a different site. Clinically useful local anaesthetics predominantly modify *h*-gating (Fig. 8.1) and, if this is visualised as due to a molecular change at site A in Fig. 8.4, the uncharged and charged moieties differ in their routes of access to the site. Thus

• *unionised* forms (e.g benzocaine) being hydrophobic enter from either side of the membrane via its lipid structure. This could account for the effectiveness of lignocaine applied externally (Table 8.4) as being due (partly—*see* below) to its uncharged fraction. The molecular change involved might be similar to that for a general anaesthetic (*see* theories, pp. 223–4)

• *ionised* forms (e.g. of lignocaine) act via a receptive area located on the inner part of the sodium channel: possibly by repulsion of *like* charges closing gates. Calcium ions can be visualised as acting at or near the same receptive area. Both with lignocaine and its quaternary derivative (QX-314), the degree of block is proportional to the rate of nerve stimulation (*frequency-dependence*). This suggests, first, that the more often the sodium channels are open, the greater the chance of these local anaesthetics reaching their effective site and, secondly, that interaction of these drugs with the *resting* ('closed') state of the channel is minimal. Lignocaine is thought to bind preferentially to the inactivated form of the channel (termed '*state-dependence*') slowing *h*-gate

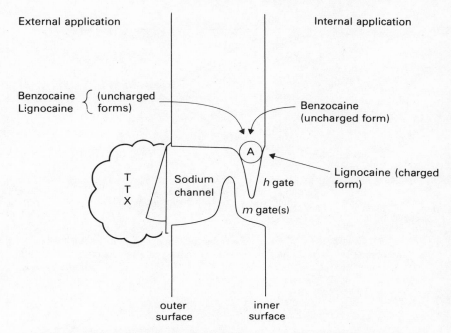

Fig. 8.4 Sites of actions of local anaesthetics on a nerve cell membrane (schematic). For tetrodotoxin (TTX), a 'lid' mechanism is illustrated (*see* text). A, supposed site of local anaesthetic action.

reopening: it is ineffective after destruction of the inactivation process with the enzyme pronase.

8.5 Ionic mechanisms of membrane labilisation

The effects produced by a *lowering* of the external calcium ion concentration (dotted lines, Fig. 8.5) are the opposite of those produced by raising the same concentration in Fig. 8.3. Again, the more rapid *m*-gate movements are predominant, resulting in greater excitability. It is an instructive pharmacological exercise to consider which of the effects of low calcium ion concentration in the extracellular fluid produce the muscular twitchings symptomatic of tetany. From Fig. 8.6 it is clear that increased excitability of the nerve is accompanied by decreased release of transmitter while the skeletal muscle membrane is labilised, though subsequent excitation–contraction coupling is diminished. Tetany would therefore appear to be mainly due to increased muscular excitability resulting in more frequent, even if less effectual, movements.

Veratrum alkaloids and batrachotoxin act similarly to a low external calcium ion concentration to move the *m*-gate voltage curve to the left (Fig. 8.5) but also inhibit inactivation so that the *h* gates remain open. Thus, repetitive responses occur (e.g. Bezold–Jarisch reflex, p. 240)

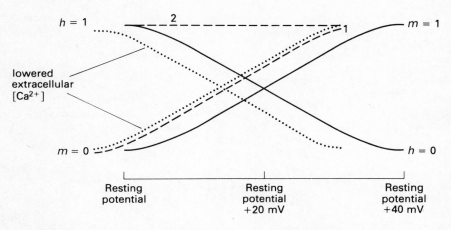

Fig. 8.5 Modification of voltage-dependence of *m* and *h* gates by illustrative membrane labilisers. Dotted lines show the effects of a low extracellular calcium ion concentration: interrupted lines 1 and 2 show the effects of *Veratrum* alkaloids. *See* caveat to Fig. 8.1 (lower).

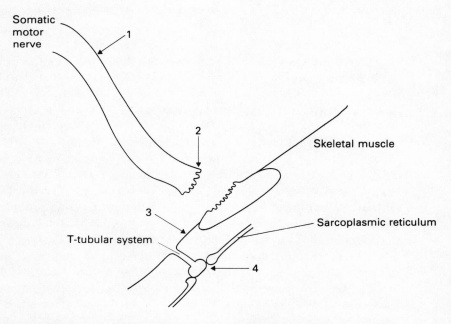

Fig. 8.6 The genesis of tetany. A low ionised calcium concentration in the plasma results in the following effects: 1, increased nerve excitability (labilisation); 2, decreased transmitter release; 3, increased muscle membrane excitability (labilisation); 4, decreased excitation–contraction coupling.

Table 8.6   Properties of neurotoxins which bind to three different sites in relation to the sodium ion channel present in nerve

Neurotoxin group	Binding site	Chemical group	Example(s)	Action General	Specific
1	At or near external orifice	Water-soluble heterocyclic guanidines	Tetrodotoxin Saxitoxin	Membrane stabilisation	Block of sodium ion channel
2	Internal*	Lipid-soluble (steroidal) amines	Batrachotoxin	Membrane labilisation	Displace *m*-gate voltage curve to the left. Inhibit inactivation
3	Probably external†	Polypeptides	α-Scorpion toxin Sea anemone toxin	Membrane labilisation	Inhibit inactivation

* Displaced competitively by local anaesthetics.
† Potentiate site 2 effects allosterically.

until, finally, a depolarisation block is produced. Alpha-scorpion (and sea anemone) toxins similarly inhibit sodium channel inactivation and potentiate batrachotoxin effects by acting at an allosteric site.

The above toxins (together with tetrodotoxin and saxitoxin) have been very useful in the isolation and characterisation of the sodium channel. Three main sites of neurotoxin action have been defined (Table 8.6) but newer toxins with different sites of attachment, e.g β-scorpion toxins, are still being discovered. Note that toxins binding at site 2 are displaced by local anaesthetics: both groups are lipophilic amines.

8.6   General anaesthesia

This is employed to produce unconsciousness immediately prior to and during a surgical operation or manipulation. The sequence of drug application is usually as follows.

Premedication. This is often given in the ward before the patient is taken to the operating theatre and consists of:
1   A *sedative*—a drug which calms without producing sleep. Usually an opioid or a benzodiazepine, e.g. temazepam (p. 229). The modern sedative has three functions (in order of relative importance)
•   to relieve apprehension before anaesthesia (and produce amnesia—benzodiazepines)

- to lessen the amount of general anaesthetic required to achieve and to maintain unconsciousness
- to sedate post-operatively

2 An *antimuscarinic drug*—usually atropine or hyoscine. The function of this agent was orginally to decrease salivary and bronchial secretions when diethyl ether (which is irritant to mucosae) was used as a general anaesthetic. With modern techniques, this is less necessary, and the antimuscarinic substance is now given mainly to prevent cardiac dysrhythmias arising from agents which can stimulate the cardiac vagus (e.g. halothane, p. 282). Additionally it might decrease postoperative vomiting (13.4) and produce amnesia (hyoscine, 2.7).

Induction. This is achieved by the i.v. injection of thiopentone, unless a very short period (a few minutes) of unconsciousness is required, e.g. to reduce a fracture of a bone or dislocation of a joint controlled by powerful muscles, such as head of femur or hip; in these cases methohexitone (Table 1.4) can be used.

Intubation. This involves the insertion of a tracheal tube so that respiration will not be embarrassed if the tongue relaxes backwards. As thiopentone tends initially to induce spasm of the vocal cords, suxamethonium is given intravenously to offset this action and facilitate intubation (Table 2.10).

Maintenance of anaesthesia. The usual agents are the gas—nitrous oxide—or the vapour—halothane. Their pharmacological properties are compared with those of the 'ideal' general anaesthetic in Table 8.7.

Skeletal muscular relaxants. Apart from the necessity for suxamethonium mentioned above, for intra-abdominal operations complete anterior wall paralysis is essential so that the smallest surgical incision will give its largest exploratory area. Some general anaesthetics (e.g. halothane, Table 2.10, p. 67) have significant neuromuscular blocking actions but, nowadays, i.v. D-tubocurarine (or usually a similarly acting drug, pancuronium, vecuronium or atracurium, p. 73) is always given to achieve this end.

For minor procedures (e.g. bronchoscopy or burn dressings) alternative i.v. methods are

- *neuroleptanalgesia*, which involves sedation with a neuroleptic (major tranquilliser, e.g. the butyrophenone, droperidol) plus analgesia (usually with an opiate agonist related to pethidine, e.g. fentanyl); this allows patient cooperation, as there is no loss of consciousness
- *dissociative anaesthesia* produces a feeling of detachment during induction. Ketamine is used and results in light sleep with strong analgesia; it probably acts on frontal association areas and subcortical

Table 8.7   Major requirements for the 'ideal' general anaesthetic compared with the properties of the two most widely used inhalational agents. For simplicity only divergencies from 'ideal' properties are mainly tabulated

Property of the 'ideal' general anaesthetic	Nitrous oxide (gas)	Halothane (vapour)
Non-flammable*		
Rapid rate of onset/recovery (*see* 1.8)	Rapid	Slower
Low concentration in inspired air adequate to maintain anaesthesia†	High (70–80%)	Low (1–5%)
Effects at anaesthetic concentrations Non-irritant to mucosae*		[*See also* malignant hyperthermia, p. 442]
No significant changes in: cardiovascular system		
blood pressure	Raised‡	Lowered§
heart rate		Slowed
sensitisation of ventricles to dysrhythmic effects of circulating catecholamines (p. 282)		Present
respiratory system		Depressed—rapid, shallow breathing‖
other organs hepatic function		Depressed¶

* Both are satisfactory in this connection.
† Essential to allow high concentrations of *oxygen* to be used if necessary. With nitrous oxide only 20% (normal air concentration)—30% O_2 can be given, so hypoxia is possible. N_2O is a useful *analgesic* when administered alone at concentrations of 50–60%.
‡ In presence of hypoxia.
§ Multifactorial in origin (including vasomotor centre, ganglionic and cardiac depression).
‖ Avoid hypercapnia by assisted respiration.
¶ Especially after repeated exposure to the anaesthetic; under such conditions an alternative is enflurane—which is slightly more depressant on the respiratory system.

sensory sites as an NMDA ion-channel blocker (p. 165). Premedication with a benzodiazepine prevents unpleasant dreams and delirium during recovery. The addictive drug phencyclidine acts similarly to produce depersonalisation, hallucinations and a schizophrenoid psychosis.

8.7   Mechanisms of general anaesthetic action

It is generally considered that these drugs act preferentially upon *synapses* rather than along nerve trunks. For example, in experiments upon the superior cervical ganglion, the synapsing fibres are blocked by a lower concentration of a drug such as pentobarbitone than are the non-synapsing fibres (Fig. 2.8).

How may this effect differentially procure unconsciousness? The obvious answer is 'by blocking the multisynaptic pathways of the

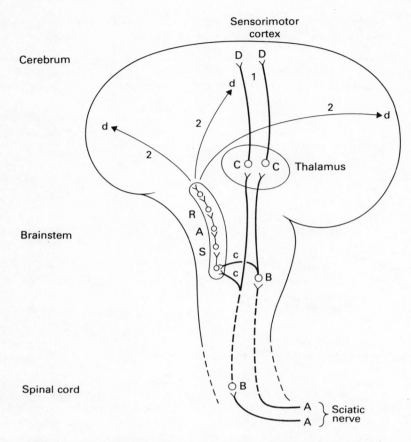

Fig. 8.7 Pathways subserving direct (1, ABCD) and delayed (2, ABcd) cerebral responses following stimulation of one sciatic nerve. Route 2 is preferentially blocked by a barbiturate. RAS, reticular activating system; c, collateral pathways.

reticular activating system'. As seen from Figure 8.7, stimulation of the sciatic nerve results in a biphasic response in the cerebral cortex as follows:

1 An initial depolarisation (latency about 10 ms) especially in the sensorimotor cortex due to bisynaptic pathways travelling via the medial lemniscus and ventroposterolateral nucleus of the thalamus.

2 A subsequent depolarisation (latency about 30 ms) over most of the cerebral cortex due to impulses travelling via collateral fibres through polysynaptic tracts in the reticular activating system (RAS).

The second route is preferentially blocked (because it has more synapses) in the presence of a barbiturate (e.g. pentobarbitone) which thus produces sleep (unconsciousness). However, recent work has suggested that such a simple explanation is not the whole story and that synaptic blockade at sites such as the limbic system, basal ganglia and/or thalamus may be equally important.

Is the block pre- or postsynaptic?

It is not a 'local anaesthetic' effect upon the finer *pre*synaptic terminals but there is evidence that barbiturates decrease transmitter release, e.g. of acetylcholine in the superior cervical ganglion or cerebral cortex. On the other hand, *post*synaptic actions may also be depressed, for example the response of some cortical neurones to glutamate is decreased by pentobarbitone or ether (but not by halothane) at concentrations which depress synaptic transmission. A further variation is that some general anaesthetics can *increase transmission at inhibitory synapses*, e.g. $GABA_A$-Cl^- ion channel complex (*see* p. 224).

Mechanism(s) of action

How, at a molecular level, pre- or postsynaptically, does the general anaesthetic interact with the membrane? There have been many theories spanning most of this century. One, frequently quoted, generalisation is that 'general anaesthetics do not show any structure–activity relationship'. Their chemical structures range from elements (e.g. xenon) via simple inorganic molecules (e.g. nitrous oxide) and simple organic molecules (e.g. halothane, diethyl ether) to heterocyclic compounds (barbiturates), more complex aromatic derivatives (propanidid) and steroids (alphaxalone). Overall the generalisation is true, although exceptions exist in some chemical series, e.g. for the lower members of the aliphatic alcohols, lipid solubility correlates well with anaesthetic potency (which probably merely indicates interaction with hydrophobic sites). Thus, non-specific mechanisms have mainly been sought

• *biochemical theories* (e.g. that barbiturates depress cerebral metabolism) have never commanded general favour

• *physical theories* (e.g. that general anaesthetics disrupt microtubular function and thereby prevent transmitter release) have been postulated. They are possible, considering the rapid aggregation and breakdown of these cytoskeletal constituents (4.13)

• *physico-chemical theories* (e.g. that, by combining with a particular chemical constituent of the membrane, physical changes are induced which lead to the desired effect) have been most popular. They have mainly concentrated on initial interactions with either hydrophilic or hydrophobic areas. An example of the former is the 'clathrate hypothesis'. This proposes that general anaesthetics form hydrates (clathrates) or 'structured water' which enclose hydrophobic areas and result in the requisite functional membrane change. Doubts that such compounds can exist at body temperature are answered by the suggestion that they are rendered stable by protein links. However, these are more serious objections: first, that some general anaesthetics are either incapable of forming clathrates (e.g. diethyl ether) or do so at 37 °C only at 'impossible' pressures (e.g nitrous oxide, >300 atmospheres); secondly, that a large increase of ambient pressure (using tadpoles, newts or mice) results in a lessening of anaesthesia ('pressure reversal'). At higher pressures, there is more stable clathrate formation so that anaesthesia should be intensified rather than diminished.

Hydrophobic interaction theories have been proposed but a precise mechanism of action is still lacking. The 'critical volume hypothesis' postulates drug (anaesthetic) combination with a hydrophobic element in the membrane which it causes to increase in size disproportionately to the volume of the general anaesthetic applied, i.e. the lipid structure becomes less condensed. *When such expansion reaches a certain ('critical') value, anaesthesia results.* An external rise in pressure would oppose the expansion and account for 'pressure reversal' of anaesthesia. However, this theory has been rendered untenable by observations that the reported expansions in red blood cell membranes (on which the theory was originally founded) do not occur. Also, 'pressure reversal' may merely be due to squeezing anaesthetic molecules from their initial target sites. Other variations suggest that primary binding at a hydrophobic site causes secondary changes in membrane fluidity (e.g. gel $\rightarrow$ liquid phase transition, p. 5) and/or protein structure to modify receptors, coupling mechanisms or ionic channels. Finally, direct transmitter (specific receptor) theories are still being promulgated for some of these drugs. For example, (3-α-hydroxy) alphaxalone is a general anaesthetic whereas the corresponding (3-β-hydroxy) isomer is not: the former, but not the latter, potentiates $GABA_A$ responses at the $GABA_A$-Cl^- ion channel complex (Fig. 7.2).

The above considerations are based upon the premise that all general anaesthetics produce their effect by an identical mechanism ('unitary theory'). That this may not be so is attested both by the difficulty of explaining the actions of all the anaesthetics similarly (*see* earlier), and by the fact that, while some anaesthetic combinations are merely additive (e.g. cyclopropane and halothane), others (e.g. alphaxalone and methohexitone) potentiate each other. However, the latter effect may well be due to pharmacokinetic considerations: it has been shown in rats that althesin (an alphaxalone preparation) prolongs the plasma half-life of methohexitone.

Part 3

Systematic Pharmacology

9 CNS Depressants and Stimulants

CNS DEPRESSANTS

Many of these have already been considered as they exert their effects upon specific functions associated with the neuraxis, for example anti-epileptics (7.1), tranquillisers (7.4), analgesics (7.9 *et seq.*) and general anaesthetics (8.6). In this chapter, the remaining major groups—hypnotics and simple aliphatic alcohols (ethanol, methanol) are discussed.

9.1   Hypnotics

These are drugs which selectively induce sleep. This natural process consists of alternating periods of (relative) unconsciousness which are divisible, by the criteria shown in Table 9.1, into two different types. The general pattern is an initial phase of non-rapid eye movement (NREM) sleep lasting approximately 60 minutes, followed by 20 minutes of rapid eye movement (REM) sleep, and continuation of a similar cycle. Both NREM and REM components appear to be necessary for a 'good night's sleep' but deprivation of the latter seems to produce more emotional upset. As many cases of insomnia have a large psychological overlay it is advisable, at the moment, to prescribe

Table 9.1   Types of sleep

	Non-rapid eye movement sleep (NREM sleep)	Rapid eye movement sleep (REM sleep)
Cortical electroencephalogram	Slow waves of high amplitude	Rapid, irregular waves of low amplitude
Associated phenomenon	Somnambulism	Dreaming
Probable site of generation	Raphe nuclei (pons/medulla)	Locus caeruleus (pons)
Activating transmitter (Fig. 9.1)	5-hydroxytryptamine	Noradrenaline

hypnotics which are stated to disturb REM sleep least, i.e. benzodiazepines and chloral hydrate. However, it is salutary to remember that all
hypnotics can only, at best, produce an 'unnatural' sleep.

The mechanisms underlying a hypnotic action might be expected
closely to parallel those inducing general anaesthesia, i.e. a selective
blockade of the multisynaptic pathways of the reticular activating
system (Fig. 8.7). This simplistic view has been modified by
• the pontomedullary mechanisms illustrated in Fig. 9.1
• the isolation from brain of 'sleep peptides' and GABA derivatives
which are hypnotic
• the concept of a brainstem reticular *inhibiting* system—which might
be preferentially antagonised by certain barbiturates and allow them to
manifest excitant and confusional actions, e.g. in the elderly (Table 1.9).

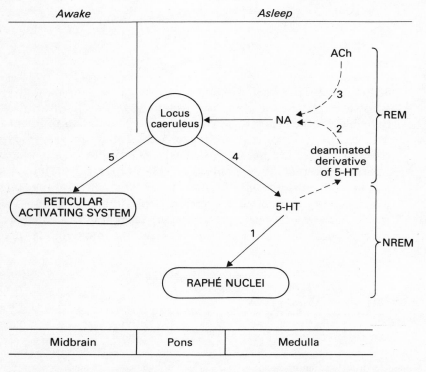

Fig. 9.1 One postulated mechanism of sleep–awake cycles in the brainstem. (1)
5-hydroxytryptamine (5-HT) acting on the raphe nuclei produces non-rapid eye
movement (NREM) sleep. The subsequent occurrence of rapid eye movement (REM)
sleep depends upon the activation of the pontine locus caeruleus (A6, Fig. 6.2) via
noradrenaline (NA), which can be achieved either by a deaminated derivative of 5-HT
(2) or by acetycholine (ACh, 3). From REM sleep, the subject either (4) re-enters the
sleep cycle or (5) awakes. Interrupted lines indicate probable pathways. Block of
brainstem histamine receptors has been postulated (to explain the sedative action of
the imipramine group of antidepressant drugs, *see* p. 182).

Note. Hypnotic effect in relation to anxiolytic and anti-epileptic actions. There is manifestly a considerable overlap of these pharmacological properties, as shown in Table 9.2. Different benzodiazepines, barbiturates and hydantoins possess varying degrees of the relevant actions which render them particularly apposite in specific clinical situations. Their sites of action in relation to the $GABA_A$-Cl^- ion channel complex are shown in Fig. 7.2.

Benzodiazepines/chloral hydrate

The most commonly used hypnotics are the benzodiazepines but (as explained on p. 178) they should only be prescribed *if absolutely necessary and then only for short periods*, e.g. 2–4 weeks.

The original benzodiazepines had long half-lives (of over a day) due either to their own persistence (e.g. nitrazepam) or to the production of a persistent active metabolite (e.g. diazepam, N-dealkylation, Table 1.7). Thus, hangover was a common concomitant. This side-effect has been significantly diminished in the newer benzodiazepines such as temazepam (3-hydroxydiazepam) which is metabolised to an inactive glycuronide and has a $t_{1/2}$ of about 8 hours.

An unusual side-effect is amnesia (? connection with memory pathways, 7.7), which may have value in pre-operative medication, 8.6.

Chloral hydrate is an alternative hypnotic, especially valuable in children and the elderly. Its exact mode of action is uncertain but the drug is rapidly reduced (by alcohol dehydrogenase) to an active derivative, trichloroethanol (Table 1.7). This results in some interesting interactions (Fig. 9.2): ethanol metabolism provides NADH to convert chloral to trichloroethanol, and the latter inhibits alcohol dehydrogenase so that less ethanol is catabolised. The overall effect is to increase the tissue concentrations both of ethanol and of trichloroethanol with a

Table 9.2 Type substances and their relative hypnotic, anxiolytic and anti-epileptic effects

Chemical group Type substance	Benzodiazepine Diazepam	Barbiturate Phenobarbitone	Hydantoin Phenytoin
Action			
Hypnotic	+	+	0
Anxiolytic	+	+	0
Anti-grand mal epilepsy	+*	+†	+

Effects: +, marked; 0, slight/negligible.
* Not all benzodiazepines are anticonvulsant.
† Phenyl substituent usually necessary (Table 1.3). Some barbiturates are actually convulsants; structure–activity relationships complicated—even differences between stereoisomers.

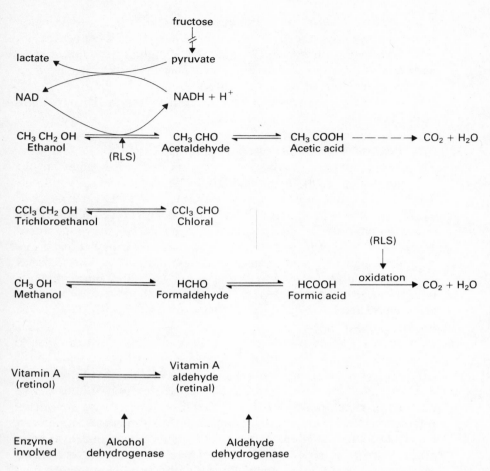

Fig. 9.2 Metabolism of three primary alcohols (ethanol, methanol, vitamin A) and the aldehyde, chloral. RLS, rate-limiting step. Dashed line indicates interconversion via acetyl CoA and the tricarboxylic acid cycle.

'knock-out' action (one type of 'Mickey Finn'). Chloral hydrate is not an easy drug to administer due to gastric irritation and a rather sickly taste. The latter can be disguised with blackcurrant syrup; an alternative to avoid stomach upsets is to give a phosphate ester (triclofos) as a pro-drug of the active agent, trichloroethanol.

9.2   Primary aliphatic alcohols: ethanol/methanol

Ethanol
Ethanol has a number of local effects—such as hardening the skin in the prevention of bedsores or as a cutaneous disinfectant (p. 395)—but here the systemic actions, particularly upon the neuraxis, are to be consi-

dered. It can be regarded as a central nervous system depressant which affects areas in inverse order to their phylogenetic development, i.e. it eliminates the most recently acquired characteristics first and the most fundamental last. Accordingly, the well known stages of intoxication are manifested as follows

• loss of cerebral inhibitory factors resulting in a freer flow of positive responses (sometimes called the 'excitement' phase): possibly valuable in the nervous after-dinner speaker requiring Dutch courage but objectionable in the brash, outspoken individual ('merry')

• loss of general motor and sensory functions ('drunk and incapable'), resulting in inability of movement and insensitivity to pain for example (hence the use of alcoholic potions prior to surgery in pre-anaesthetic days)

• finally, depression of the vital centres regulating respiration and circulation: death is a real possibility not sufficiently appreciated by idiots who wager that they can drink a whole bottle of spirits.

Ethanol manifests strong hydrophilic *and* lipophilic qualities, independently of pH. Accordingly it

• is useful for the solubilisation and administration of hydrophobic compounds

• is rapidly absorbed following oral ingestion both in the stomach and small intestine

• is fairly quickly distributed throughout the total body water.

Its metabolism is shown in Fig. 9.2 and this accounts for over 90% removal of the active agent. But, because the rate-limiting step is the conversion of ethanol to acetaldehyde, the remaining small amounts of the alcohol excreted in the breath or in the urine are accurate estimates of the blood level and, therefore, useful forensically. The rate limiting step is a first-order reaction only when unusually small amounts of ethanol (e.g. an eggcupful of beer) are imbibed. Above that, the reaction becomes *zero-order* due to saturation of the processes regenerating nicotine adenine dinucleotide (NAD) from its reduced derivative. The metabolic rate usually lies between 0.1 and 0.15 g kg^{-1} *per hour* (though ethnic and genetic variations exist) but can be increased moderately by the induction of hepatic alcohol dehydrogenase in chronic users. The ability of many of the latter to remain apparently sober in the presence of relatively high blood ethanol concentrations undoubtedly also displays considerable pharmacodynamic tolerance (p. 188).

In acute ethanol intoxication, the lethal implications are due to central nervous system depression of vital functions—respiration and circulation—the latter exacerbated by the peripheral vasodilation accompanying alcoholic excess. Thus, breathing and blood pressure must be maintained and loss of body heat prevented (i.e. keep the patient warm). The enhancement of ethanol catabolism using pyruvate precursors (e.g. fructose, Fig. 9.2) is not sufficient in practice to warrant its use and can actually exacerbate any tendency to metabolic acidosis (caused by the low NAD/NADH ratio slowing several stages in the Krebs' cycle, Fig. 14.5).

Alcoholism

Chronic alcoholism is a serious problem in our time. Drinking affords an easy release from the pressures exerted by modern society. There are many degrees from true 'social drinking' to the most severe physical dependence. The greatest success has undoubtedly been achieved by example (e.g. Alcoholics Anonymous); therapy has been less effective.

One interesting pharmacological approach has involved the use of inhibitors of the enzyme, aldehyde dehydrogenase—type substance, disulfiram. This is a pro-drug (activated in the liver to diethyldithiocarbamic acid) which, by chelating cupric ions, not only prevents the conversion of acetaldehyde to acetic acid (and hence its rapid removal) but also blocks the action of dopamine-β-hydroxylase (Fig. 3.3), so that dopamine collects in preference to noradrenaline in noradrenergic terminals. The rationale is to inhibit the enzymes sufficiently so that, when the patient drinks a *small* amount of ethanol (test dose), mild symptoms of acetaldehyde and dopamine excess are experienced, namely vasodilation (skin flushing), palpitations and headache. These are usually discouraging enough to prohibit further intake of ethanol while on the medication. Such treatment must be closely supervised since serious reactions—dyspnoea, cardiovascular collapse and even death—have occurred. Disulfiram has the trade-name Antabuse®, and a similarly acting drug is calcium carbimide (Abstem®). Some other drugs, e.g. sulphonylureas (Table 14.9), griseofulvin (18.7) and metronidazole (p. 413) may act similarly, so patients should be warned accordingly.

Ethanol can show synergism with other CNS depressants (p. 439) including anti (H_1)-histamines which cross the blood–brain barrier (p. 135): and it can produce hypoglycaemia in diabetic patients (p. 347). Great care is necessary when prescribing drugs in cirrhotic cases (p. 34).

Methanol

The central nervous system actions are similar to those of ethanol.

Metabolically, the same series of reactions takes place (Fig. 9.2) but with the following important differences
- the overall rate is only one-fifth (0.02–0.03 g kg^{-1} h^{-1}). Thus, coma can persist for days and treatment must be correspondingly extended
- the rate-limiting step is the oxidation to carbon dioxide and water. So, high concentrations of toxic metabolites—formaldehyde and formic acid—collect in the body. This is especially liable to occur in the retina where (as shown in Fig. 9.2) much alcohol dehydrogenase is

present to carry out the physiological conversion of retinol (vitamin A, a primary alcohol, 16.2) to the corresponding aldehyde, retinal. This may account for the optic atrophy which occurs in chronic methanol poisoning.

In the acute toxic situation, vital respiratory and circulatory functions must be maintained and the metabolic acidosis corrected with intravenous sodium bicarbonate solution. The suggestion that the administration of ethanol (which has a greater affinity for alcohol dehydrogenase) will lessen the formation of toxic methanol metabolites is theoretically attractive but requires careful consideration because
• ethanol depression of the neuraxis and tendency to produce metabolic acidosis will summate with that of methanol
• most 'methanol' addicts drink methylated spirits (which consists of 90 *ethanol* and 9.5% methanol), so that the putative antidote is already present in high concentration.

'Antifreeze' often contains methanol in addition to the standard ingredient *ethylene glycol* which has similar actions, catabolism and toxicity.

CNS STIMULANTS
Many of these have already been considered: antidepressants (7.5), agonists of excitatory transmitters (e.g. glutamate, 6.4), and antagonists of depressant agents (e.g. picrotoxin, bicuculline, 6.4).

In general the neuraxial stimulants are most simply classified, especially with respect to their motor effects, according to their major (primary) site of action upon the central nervous system, as shown in Table 9.3. It must be stressed that, as the dose of the agent is increased
• the action at the primary locus becomes more intense
• the effect irradiates (i.e. becomes more widespread) to involve other areas of the neuraxis (e.g. caffeine can stimulate medullary centres, picrotoxin can produce clonic convulsions).

9.3   **Methylxanthines**
Drinks such as tea, coffee and cocoa contain varying amounts of xanthine (2.6-dioxypurine) derivatives: caffeine (1,3,7,-trimethyl), theophylline (1,3-dimethyl), and theobromine (3,7-dimethyl). The latter is not very important pharmacologically, so a meaningful comparison is as follows.

Central nervous system actions (caffeine ⩾ theophylline)
• increased ability for substained mental and physical activity with, sometimes, slight emotional dependence
• strong coffee as the traditional analeptic (9.6)
• nausea and vomiting as a side-effect at high dosage
• cardiovascular actions (*see* Table 9.4).

Table 9.3   A classification of central nervous stimulants, particularly in relation to motor actions

Agent	Major site(s) of action		
	Forebrain	Brainstem	Spinal cord
Methylxanthine			
caffeine	+ +	+	
theophylline	+		
Amphetamine	+ +		
Picrotoxin		+ +	
Doxapram		+ +	
Strychnine			+ +
Tetanus toxin			+ +
Main therapeutic manifestation	Wakefulness	Respiratory and cardiovascular stimulation	
Major central nervous system Side-effects	Restlessness	Hyperpnoea; hypertension; hypersalivation	
Toxic effects	Clonic convulsions	Convulsions of 'brainstem type'	Tonic convulsions
• purposive	Yes	Not usually	No
• reciprocal inhibition	Present	Present	Absent
• examples	Chewing movements; alternating flexion and extension of limbs	Clawing in cats; scrabbling in rabbits*	*See* text, 9.7

+ +, marked; +, present.
* Only seen in experimental animals.

Peripheral actions (theophylline>caffeine)
• bronchodilation (useful in asthma, 11.5)
• increased cardiac output. This is mainly due to the positive inotropic effect and can be used in failure especially of the left ventricle, where the associated bronchodilation also helps. Heart rate and total peripheral resistance changes are often insignificant as the direct actions are diametrically opposed by CNS effects (Table 9.4). Beneficial cardiac relief only occurs if the drug is given (as a soluble complex with ethylenediamine = aminophylline) i.v. but slowly, otherwise, there may be circulatory collapse due to ventricular dysrhythmias (like isoprenaline, Table 10.5) and/or peripheral vasodilation.
• diuretic, weak and obsolete (12.3 and footnote to Table 12.2)
• increased gastric acid secretion: methylxanthine-containing drinks are interdicted in peptic ulcer patients (p. 321).

Table 9.4 Effects of caffeine and theophylline on the circulatory system

	Direct action	Central nervous system action
Heart		
force	Positive inotropic effect	
rate	Positive chronotropic effect on sinu-atrial node	Negative chronotropic effect by stimulation of cardio-inhibitory centre (Fig. 10.7)
toxic	Ventricular dysrhythmias	
Peripheral resistance	Vasodilation of blood vessels (predominates)	Vasoconstriction by stimulation of the vasomotor centre

Many of the direct responses to methylxanthines (e.g. positive inotropic and positive chronotropic actions) were originally explained as due to phosphodiesterase III inhibition resulting in cAMP persistence but adenosine antagonism (at P_1 receptors) is evident at much lower (theophylline) concentrations in a number of preparations (footnote to Table 5.8). Block of P_1 (A_1) purinoceptors — which mediate a negative inotropic effect (*see* Table 5.8 and Fig. 10.13) — would account for the positive inotropic response. However, the 6-thio derivative of caffeine—which is both a phosphodiesterase inhibitor and P_1 antagonist—produces *negative* inotropic and chronotropic effects. The positive inotropy of methylxanthines *is* dependent on an increase in cytoplasmic Ca^{2+} ions and caffeine *can* release these from the cardiac sarcoplasmic reticulum (p. 263).

Caffeine and theophylline (as free bases or salts) are well absorbed following oral administration and distributed into the total body water. They are mainly broken down by demethylation and oxidation to less methylated xanthines and uric acids: any amounts of free xanthine leading to uric acid production (Fig. 12.5) are insufficient to interdict the use of these drugs in patient with a gouty diathesis.

9.4 Amphetamine

As indicated in Table 3.2, this drug has an indirect sympathomimetic effect peripherally but is also able to penetrate the blood–brain barrier and exert a marked central stimulant action, especially in its dextroconfiguration (i.e. Dexedrine®). Before their great potential to induce psychoses (Table 7.9) was realised, dexamphetamine (and the similarly acting drug methylphenidate) were extensively used (*see* later) and became twin menaces in the 'drug scene'. Now their indications are strictly limited to the treatment of
- narcolepsy: this is an uncommon condition in which REM sleep (9.1) occurs too early and these drugs delay its premature onset
- hyperkinetic syndrome in children. Some agents act paradoxically in the young—e.g. anti-(H_1) histamines can excite, Table 5.5 footnote—

and this is a further example: in this condition, amphetamine causes depression.

Harmful responses to amphetamine occurred because of its use
• as an appetite suppressant (*see* 9.5). This was popular in the late '30s and early '40s before the dangers of this drug and the fact that tolerance to its anorexiant effects rapidly developed (not unexpectedly in an indirectly acting substance) were fully appreciated
• in decongestant inhalers (which led to many cases of physical dependence and its replacement with less dangerous compounds, 11.10)
• by athletes to lessen fatigue. This resulted in the deaths of some international cyclists due to hyperpyrexia (Table 7.10) and circulatory overstimulation followed by collapse, and illustrates the very serious nature of amphetamine abuse.

Amphetamine is largely excreted unchanged via the kidney (p. 12) and, as it is a base, removal is expedited if the urine is made acid. As might be expected of a molecule containing a benzene ring, part of the drug is (para)hydroxylated in the liver (p. 31).

9.5   Feeding: treatment of obesity

Excluding genetic factors, the basic physiology of appetite is as follows. A feeding centre in each lateral hypothalamus is inactivated by a satiety centre in the ventromedial nucleus of the hypothalamus (probably responding to its own cellular level of glucose utilisation, Fig. 14.3, legend) but also to signals in the blood activated by food intake, e.g. satietins (α_1-glycoproteins), cholecystokinin. Other CNS centres, particularly in the limbic system and raphe nuclei, are additionally involved.

Pharmacologically, there is uncertainty about the transmitters involved at all these sites: catecholamines and 5-hydroxytryptamine have been major candidates. Amphetamine is considered to act as an appetite suppressant by the release of catecholamines at inhibitory synapses but is not used because of its high abuse potential. Fenfluramine has a similar anorexiant action with less abuse potential and is sedative. It varies from amphetamine in affecting 5-hydroxytryptamine rather than catecholamine levels. It is only indicated as adjuvant therapy in severe cases of obesity.

Weight loss is indicated in a number of pathological conditions (e.g. non-insulin-dependent diabetes, hypertension), or as a vital adjunct to more specific treatments. The methods used are:
1 *Reduction of (kilo)calorie intake.* This is by far the single most important factor and many regimes are available: most provide about 1000 calories per day.
2 *Exercise.* The number of calories dissipated by physical activity (suitable for the overweight) is relatively small but there is no doubt that lack of exercise is a major element in the development of obesity. Conversely, regular muscular routines (even walking or cycling to work,

instead of driving) result in appreciable weight losses—possibly due to psychological as well as physiological factors.

3 *Drugs.* These are a poor third in this connection. They are indicated for short periods (weeks) at the beginning of therapy in patients who are urgently required to lose weight but have insufficient moral fibre to achieve this unaided.

9.6 Analeptics

These are drugs which produce 'recovery from the dead' (Gk: *analepti-kos*, restorative), i.e. they stimulate the vital centres for respiration and circulation in the brainstem. Caffeine (strong coffee) is useful in minor forms of central nervous system depression, e.g. moderate ethanol intoxication. Picrotoxin—which was once used to promote respiratory activity in *severe barbiturate poisoning*—has now been replaced in this situation by artificial respiration, oxygen (11.6), maintenance of blood pressure and care of the unconscious patient (p. 445). As mentioned in 11.7, doxapram can be useful in chronic bronchitis.

9.7 Spinal cord stimulants and their antagonists

Agents which act primarily to stimulate the spinal cord are only of toxicological interest. Significant ones are strychnine and tetanus toxin which both interrupt glycine-mediated inhibitory pathways (6.4).

Strychnine poisoning illustrates the classic train of events produced by a *spinal* convulsant. Initially, there are exaggerated responses to afferent stimuli with loss of reciprocal inhibition, so that tonic fits occur in which both agonists and antagonists are contracted. Next, there is irradiation of the response to stimulate progressively larger cord areas until there is total spinal motor activation. During a fit, the posture adopted depends upon the relative strengths of, for example, flexor and extensor muscles and varies with the species: in humans there is opisthotonos (Gk: *opistho*, back; *tonos*, tension), i.e. predominant extension of the back muscles so that the body is arched with the head and heels touching the floor, the arms are flexed across the chest and the lower limbs are extended, adducted and medially rotated. A more serious consideration, however, is fixation of the respiratory muscles. As hypoxia develops, the musculature is unable to maintain its tetanic state so that the fit subsides and normal respiration ensues. Further afferent stimuli then initiate a repetition of the cycle: so, nurse in a quiet, dark room. The victim usually succumbs during one of the hypoxic episodes, probably due to paralysis of vital brainstem centres. In most cases death is rapid. Treatment of milder cases is symptomatic—i.v. thiopentone or an anticonvulsant (e.g. diazepam) followed by intubation and artificial respiration.

Note the retinal sensitivity change produced in humans by low doses of strychnine (18.3).

10 Cardiovascular System

10.1 Physiological background

The most commonly measured variable is the systemic arterial blood pressure and it is important to appreciate (Fig. 10.1) that the major (though not the only) determinant of the

- *systolic pressure* is the cardiac output (rate *times* stroke volume). The latter is primarily dependent on the venous return to the heart (which is *in*creased by venoconstriction) manifested as a change in ventricular end-diastolic volume (VEDV). Inotropic effects (e.g. of sympathetic activation, Fig. 10.2) also alter stroke volume
- *diastolic pressure* is the total peripheral resistance. The greatest contribution is from the arterioles but there is some immediate postcapillary resistance in the smaller venules (r, Fig. 10.2).

The heart consists of two pumps in series and its relationship to the systemic circulation is illustrated in Fig. 10.2. The (normally) tonic effects of autonomic stimulation are:

1 *Parasympathetic*
- slowing of the heart rate (negative chronotropic effect, NCE):
- however, other marginal actions may become significant under particular circumstances (*see* acetylcholine, Table 10.5).

Vagal tone is important in determining the *rate* of the resting heart: it is slight in infants and the elderly (p. 56).

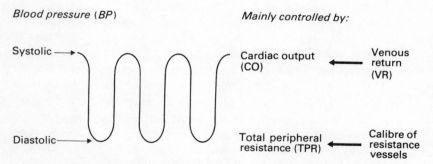

Blood pressure (BP)   *Mainly controlled by:*

Systolic →   Cardiac output (CO) ← Venous return (VR)

Diastolic →   Total peripheral resistance (TPR) ← Calibre of resistance vessels

Fig. 10.1 Chief factors determining the systolic and the diastolic arterial blood pressures.

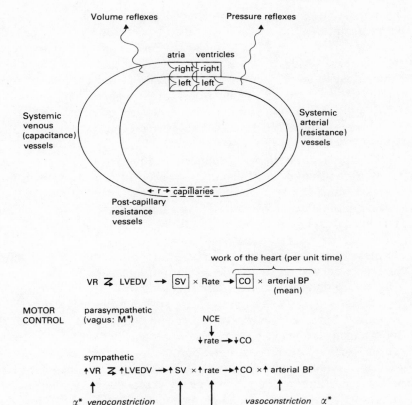

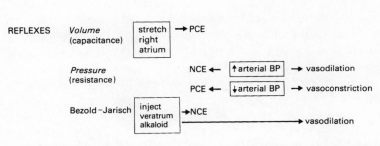

Fig. 10.2 Basic physiology of the systemic cardiovascular system (changes in the pulmonary circuit are ignored) thus the zigzag arrows indicate that the venous return (VR) to the right atrium only affects the left ventricular end-diastolic volume—LVEDV—indirectly. SV, stroke volume. The main effects produced by autonomic stimulation (predominant receptor types asterisked; pathways, Fig. 10.7) are detailed below the figure (↑, increased, ↓, decreased) and followed by the major reflexes (stimulus enclosed in rectangle). On the venous (capacitance) side are reflexes whereby expansion of the atria (increased venous return) elicits a tachycardia; on the arterial (resistance) side, a group of baroreceptor reflexes produces vasodilation and decreased cardiac output as a response to raised systemic blood pressure, and *the reverse effects when the pressure is lowered.* For Bezold–Jarisch reflex, *see* text.

2　*Sympathetic*

- venoconstriction (decreased capacitance) resulting in enhanced return and therefore, by Starling's law, an augmented stroke volume (A → B, Fig. 10.11)
- increased force of myocardial contraction at the same end-diastolic volume (B →C, Fig. 10.11); positive inotropic effect, PIE

A → C is the result of the above *two* effects occurring together.

- increased rate of the heart beat (positive chronotropic effect, PCE) by a direct action on the sinu-atrial node.

The above *three* changes produce a rise in systolic blood pressure.

- vasoconstriction of resistance vessels which results in a raised diastolic blood pressure

Finally, release of adrenaline from the adrenal medulla will additionally activate β_2-adrenoceptors, (10.2).

Cardiovascular reflexes which modify autonomic efferent pathways in the brainstem and are of pharmacological interest are also shown in Fig. 10.2: they will now be briefly described.

1　*Volume (capacitance) reflexes*, e.g. stretch of either atrium or the sinu-atrial junction (venous congestion in the clinical situation) produces a tachycardia (PCE), *especially if the initial heart rate is low*; also causes release of atrial natriuretic peptides (atriopeptins).

2　*Pressure (baroreceptor, resistance) reflexes*, e.g. an increased blood pressure exerts a reflex fall in pressure mediated by a decrease in sympathetic and an increase in parasympathetic efferent nerve activity (*see also* Fig. 10.7). These reflexes can work in the opposite direction when activated by decreases in pressure. In the normotensive individual, they show maximum sensitivity around the mean blood pressure, the effects falling off at higher or lower values and becoming negligible at mean ± 40 mmHg. In the hypertensive patient, they peak around the *raised* mean pressure.

While the above reflexes are important in acute control, other factors are involved in the long term, particularly the *renin–angiotensin–aldosterone* system, controlling circulating blood volume. This, in turn, suggests alternative methods for the treatment of hypertension (10.5).

3　*Bezold–Jarisch reflex.* This is probably a pharmacological curiosity rather than a physiological entity. It is elicited by the intravascular injection of veratrum alkaloids (membrane labilisers, 8.5: which produce a maximum response if injected into the coronary circulation), 5-hydroxytryptamine (p. 132) or prostaglandin I_2. The afferent fibres are in the vagal and glossopharyngeal nerves and the reflex produces slowing of the heart and vasodilation.

Important situations which modify sympathetic activity to the heart and blood vessels are collated in Table 10.1. Note particularly the increase associated with heart failure (*see* 10.11).

Table 10.1 Some factors modifying efferent sympathetic activity to the cardiovascular system

	Resultant effect	
Modifying factor	Increased sympathetic response	Decreased sympathetic response*
Physiological		
Arterial blood pressure: (baroreceptor)		
decrease	+	
increase		+
Atrial stretch: (capacitance/volume)	+(PCE only)	
Exercise	+	
Pathological		
Heart failure	+	
Pharmacological		
Stimulation of CNS α-adrenoceptors†		+
Block of CNS β-adrenoceptors†		+
Bezold–Jarisch reflex		+

+, present.
* Usually accompanied by increased vagal activity.
† For CNS effects *see* pp. 248–9.

10.2   Adrenoceptors (postsynaptic) in the peripheral cardiovascular system

First, look at Fig. 10.7, Autonomic.

The graphs shown in Fig. 10.3 were obtained by comparing the maximum systolic and diastolic blood pressure responses in anaesthetised cats following i.v. injections of the three agonists in the absence and in the presence of concentrations of antagonists which completely blocked α-, β_1- or β_2-adrenoceptors, given singly or in combination, *in any order*. The fact that many different blockers (including reputed α_1- and α_2-selective antagonists, Table 3.5) gave similar results indicates that *pre*synaptic receptors are negligibly involved. The agonists used do not significantly cross the blood–brain barrier, so *central* effects can be ignored.

Important consequences of the data shown in Fig. 10.3 are

• adrenaline in low doses (e.g. X in Fig. 10.3) or at very slow rates of infusion—such as have been used experimentally in humans—can give a fall in (especially diastolic) pressure due to β_2-adrenoceptor activation. This is not possible with noradrenaline as its threshold for a β_2-receptor effect is well to the right of the diagram (a similar situation exists for *adrenaline* in most rabbits and chickens)

• at higher dosage (e.g. Y in Fig. 10.3), noradrenaline produces a greater rise in blood pressure than adrenaline, because the quantitatively similar α- and β_1-effects are not opposed by any significant β_2-

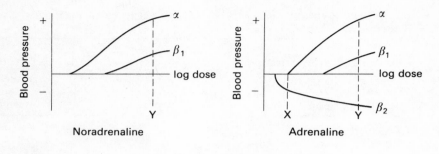

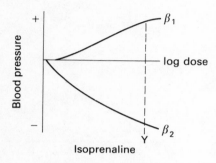

Fig. 10.3 The relative contributions of α-(vasoconstrictor), β_1-(positive inotropic and chronotropic) and β_2-(vasodilator) adrenoceptors to the blood pressure responses ($+$, increased; $-$, decreased) elicited by three catecholamines; noradrenaline, adrenaline and isoprenaline, respectively, given as i.v. doses to anaesthetised cats. *The scales of all the graphs are identical.* For X and Y *see* text.

action (in most rabbits and chickens the pressor responses of noradrenaline and adrenaline are similar)
• finally, note that with adrenaline the depressor effect of β_2-activation is always greater than the pressor β_1-response. Accordingly, in the presence of *total* α-blockade, a pressor effect (Y in Fig. 10.3) is converted to a depressor response. Such 'adrenaline reversal' cannot occur in most rabbits and chickens with adrenaline or in *any species* with noradrenaline (rarely the exceptional cat or rabbit is found which will produce a fall in blood pressure at low dosage and these—*and only these animals*—can manifest noradrenaline reversal). The blood pressure effects of the three catecholamines are straightforward from Fig. 10.3, and the resultant alterations in total peripheral resistance are mirrored, especially in the diastolic changes.

In summary (*see also* Table 10.4)
1 Noradrenaline invariably produces a rise in systolic, mean and diastolic blood pressures (except for the exceptional cat or rabbit, *see* above).
2 Adrenaline, at low concentrations, may show predominantly vasodilation which can persist (as a fall in diastolic pressure) with slightly higher doses: otherwise, it increases systolic, mean and diastolic pressures.

3 Isoprenaline gives, as its overall action, falls in both mean and diastolic blood pressures but the systolic pressure can be unaffected or even slightly raised, due to the massive increase in cardiac output.

Although these three catecholamines are very important to illustrate pharmacological principles, they are relatively insignificant therapeutically because they are very potent drugs with correspondingly inherent dangers.

Indications

Noradrenaline. As an alternative to adrenaline for combination with local anaesthetic solutions (*see* Table 8.2, footnote).

Adrenaline
• With local anaesthetic solutions (as just described)
• As a functional antagonist to histamine in anaphylactoid reactions and severe angioneurotic oedema (Table 5.4)
• In cardiac arrest (in hospital) direct injection into the ventricular myocardium to produce fibrillation (p. 280), which is then converted by electrical shock into normal, sinus rhythm.

Isoprenaline
For conditions in which heart conduction is greatly depressed (e.g. Stokes–Adams attacks, *see* Table 10.5).

Excitation–contraction coupling in vascular smooth muscle. The common final regulation is *via* cytoplasmic Ca^{2+} ions which can be generated by any of the mechanisms illustrated in Figs. 4.8 and 4.9.

For *vasoconstriction* this can be exemplified by the actions shown in Fig. 10.4.
1 Noradrenaline can produce
• an increase in intracellular calcium release (α_1-receptor-mediated hydrolysis of phosphatidyl inositol diphosphate)
• an increase in calcium ion entry from the extracellular fluid by a *delayed* depolarisation (slow excitatory junction potential) activating *voltage-operated* channels and/or via *receptor-operated* channels.
2 Sympathetic stimulation (to vessels which respond with vasoconstriction) gives
• noradrenaline release, with effects as above
• liberation of co-transmitters. The one illustrated in Fig. 10.4 is ATP which, *via* P_2-purinoceptors causes an *immediate* depolarisation (fast e.j.p.) with resultant entry of calcium ions into the smooth muscle cell.
The relative proportions of the above effects vary both with the species and the particular vascular smooth muscle tissue involved.
Finally, to confirm that depolarisation results in vasoconstriction it

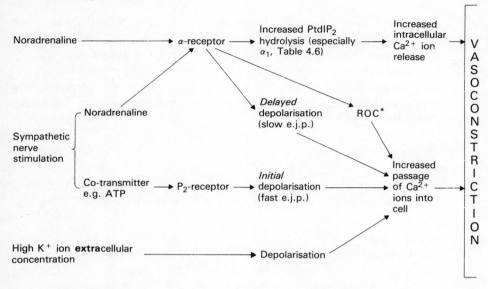

Fig. 10.4 Vasoconstrictor mechanisms. *See* text for explanation. PtdIP$_2$, phosphatidyl inositol diphosphate; e.j.p., excitatory junction potential. ROC, receptor-operated channel; *, in some vascular tissues independent of an α_1-adrenoceptor.

can be shown that raising the extracellular potassium ion concentration (a depolarising manoeuvre) does cause contraction.

See also endothelium-derived contracting factor(s), p. 247.

For *vasodilation, see* p. 245 and Fig. 10.5.

10.3   Changes in blood vessel calibre

Commonly used methods for their determination are as follows (for single cell preparations, *see* p. 263).

Isolated vessels. These usually lack tone and, therefore to show vasodilator activity, it is necessary first to induce a contracted state with noradrenaline (or another constrictor). Larger vessels (arteries, veins) are often spirally cut (to allow registration of effects upon both circular and longitudinal components—though some preparations allow these to be recorded separately). Vessel preparations are valuable for, e.g., dose–response curves and electrophysiological recordings, but the responses obtained are not necessarily indicative of drug actions in whole animals. Umbilical vessels are not innervated and their use eliminates effects upon intrinsic nerves plexuses; but they may respond differently to other systemic vessels with some drugs.

Isolated organs (e.g. cat hind-limb, rabbit ear). Again, these are often lacking in vessel tone but enable a distinction to be made between:

1   *Capacitance* actions—which results in changes in *volume* (measured with a plethysmograph).
2   *Resistance* effects—which result in changes in *flow*: this can be determined under conditions of
- constant pressure (height of perfusing fluid); measure flow
- constant flow (by perfusion pump); measure pressure in side-tube proximal to the preparation.

Whole animal. Simultaneous recording and (if necessary, good control) of blood pressure are needed to separate *active* responses (i.e. directly on the vessels) from *passive* effects (i.e. due to changes in blood pressure or differing external pressures on the vessel wall, e.g. on skeletal muscle vasculature during exercise). Similar methods are used to those for isolated organs, with the addition, for resistance effects, of flowmeters (internal for larger, external for smaller vessels; both are expensive) and the use of the Fick principle for particular circulations which add or subtract specific markers. Intravascular injection of radio-labelled microspheres allows the distribution of vaso-activity between different organs to be determined.

Human. Plethysmographic and Fick principle methods are those most commonly used. In certain circumstances, direct methods may be possible such as photography of retinal vessels or determination of *either* skin colour (red, for example, indicates vasodilation of capillaries and subpapillary venous plexuses) *or* skin temperature (a raised temperature indicates vasodilation, mainly of arterioles). Some isolated vessels are available, e.g. saphenous veins obtained from patients undergoing coronary bypass operations.

Capillaries demand further attention because of alterations in permeability consequent upon their change in calibre. This can be monitored by the unnatural escape of recognisable substances when permeability is increased (e.g. Evans' blue or ^{131}I-labelled serum albumin).

Endothelium-derived factors
Many vasodilator actions—classically acetylcholine acting via muscarinic receptors—not only need significant tone to be present in isolated vessels (p. 244) but also require intact endothelia. If the latter are removed by rubbing, collagenase or a detergent, e.g. deoxycholate, the vasorelaxant responses are unobtainable. The muscarinic vasodilator action is associated with *an increase in cyclic GMP* and *hyperpolarisation*—which are now considered to be generated via two separate endothelium-derived factors (EDRF and EDHF, respectively) as illustrated in Fig. 10.5.

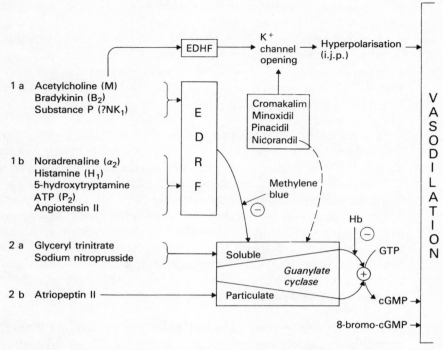

Fig. 10.5 Vasodilator mechanisms (*see* text for explanation). EDRF, endothelium-derived relaxing factor; EDHF, endothelium-derived hyperpolarising factor; Hb, haemoglobin; i.j.p., inhibitory junction potential. All arrowed lines indicate excitatory actions, unless accompanied by ⊖ when inhibitory effect. Interrupted line indicates possible additional action of nicorandil due to its .NO_2 group.

Endothelium-derived relaxing factor (EDRF)

Experimental analysis has revealed several categories of vasodilator mechanism which are preceded by an *increase in cGMP* (Fig. 10.5) namely

1 EDRF required

a for major action

b for minor action. These autacoids predominantly produce vasoconstriction (via the relevant postsynaptic receptors) but this can be *in*creased—if not already maximal—by endothelial removal.

2 EDRF not required

a by direct activation of *soluble* (cytoplasmic) guanylate cyclase: EDRF has been identified with nitric oxide (NO) — see below — and it is suggested that 'nitrites' (p. 268) and sodium nitroprusside (p. 258) generate NO directly.

b by direct activation of *particulate* guanylate cyclase, e.g. with atriopeptin II.

Bypassing of either of these stages by the administration of 8-bromo-cGMP (a stable analogue of cGMP) results in vasodilation due to a decrease in 'free' (cytoplasmic) Ca^{2+} ions available to interact with the muscular contractile elements (activator calcium, *see* Fig. 10.9) brought about by *multiple* actions which lower both intracellular calcium ion release and entry from the extracellular fluid via ion channels (particularly if these have been increased by prior administration of, for example, noradrenaline, Fig. 10.4).

Properties of EDRF
- it has a very short life (less than a minute)
- it is released spontaneously from healthy vascular endothelia, especially in the presence of vasoconstriction
- it is also anti-aggregatory as well as vasodilator: similar properties to those of another endothelial product, prostacyclin.
- a major constituent is considered to be nitric oxide (NO) — possibly derived from L-arginine — or a related, labile, nitro-compound.

Endothelium-derived hyperpolarising factor (EDHF)
Hyperpolarisation of vascular smooth muscle will cause vasodilation by closure of voltage-dependent calcium channels. This is the case with the potassium channel openers (p. 259), e.g. cromakalim whose effect is associated with an increase in ^{86}Rb efflux (taken as a measure of K^+ ion permeability) and opposed by a raised *extra*cellular potassium concentration. The action of acetylcholine (via muscarinic receptors) in producing hyperpolarisation in vascular smooth muscle is similar but differs in two respects—it is transient and *it is endothelium-dependent*. The conclusion is that acetylcholine produces vasodilation initiated via EDHF but maintained via EDRF.

Several endothelium-derived *contracting* factors—endothelins (ETs)—have been associated with hypoxia and reported to be necessary for vasoconstriction produced by, for example, calcimycin. ET-1 is a 21 amino acid peptide (with *two* disulphide bonds linking cysteine residues) generated from vascular endothelial cells by the action of an endothelin converting enzyme. It activates a *specific* phospholipase C to induce phosphatidyl inositol diphosphate hydrolysis and is a *very potent vasoconstrictor. See also* epithelium-derived factor(s) in relation to airways smooth muscle responses to drugs (p. 290).

Vasodilator drugs
It is useful to recognise the three broad categories shown in Fig. 10.6

Capacitance dilation has a *major* effect upon systolic pressure but, in addition, causes postural hypotension, i.e. there is a fall of blood pressure on standing up from a recumbent position. Normally under such circumstances the diminished venous return (due to the effect of gravity on the flow from the infracardiac tissues) is instantaneously corrected via the baroreceptors (10.1), particularly by constriction of the capacitance vessels. This is not possible if any efferent part of the reflex pathway is out of action (e.g. ganglion or adrenergic neurone

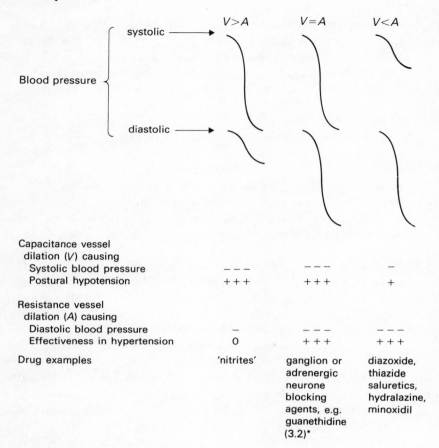

Blood pressure {
  systolic ⟶
  diastolic ⟶
}

	V > A	V = A	V < A
Capacitance vessel dilation (V) causing			
Systolic blood pressure	– – –	– – –	–
Postural hypotension	+ + +	+ + +	+
Resistance vessel dilation (A) causing			
Diastolic blood pressure	–	– – –	– – –
Effectiveness in hypertension	O	+ + +	+ + +
Drug examples	'nitrites'	ganglion or adrenergic neurone blocking agents, e.g. guanethidine (3.2)*	diazoxide, thiazide saluretics, hydralazine, minoxidil

Fig. 10.6 Three types of vasodilator drug acting on capacitance vessels more strongly than, similarly to or less than on resistance vessels. *V*, capacitance vessel dilation; *A*, resistance vessel dilation. *Note*: – – –, marked fall; –, slight fall; + + +, marked; +, slight; 0, none.
*All obsolete in treatment of hypertension.

blocking agents) or if the veins are directly dilated (e.g. with 'nitrites').

Resistance dilation particularly lowers diastolic blood pressure, which is an essential prerequisite if the drug is to be useful in the therapy of hypertension, but some decrease in the systolic BP is also important (*see* below).

10.4   Drugs which affect the blood pressure

Pharmacologically, very many drugs produce cardiovascular changes, either as major or side-effects. Possible sites of action are illustrated in Fig. 10.7 and typical drugs stimulating or depressing them are shown in Table 10.2 (pp. 250–1); add further examples yourself.

A word on the central mechanisms shown diagrammatically in Fig.

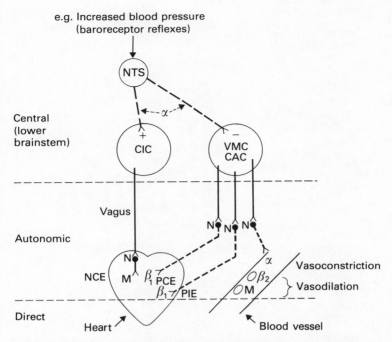

Fig. 10.7 Possible sites of action of drugs which modify blood pressure. *Central*: a rise of blood pressure elicits the baroreceptor reflexes which, via the nucleus tractus solitarius (NTS) and associated centres (*see* text), and subsequent pathways (stimulated by α-adrenoceptor activity), depress ($-$) the vasomotor/cardioaccelerator centre (VMC/CAC) and activate ($+$) the cardioinhibitory centre (CIC). *Autonomic*: Acting in relation to the peripheral autonomic nervous system on α- or β_1-adrenoceptors or at postganglionic sympathetic nerve terminals (adrenergic neurone blocking drugs) or on nicotinic (N) or muscarinic (M) cholinoceptors. Continuous lines indicate cholinergic, and interrupted lines noradrenergic, fibres. Note that on blood vessels β_2-adrenoceptors are not innervated (and M-cholinoceptors rarely so) and, thus, are only affected (directly) by circulating agents. *Direct*: the action (arrowed) is either on the heart or on the vasculature independently of innervation.

10.7. Transmitters involved at the lower brainstem level are *noradrenaline* (e.g. nucleus tractus solitarius is in the A2 group, Fig. 6.2), *adrenaline* (at neurones in the C1 group, p. 161), *5-hydroxytryptamine* (parts of the B3 group) and, probably, GABA and glutamic acid. Agonist and antagonist applications by microiontophoresis show that α-adrenoceptors exist but probably on *modulating*, rather than on direct pathways: this leads to the corollary that centrally acting (α-agonist) antihypertensives cause little postural hypotension, i.e. they do not block the executive reflexes. Beta-adrenoceptors are present but their role is even less certain. However, β-blockers, e.g. propranolol (centrally applied), do lower efferent sympathetic discharge to the heart.

Figure 10.7 provides a convenient framework for blood pressure analyses but is not exhaustive. Other actions include

Table 10.2 Blood pressure responses produced by illustrative drugs acting at the various sites depicted in Fig. 10.5. Drugs used clinically are shown in **bold** type

Reference	Depressor drug	Site of action		Pressor drug	Reference
		General	Specific		
		Central			
10.5	**Clonidine**	+ ⎱	α-Adrenoceptor		
10.5	**Methyldopa**	+ ⎰ (*see text*)	α-Adrenoceptor		
10.5	**Propranolol**	−	(?) β-Adrenoceptor		
Table 7.15	Morphine (high dose)	− VMC	(?)-Receptor(s)	+ Picrotoxin	Table 9.3
9.6	Barbiturates (high doses)	− VMC	(?)-Receptor(s)		
10.1	Veratrum alkaloids	+ (Reflex)	Bezold-Jarisch		
		Autonomic			
2.8	Hexamethonium	−	Ganglion	+ Acetylcholine (higher dose)	2.4
				+ Nicotine (lower dose)	2.5
				+ DMPP	Table 2.4
3.2	Guanethidine	−	Postganglionic (nor)adrenergic ending	+ Tyramine	3.2
10.5	**Prazosin**	−	α-Adrenoceptor (vascular)	+ Noradrenaline	10.2
				+ Adrenaline	10.2
				+ Ergotamine	15.6
10.5	**Propranolol**	−	β₁-Adrenoceptor (cardiac)	+ Noradrenaline	10.2
				+ Adrenaline	10.2
				+ **Dobutamine**	p. 267
10.5	**Propranolol**	−	β-Adrenoceptor (renin release)		
10.5	**Labetalol**	−	α- and β-Adrenoceptor		

Table 10.2 — *Cont'd*

Reference	Depressor drug	Site of action		Pressor drug	Reference
		General	Specific		
10.2	Isoprenaline	+	β_2-Adrenoceptor (vascular)		
10.2	Adrenaline (low dose)	+			
Table 3.1	Salbutamol	+			
2.4	Acetylcholine	+	M-cholinoceptor (cardiac and vascular)		
Table 2.4	Methacholine	+			
		Direct (blood vessel wall)			
10.5	**Captopril**	−	Angiotensin converting enzyme		
Table 4.8	**Nifedipine**	−	Calcium L-channels		
10.5	**Thiazide saluretics***				
10.5	**Hydralazine**				
10.5	**Minoxidil**				
10.5	**Diazoxide**				
10.5	**Sodium nitroprusside**				
10.5	**Pinacidil**	+	Potassium channel (opener)		
10.10	**'Nitrites'**				

(?), uncertain; +, stimulation; − depression; VMC, vasomotor centre.

* Saluretic effect also produces some depressor action in early stages of therapy, *see* text.

- *central*: higher centres, especially cortical and hypothalamic, mediating alterations in sympathetic tone. Other reflexes, e.g. Bezold–Jarisch reflex (p. 240)
- *autonomic*: changes in release both of *catecholamines* from the adrenal medulla (e.g. increased by splanchnic nerve activation; nicotine, 2.5; histamine or 5-hydroxytryptamine, Table 5.2) and of *renin* via β-adrenoceptors (p. 117)
- *circulating blood volume alterations*—primarily affecting venous return, e.g. via the renin–angiotensin-aldosterone system (? also atrial natriuretic peptides). These are the main physiological means of controlling blood pressure *in the long term.*

While the above considerations are important, e.g. in experimental analysis of mechanisms and sites of action, e.g. with regard to possible side-effects of drugs used for other therapeutic purposes (remember that there can be species variations), the major clinical indications demand actions which are relatively specific, with minimal side- (including long-term) effects. These are indicated (by **bold** type) in Table 10.2 and most are discussed in detail in the next section (*see also* treatments of: low blood pressure (p. 267), angina pectoris (10.10) and heart failure (*see* 10.11).

10.5   Drugs used in the treatment of hypertension

If the rise in blood pressure is due to an increase in circulating catecholamines, e.g. phaeochromocytoma, e.g. monoamine oxidase inhibitor–tyramine crisis (p. 184); give combined α- and β-adrenoceptor blockade (phentolamine plus propranolol, or labetalol, p. 258).

Primary (essential) hypertension

Treatment is always indicated if this is liable to lead rapidly to severe pathological complications—malignant (accelerated) hypertension—or is already producing central nervous system symptoms (hypertensive encephalopathy).

In the much more common benign, essential hypertension, the vital consideration is whether the proposed therapy (which, if started, is often lifelong) will procure a significantly greater life expectancy and avoidance of disagreeable symptoms than if only adjunctive treatment (weight reduction, moderate exercise, low saturated fat diet and low salt intake) was given. Thus patients for antihypertensive therapy have to be carefully selected on a basis of the average prognosis for their age, sex and systolic/diastolic pressures (the aim is to lower both of these); and the drug(s), taken orally, must be both effective and safe during long-continued usage.

Therapy is nowadays* begun with *either*

• a β-blocker such as propranolol titrated (if necessary) to a maximum effect (pulse not less than 55–60 beats min^{-1}, p. 87) without serious side-effects; if the blood pressure is still too high, add a thiazide (*see* next point) *or*

• a saluretic vasodilator (e.g. chlorothiazide, Table 12.4). This has a shallow dose–response curve (Fig. 12.4) so that, if it is inadequate, rather than increasing the dosage, add a β-blocker. Thiazides takes 2–3 days to exert an effect with a maximum response at 2–3 weeks.

If neither regime is wholly satisfactory, add a different kind of vasodilator, usually a calcium-channel blocker, an angiotensin converting enzyme (ACE) inhibitor (also decreases aldosterone release) or hydralazine.

The advantages of such combination therapy are that as these agents:

1 Act by different mechanisms, they activate different compensatory processes which are often blocked by other drugs in the combination; for example

• β-blockade of cardiac action by propranolol produces reflexes resulting in α-adrenoceptor-mediated vasoconstriction; that is opposed by the vasodilator effects of the other components

• *vasodilation* induces reflex tachycardia (which is prevented by the β-blocker) and/or increased renin secretion with retention of salt and water (which is prevented by the β-blocker and opposed by the diuretic or ACE inhibitor) respectively

• *saluresis* caused by the thiazide results in renin secretion, this is prevented by the β-blocker.

2 Can be used in relatively smaller dosages, the frequency of their individual side-effects is significantly diminished.

β-blockers

Although these drugs are used extensively in the therapy of hypertension, their exact mode of action is still uncertain. Possibilities (not necessarily exclusive) are as follows.

Central mechanisms
Central nervous system β-antagonist. Animal experiments indicate that this is feasible but there is poor correlation between the ability of a β-blocker to cross the blood–brain barrier and its relative antihypertensive potency. Another possibility is a drug-induced change in the baroreceptor reflex sensitivity.

*Recent reports that β-blockers and thiazides can adversely affect serum lipids while calcium channel blockers and ACE inhibitors do not suggests a possible future change here: but the two former are *well-tried* drug groups.

Autonomic mechanisms

1   *Cardiac β_1-adrenoceptor antagonist.* It is visualised that the fall in blood pressure is due to depression of heart activity. However, this results, *acutely*, in reflex vasoconstriction but proponents of this hypothesis suggest that, with time, circulatory adjustments (e.g. vascular autoregulation) are made so that eventually a decreased cardiac output unaccompanied by a raised blood vessel tone is achieved. This is probably a major mechanism, as it is in angina pectoris treatment (10.10). However, β-blockers (e.g. pindolol) with marked intrinsic sympathomimetic activity (Table 3.4) and thus relatively little cardio-depressant action, are effective antihypertensive agents. This suggests that multiple factors are involved.

2   *Prevention of renin release by β-antagonism.* This could obviously benefit those benign hypertensive patients (about 20%) who have high circulating renin levels, but it is stated to be an unlikely mechanism in all cases as the doses of some β-blockers required to reduce plasma renin to insignificant levels are often *well below* their antihypertensive doses.

3   *Vascular.* Beta$_2$-*pre*synaptic adrenoceptors are considered to increase transmitter release (p. 88) in vasoconstrictor fibres so that β-block should decrease α-mediated vasoconstriction. This idea conflicts with the hypothesis advanced for the occurrence of cold limbs (*see* side-effects).

Direct mechanisms

There is no correlation between membrane-stabilising and antihypertensive activities: thus sotalol, which lacks the former, possesses the latter. Other hypotheses whereby vasodilation is directly induced have been advanced with little firm evidence to support them, as yet.

Side-effects

As detailed on p. 87 (special care is required in asthmatics and diabetics—avoid in heart failure). Reflex α-adrenoceptor-mediated vasoconstriction (blocked by labetalol, Table 10.3) can cause decreases in skin and skeletal muscle blood flows resulting in cold extremities, especially in females. This effect is stated to be less common with β_1-selective blockers or partial agonists, which allow or induce mitigating postsynaptic β_2-adrenoceptor-mediated vasodilation. Impotence in the male has been reported.

Thiazide saluretics

These are the alternative first-line group in the treatment of hypertension. There are two main actions here.

1   *Saluretic.* Undoubtedly water and sodium chloride removal (like a

Table 10.3 Alternative drugs used in the treatment of hypertension

General site	Drug	Major mechanism	Most common side-effect(s)	Main disadvantage(s) on chronic usage	Route and role in treatment of hypertension*
Central	Clonidine	α-Adrenoceptor agonism	Drowsiness Dry mouth	Sympathetic overactivity on abrupt withdrawal	Oral in essential
	Methyldopa	α-Adrenoceptor agonism (after conversion to α-methylnoradrenaline)	Drowsiness Dry mouth Loss of ejaculation	Type II allergic blood disorders (Table 20.1) Hepatic impairment	Oral in essential
Autonomic	Labetalol	α- and β-adrenoceptor blockade	Similar to those of β-blockers but cold extremities uncommon (*see text*)		Oral in essential; i.v. infusion in emergency
	Prazosin	α-Adrenoceptor blockade (possibly, also, direct vasodilator)	Less than those of most α-blockers (3.4); drowsiness		Oral in essential
Direct	Minoxidil	Vasodilation (resistance greater than capacitance)	Tachycardia Oedema	Hair growth (especially of face in females)	Oral in refractory essential
	Diazoxide	Vasodilation (resistance greater than capacitance)	Tachycardia Oedema Hyperglycaemia	Not applicable (*see text*)	i.v. bolus in emergency
	Sodium nitroprusside	Vasodilation (resistance *and* capacitance vessels)	†	Not applicable (*see text*)	i.v. infusion in emergency

* Treatments: 'oral in essential' indicates use in benign type; i.v. in very severe accelerated (malignant) type or other emergency.
† Too rapid infusion can cause dizziness, retching, palpitations, chest pain—if so, slow the rate.

low salt diet) lowers the blood pressure, opposed to some degree by compensatory renin release. This might account for the fact that 'moderate strength' saluretics (e.g. thiazides) lower blood pressure better (except in chronic renal failure, Table 12.4) than 'high-ceiling' diuretics (such as frusemide) which engender more renin production (12.5). Initially, if the plasma volume is maintained experimentally by fluid infusion, the antihypertensive effect is prevented. Later, however, this is not the case, which suggests that some other mechanism is now responsible for the fall in blood pressure (*see* next).

2   *Peripheral vasodilation.* This is probably a similar effect to that of the related drug, diazoxide (which produces mainly resistance vessel relaxation (Fig. 10.5) but is unsuitable for chronic use, *see* p. 258).

Side-effects
These are detailed in Table 12.4. Contra-indicated in patients with diabetes mellitus or gout. Impotence can occur.

Calcium channel blocking drugs
Their properties are described in 4.11. Though all groups have been used in the treatment of hypertension (Table 4.8), *nifedipine* is the type substance as a vasodilator.

Angiotensin converting enzyme (ACE) inhibitors
These inhibit the formation of angiotensins II and III (*see* Fig. 5.5)—so preventing vasoconstriction and aldosterone release (with its consequent retention of sodium chloride and water in the body). The antihypertensive action is particularly marked in patients with initial high plasma renin activity but can work in other cases. One suggestion to explain the lowering of blood pressure in these latter cases is that the ACE inhibitor prevents angiotensin II formation not only in the plasma *but also in the tissues* (e.g. heart, blood vessels) and thus its potentiating effects (*see* p. 139) on the sympathetic innervation to these organs is lost. The type substance, *captopril*, can cause hypersensitivity reactions, a persistent dry cough (for possible genesis, *see* 5.9) and abnormalities of taste (dysgeusia). Albuminuria, neutropenia and hyperkalaemia (due to decreased aldosterone production) are more common if there is renal impairment: monitor if necessary.

Several *renin inhibitors*, which block the angiotensin cascade (*see* Fig. 5.5) at an earlier stage than the ACE inhibitors, are being investigated.

Hydralazine
This is representative of a miscellaneous group loosely termed 'vasodilators'. It does not require EDRF (p. 246) to produce relaxation of

resistance more than capacitance vessels (Fig. 10.6) but the mechanism of action is not known. The side-effects experienced when it was given by itself—e.g. palpitations, oedema—have largely been eliminated by combination therapy with a β-blocker and a thiazide saluretic. The occurrence of systemic lupus erythematosus (type III hypersensitivity; particularly in 'slow' acetylators, Table 20.4,2) is minimal at the lower dosage now used and reversible on discontinuance of the drug.

Alternative drugs
Other drugs used in the treatment of hypertension, with their particular characteristics and indications, are shown in Table 10.3. Brief notes on each follow.

Centrally acting agents
Clonidine. This drug lowers the blood pressure by decreasing efferent sympathetic activity (including release of catecholamines from the adrenal medulla) by acting as a CNS α-adrenoceptor agonist on either noradrenergic and/or adrenergic synapses (p. 249). Classically, it is α_2-selective (Table 3.5) but effects on α_1- (and other) receptors have been implicated in its actions. Additionally clonidine inhibits dopamine-β-hydroxylase and phenylethanolamine N-methyltransferase (PNMT) activity in CNS noradrenaline and adrenaline neurones associated with cardiovascular control. For example, the depressor action of clonidine is accompanied by decreased PNMT activity (and therefore adrenaline synthesis) in C1 neurones (p. 249) where adrenaline could be exerting pressor effects.

It is not commonly used because, if the patient inadvertently forgets to take a dose, circulating levels of catecholamines rise with resultant sympathetic actions ranging from sweating and tachycardia to more dangerous cardiovascular effects. One suggestion is that by a peripheral, presynaptic α_2-agonism (Table 3.5) clonidine normally inhibits catecholamine release which, accordingly, increases on drug discontinuance. Another idea is that the return to normal of PNMT activity on withdrawal of clonidine produces sufficient adrenaline in C1 neurones (*see* above) to increase efferent sympathetic discharge.

Methyldopa (α-methyldopa). Previous ideas that this drug has peripheral actions which produce the fall in blood pressure have been discounted. It is given in this form merely to cross the blood–brain barrier. Once inside noradrenergic (or adrenergic) brainstem neurones, it is converted (Fig. 3.3) successively to α-methyldopamine and α-methylnoradrenaline (and α-methyladrenaline). The depressor action is due to one or both of the latter two compounds because, if their formation is prevented by pretreatment with the relevant enzyme inhibitors which can cross the blood–brain barrier, the antihypertensive effect is lost. This drug will certainly lower the blood pressure as required but it causes too much sleepiness for routine use. It can also produce allergic type II reactions (Table 20.1—circulating IgG antibodies give a positive Coombs' test, though haemolytic anaemia is uncommon).

Autonomically acting agents
Labetalol. This drug combines a non-selective β-adrenoceptor blocking action with peripheral, postsynaptic α-adrenoceptor blockade (p. 85). The results are
• an intensification of the hypotension produced by each mechanism, because compensatory processes (*see* earlier) are diminished: yet, postural hypotension is relatively uncommon
• a more rapid onset of the β-antagonist depressor effect (as *immediate* reflex α-vasoconstriction is reduced)
• a negligible incidence of cold extremities as α-vasoconstriction is blocked (p. 254).

Prazosin. This peripheral, postsynaptic α_1-adrenoceptor selective blocker (Table 3.5) produces
• some drowsiness
• postural hypotension: it dilates both capacitance and resistance vessels
• only slight reflex tachycardia.
    All these suggest that other mechanisms of action may be involved, particularly direct vasodilation, and this drug is often classified in the next group.

Directly acting vasodilators
Sodium nitroprusside. This gives a strong vasodilation (of both capacitance and resistance vessels) via activation of guanylate cyclase (Fig. 10.5) which it achieves by the formation of nitric oxide (NO) or a labile nitro-containing compound. Its chemical formula $[Fe.(CN)_5NO]^{3-}$ should enable you to see that it can form NO and understand that it can be converted via cyanide (below toxic concentrations unless there is poor liver function) to the relatively inactive thiocyanate ion. Thus, given by i.v. infusion, its effects have both a rapid onset and offset.

Diazoxide. Related chemically to the thiazide saluretics, it produces a much stronger (predominantly resistance vessel) dilation which is useful for the acute lowering of blood pressure. Then, it must be administered by rapid i.v. (bolus) injection because of heavy plasma protein binding (p. 16) but the effect then lasts for several hours. Diazoxide is unsuitable for longer-term lowering of blood pressure because it causes retention of sodium chloride and water (due to renin release) and also a much greater depression (than thiazides) of insulin secretion from the β-cells of the pancreatic islets (Table 14.6). This latter action is due to the opening of ATP-activated K^+ ion channels (Fig. 14.4)—might a similar effect account for the vasodilation? (*see* below).

Minoxidil. A powerful relaxant—mainly of resistance vessels —which causes reflex tachycardia and oedema (due to renin release) unless given with a β-blocker and a thiazide saluretic. Hirsutism is an unwanted side-effect of prolonged therapy. This drug has been shown to open K^+ ion channels (*see* below).

Potassium channel openers (Fig. 10.5). This group—in addition to minoxidil—includes future possible antihypertensive drugs cromakalim, pinacidil and nicorandil (the latter *also* contains a nitrite group). They hyperpolarise the vascular smooth muscle membrane which also decreases (voltage-dependent) calcium channel opening. The most likely *potassium* channels involved appear to be the calcium-activated ones—the high conductance subgroup as they are apamin-insensitive (Table 4.9, 5). The potassium channel openers also produce a negative inotropic effect in stimulated heart muscle which could be mediated through the same channels because this action is antagonised by tetraethylammonium.

10.6 Migraine and its treatment

This relatively common condition shows a strong hereditary diathesis. It consists of attacks which often begin with visual disturbances (aura) and rapidly progress to a unilateral, throbbing headache accompanied by nausea and vomiting. Usually, the episode is precipitated by a triggering factor: these show a wide variety (physical, e.g. glare; psychological, e.g. anxiety; hormonal, e.g. premenstrual; *commonly* a food) but are often constant for a particular individual. Dietary factors implicated (apart from ethanol) frequently contain amines, e.g. tyramine, and it has been shown that some migraine sufferers have a low capacity to conjugate (inactivate) this substance. It is agreed that the manifestations are due to vascular changes in the head region but whether these are extracerebral and/or intracerebral, and whether they involve vasodilation or vasoconstriction, are contested. In the absence of a satisfactory experimental model, attention has been turned to the possible modes of action of drugs known to be therapeutically useful, especially against the headache. The keystone of treatment—ergotamine—is well known as an α-adrenoceptor antagonist (for instance it readily produces 'adrenaline reversal', 10.2) but its relaxation of vessels is mainly shown if they are initially contracted: when applied to a dilated vessel (such as may be causing the migraine headache), ergotamine induces constriction (possibly the relieving effect), due either to *partial* α-adrenoceptor or 5-HT agonism or by direct contraction (Table 15.5). Methysergide—only used in very severe, refractory cases of migraine—and its more commonly used replacement pizotifen (US: pizotyline) primarily act as antagonists at the 5-HT$_2$ receptor, which normally mediates vasoconstriction (Table 5.3). Conversely, a 5-HT$_1$ *agonist* is considered to be beneficial by producing *extra*cerebral vasoconstriction. This again suggests the involvement of 5-HT in the pathogenesis (remember, also, that there is considerable overlap between blockers at α-adrenoceptors and 5-HT receptors). Present theories ascribe the ameliorating effects of drugs to modifications of 5-HT (and possibly noradrenaline and/or prostaglandins) functions on *blood vessels* (directly or via their nervous control, Fig. 10.7) and/or *pain mechanisms* (directly or via central—Fig. 7.5—or peripheral nervous pathways). The latter possibility could account for the trials of 5-HT$_3$ antagonists (Table 5.3) in migraine. During an attack, platelet aggregation is a likely source of 5-HT (and eicosanoids) which is prevented by low doses of aspirin, p. 381—could this help its analgesic action against migraine?

Treatment
Avoidance of triggering factors.
Prophylaxis. Drugs commonly used are
• pizotifen (US: pizotyline), primarily a 5-HT$_2$ antagonist, which has replaced methysergide due to the latter's fibrotic side-effects (5.8)
• propranolol. β-block can potentiate ergotamine vasoconstriction
• amitriptyline: ? related to antidepressant action

All the above can interact with 5-HT and/or adrenergic functions.

• feverfew (mechanism unknown) is often helpful.

Acute attack
• rest in darkened, quiet room
• analgesia: aspirin (? additionally preventing release of 5-HT from platelets, 17.2) or paracetamol
• anti-emetic: metoclopramide (p. 317); also quickens gastric emptying so that orally given drugs are more rapidly absorbed
• ergotamine; orally, rectally or by inhalation. Oral preparations usually also contain an anti-emetic (e.g. cyclizine) and often caffeine, which (by vasodilation, 9.3) promotes more rapid absorption from the gut. The major side-effects of ergotamine (Table 15.5) are vomiting (covered by the anti-emetic) and widespread vasoconstriction, which contraindicates its use in cases of ischaemic heart disease, peripheral vascular disease or prophylactically.

THE HEART

10.7 Physiological basis

The four fundamental aspects of cardiac activity and their association with particular areas of the organ, together with the shapes of their respective action potentials, are shown in Fig. 10.8.

Inotropic (Gk: *is, inos*, fibre) actions are generated as shown in Fig. 10.9 for *mammalian* heart muscle. The action potential, passing along the surface of the myocardium, progressively depolarises successive T-tubular systems and their longitudinal extensions (unlike skeletal muscle where the sarcoplasmic reticulum plays the major role in rapidly activating the 'deeper' parts of the muscle, *see* Fig. 8.6). Depolarisation results in the passage of calcium ions into the myocardial cell. However, the amount entering is inadequate for excitation–contraction coupling, so this 'trigger' calcium mobilises sufficient 'activator' calcium both from intracellular stores and by activating enzymes which can induce

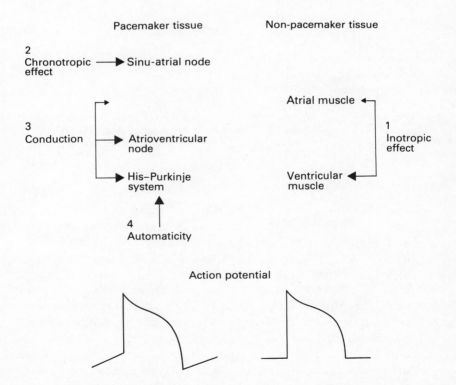

Fig. 10.8 Four facets of cardiac action—size of arrowheads represents importance—with (*below*) diagrammatic representation of action potentials in the two types of tissue (pacemaker and non-pacemaker).

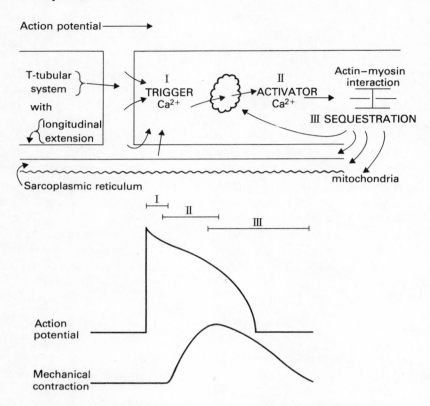

Fig. 10.9 (*Above*) Excitation–contraction coupling in *mammalian* heart muscle (schematic). (*Below*) Phases of calcium ion movements delineated in relation to the excitation (action potential) and to the mechanical contraction and relaxation, respectively (*see also* Fig. 4.10).

more calcium channel opening (Figs 4.8 and 4.9). Combination of the free ions with troponin C—a homologue of calmodulin (4.12)—produces an allosteric change in tropomyosin which allows interaction between myosin and actin resulting in mechanical contraction of the heart muscle (systole). Next, the calcium ions undergo a third process, i.e. return to their stores; this is termed sequestration and results in relaxation of the muscle (diastole). The phases of calcium ion changes are correlated temporally with the corresponding action potential (*see* 10.12) and mechanical contraction recordings (e.g. in a papillary muscle) in Fig. 10.9. It is instructive to consider the changes induced in the *mechanical* contraction by the action of a β_1-adrenoceptor agonist, such as adrenaline, which intensifies all the calcium ion movements. Fig. 10.10 illustrates that the catecholamine addition causes a more intense and greater mobilisation of free calcium ions, resulting in a more rapidly developed and enhanced contraction (positive inotropic

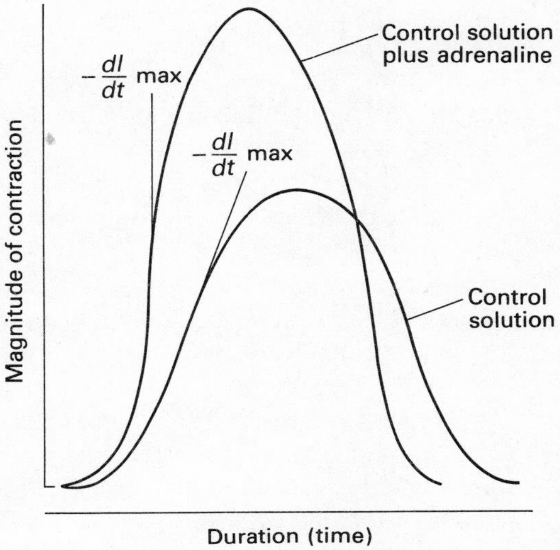

Fig. 10.10 The effect of adrenaline (compared with control) on the mechanical contraction of a strip of ventricular muscle or an isolated papillary muscle, under isotonic conditions. Measure maximum contraction, duration and maximum rate of shortening—the latter by differentiation of steepest part of upstroke ($-\dfrac{dl}{dt}$ max: minus as length, l, is decreasing).

effect) but, due to increased sequestration, of shorter duration. This latter change is necessary because otherwise, due to the concomitant direct positive chronotropic effect (*see* Table 10.4), there would be insufficient diastolic filling time.

Calcium ion transport into the sarcoplasmic reticulum is achieved by a Ca^{2+}-dependent ATPase (p. 112) *which in cardiac muscle* is activated by the phosphorylation of a receptor protein (phospholamban) by either cAMP-dependent phosphokinase or Ca^{2+}-calmodulin phosphokinase (Fig. 4.8). As both of these phosphokinases are stimulated by adrenaline, it will therefore increase sequestration of calcium ions into the sarcoplasmic reticulum. Caffeine promotes calcium ion release from the sarcoplasmic reticulum and ryanodine (p. 113) opposes this.

10.8 Methods for the determination of cardiac muscle contraction

The available preparations have ranged from isolated myocardial cells (tissue-cultured) which beat spontaneously and are devoid of nervous elements to the hearts of conscious humans (strain gauges fixed to ventricular myocardia of patients undergoing repeated open-chest operations). Commonly used techniques are as follows.

Single cell preparations

Tissue culture or collagenase treatment of whole preparations can be used to produce isolated cells. High resolution single-channel current recordings can then be made using the patch-clamp gigohm-seal technique (p. 108).

Isolated myocardial preparations
Papillary muscle. Thin specimens (to make sure of adequate oxygenation) from, for example, the right ventricle of a guinea-pig are suspended horizontally in a warmed bath through which a nutrient, buffered solution saturated with oxygen is continuously passed. The muscle requires rhythmical (electrical) stimulation. Under isometric or isotonic conditions the tension or contraction, respectively, that develops may be measured (Fig. 10.10). The preparation allows simultaneous registration of the action potential (Fig. 10.14) via a microelectrode (nowadays, single-channel recordings are preferred to monitor electrical events—*see* above).

Atrial preparations are often used side by side in the same organ bath. The left atrium is electrically driven ('paced') and recordings show *mechanical* effects; the right atrium beats spontaneously and shows *rate* effects. Increased rate produces its own gradual increase in mechanical contraction ('positive staircase') probably by facilitation of excitation–contraction coupling, except in the rat where the opposite occurs ('negative staircase'). Thus, true mechanical effects are only obtained in *paced* preparations.

Isolated whole heart
Langendorff preparation. The perfusing cannula is inserted into the stump of the aorta so that the oxygenated fluid is delivered at constant pressure (maintained level in overhead reservoir)—not into the left ventricle (as the flow closes the aortic valves), but into the coronary vessels with eventual escape via the coronary sinus. The perfusion is thus *through* the myocardium. Nevertheless, this is a sturdy and valuable preparation for class-work.

Heart–lung preparation. Perfusion fluid (at constant temperature) passes through the heart chambers normally and then goes round an 'artificial' circulation, which allows changes in total peripheral resistance and/or venous return to be made. The heart is effectively denervated during the surgical preparation, so the rate is constant, thus avoiding any 'staircase' effects. Figure 10.11 can now be obtained by varying venous return and taking simultaneous measurements of *stroke volumes* (flows into the external circuit at constant peripheral resistance) and of *ventricular volumes* (directly, by means of a plethysmograph—termed a cardiometer—which encloses both ventricles). For technical reasons, this preparation is usually 'failing' gradually all the time and, accordingly, is useful to demonstrate the positive inotropic effect (PIE) of a drug such as digoxin which is used in heart failure. Otherwise it has been superseded by more 'physiological' preparations (*see* below).

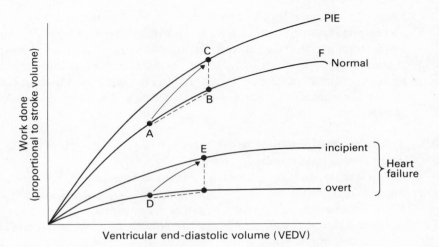

Fig. 10.11 Work–volume relationships for the heart, using a heart–lung preparation. Work is proportional to stroke volume, as peripheral resistance and rate are maintained constant. For normal and PIE lines *see* text. In cardiac failure the curve is depressed (as shown) so that dilation of the heart does not result in any significant increase in the force of contraction; but reflex sympathetic stimulation may partially alleviate the situation (D → E). Therefore, β-blockers can precipitate overt from incipient heart failure (E → D; *see also* 3.5).

Whole heart preparations in situ

There have been a number of these increasing in complexity up to freely moving animals with telemetric recording from implanted instruments. In all, efferent nerves are intact (so that effects following their stimulation or blockade can be studied), and pacing can be applied if necessary; in many, afferent nerves are functional so that homeostatic reflexes may also come into play. Ventricular pressure (P)—rather than volume—measurements are taken (they need much less surgical interference) and differentiation of similar recordings to those shown in Fig. 10.10 allow *dP/dt* max to be used as a measure of maximum systolic activation.

Now return to Fig. 10.11. Along the 'normal' line, an increase in ventricular end-diastolic volume (VEDV) produces an enhanced contraction (A → B; Starling's law). This is analogous to the similar response in skeletal muscle and can most simply be rationalised as being due to the initial stretch making more actin and myosin combination sites available on activation—with an obvious limit (F) to this process when the strands become too separated (over-dilated heart). *Any change in the stroke volume which the cardiac muscle is able to achieve at any given VEDV is termed an inotropic effect.* Thus, B → C represents a positive inotropic effect (PIE) which could be induced, for example by adrenaline or digoxin. A suggestion has been made that A → B is also an inotropic effect: it could be considered a 'volume' inotropic effect, such as would be produced by adrenaline because of its venoconstrictor action increasing venous return (10.1). However, in the 'most physiological' whole heart preparations at constant heart rate, increased venous return (within limits) has a negligible effect upon dP/dt max; i.e. in the whole animal, 'volume' inotropic effects are largely neutralised by homeostatic mechanisms. Thus it is legitimate to define an inotropic effect (IE) as above.

10.9   Sympathomimetic actions on the heart
(For changes in automaticity *see* p. 279 *et seq.*)

General circulatory actions of representative catecholamines with respect to their influences on blood pressure are correlated in Table 10.4. The peripheral vessel responses have already been discussed (10.2) and the corresponding blood pressure changes designated. These have some important cardiac consequences. Due to the fact that noradrenaline produces a greater rise of blood pressure than an equal dose of adrenaline, it causes the greater reflex bradycardia so that noradrenaline actually *slows* the innervated heart. This, in turn, means

Table 10.4   Effects of noradrenaline, adrenaline and isoprenaline on the cardiovascular system (*see also* isoprenaline, Table 10.5)

	Noradrenaline	Adrenaline	Isoprenaline
Peripheral circulation			
Vasoconstriction (α)	+++	+++	0
Vasodilation (β_2)*	0	--†	----
Total peripheral resistance (at Y, Fig. 10.3)	+++	+	---
Heart			
Positive inotropic effect direct (β_1)‡	++	++	+++
Chronotropic effect direct, positive (β_1)‡	++	++	+++
reflex	---	-	+
net result	-	+	++++
Cardiac output	+	++	++++

Factors tending to raise blood pressure: ++++, very marked; +++, marked; ++, present; +, slight; 0, negligible.
Factors tending to lower blood pressure: ----, very marked; ---, marked; --, present; -, slight; 0, negligible.
* Coronary vasodilation undoubtedly occurs with all three catecholamines; however there is controversy over the exact contributions made by direct β_2-stimulation and 'relative myocardial ischaemia' due to increased heart work (*see* 10.10). But in all other vascular beds vasodilation with noradrenaline is negligible.
† Exceptions: most rabbits, chickens (10.2).
‡ Using isolated or denervated whole heart preparation: the direct positive inotropic effect threshold is just slightly below that for the direct positive chronotropic effect (Table 10.5)—but usually both actions occur together.

that noradrenaline has little effect upon the cardiac output in the whole animal, although its positive inotropic and chronotropic effects are about equal to those of adrenaline on isolated or other denervated preparations.

Antihypotensive therapy

Raising the foot of the *bed* to provide adequate cerebral circulation is a useful first-aid measure.

Broadly, low blood pressure may be due to a decrease in one or more of several factors

- *cardiac output* ('cardiogenic shock')—this requires specialised treatment depending on the cause, including dobutamine (*see* below)
- *circulating blood volume* ('hypovolaemic shock')—give cross-matched blood or other plasma-expanding fluids
- *peripheral resistance* ('peripheral circulatory failure')—this would appear to constitute a clear indication for a vasoconstrictor drug, but caution is necessary. In a severe case, there will probably already be maximal vasoconstriction (either neurally or hormonally mediated; *see* 5.11 for role of the latter in the genesis of 'irreversible' shock). The preferred drug at the moment is *dobutamine* (Fig. 10.13), given by i.v. infusion since it has a very short plasma half-life. This derivative of dopamine is mainly a β_1-adrenoceptor stimulant whose inotropic effect is stated to be greater than its chronotropic effect; this is useful, as tachycardia is already present. The divergence of cardiac actions could be due to different isoreceptors or less reuptake in the myocardial tissue than at the sinu-atrial node (which *has* more uptake$_1$ sites).

10.10 Coronary circulation: treatment of angina pectoris

The major determinants of coronary flow are

- *input hydrostatic pressure* (average usually taken as mean aortic blood pressure because most of the flow occurs during diastole due to passive factors, *see* below)
- *calibre of coronary resistance vessels* (depends principally on the interaction between passive and active factors).

Passive factors

The most important is the intramyocardial pressure which is so great during systole that it occludes vessels in the endocardial half of the myocardium: during diastole the balance is adjusted by a corresponding increase in the endocardial to epicardial flow-ratio. Heart rate is also important here by modifying diastolic filling time.

Active factors

1 *Neural or neurohumoral.* Cholinergic effects are minimal. Alpha-adrenoceptors which are vasoconstrictor are present in the larger vessels but the predominant sympathetic effect is vasodilation via β_2-adrenoceptors in all vessels (however, *see* below).

2   *Metabolic.* The cardiac muscle extraction of oxygen from the blood is normally very high with the result that, when the heart work increases, a relative hypoxia rapidly ensues. This, in turn, releases metabolites which cause local vasodilation thus restoring the balance between oxygen required and oxygen available. Adenosine and prostaglandins are the most likely endogenous vasodilators to be involved.

It is possible to separate these active factors experimentally but there is not general agreement regarding the findings. It is much more profitable to appreciate that

• *beta-adrenoceptor stimulants* all dilate coronary vessels (Table 10.4, footnote*) but are useless in angina pectoris because they simultaneously increase the cardiac oxygen requirement

• conversely, *β-adrenoceptor antagonists* are valuable in angina pectoris.

Angina pectoris is a spasmodic, suffocating attack accompanied by a midline chest pain which radiates down the left arm. It is due to a relative myocardial ischaemia caused by coronary atherosclerosis and/or spasm ('variant angina'—rare). It is often associated with exertion ('angina of effort') but in more severe cases can occur at rest (e.g. due to excitement). Primary angina (i.e. not secondary to other conditions, such as anaemia) is often associated with hypertension and is the common precursor of a myocardial infarct. Apart from changes in lifestyle—stop smoking (Table 2.5), lose weight (decreases heart work), gentle exercise (slight, gradual increase of heart work)—the mainstays of treatment are

• *glyceryl trinitrate* by sublingual administration (acts in about 2 minutes, lasts about 30 minutes) taken prophylactically just prior to possible precipitating causes or therapeutically at the onset of an attack. It can also be given by transdermal patch or skin ointment (slower but more prolonged action, p. 394). Longer-acting 'nitrites' (e.g. isosorbide dinitrate) are also used in prophylaxis.

• *beta-adrenoceptor antagonists* or *calcium channel blocking agents* taken regularly orally have a prophylactic effect.

'Nitrites'

This term encompasses all nitrites plus organic nitrates: type substance, glyceryl trinitrate (US: nitroglycerin). Their pharmacological actions are, almost exclusively, relaxation of smooth muscle—most probably due to activation of soluble guanylate cyclase resulting in increased cGMP with a consequent deficiency of calcium ions for excitation–contraction coupling (Fig. 10.5)—with a marked effect on blood vessels, capacitance and capillary more than resistance elements (Fig. 10.6). With glyceryl trinitrate, postural hypotension can occur. However, because the overall falls in diastolic and mean blood pressures are not too large, a satisfactory head of aortic pressure is maintained and there is insignificant reflex tachycardia.

The effective mechanisms of 'nitrite' actions in the relief of angina pectoris (*in relative order of importance*) are

1 Venodilation, decreasing the venous filling pressure (preload) of the heart—which, accordingly, has less work to perform.

2 Resistance vessel dilation (to a smaller degree) decreasing the arterial blood pressure (post- or afterload of the heart).

3 Coronary vessel vasodilation. Undoubtedly, this effect occurs in normal vessels. But it cannot take place in atherosclerotic vasculature, so it could only affect any *healthy* vessels remaining in the myocardium of the anginal patient. However, ischaemia-induced metabolites, such as adenosine, are already dilating some of these, namely the smaller resistance vessels. This accounts for the observation that, while dipyridamole (which prevents adenosine reuptake) can potentiate the coronary vasodilator effect of exogenous adenosine given to young animals (i.e. with normal vasculature), this drug is only weakly active in the anginal patient where maximum dilation of smaller resistance vessels in hypoxic areas has already been produced by the release of endogenous metabolites. 'Nitrites' *can* dilate any smaller resistance vessels which are unaffected by (remote from) ischaemia and larger (so-called 'conducting') healthy, collateral coronary vessels: the latter fact has been confirmed by radiography in anginal patients.

Side-effects of 'nitrites' are due to vasodilation in inappropriate situations and may cause headache (intra- and extracerebral vessels; relatively common) or flushing in 'blush areas' (menopausal females resent this). Tolerance to these effects usually develops on regular use.

Toxic effects are unlikely unless massive doses of conventional 'nitrites' are taken but may occur insidiously, e.g. if drinking water is contaminated by excessive use of nitrates as fertilisers. (Their conversion to carcinogens represents a long-term danger in this connection, p. 443.) A major manifestation of 'nitrite' overdose is *methaemoglobinaemia*. This is an overall oxidation produced by a complex series of reactions and results in a patient who is 'blue' and lacking in erythrocyte oxygen-carrying capacity. Methylene blue should be given to reduce the ferric to ferrous iron (p. 387).

Beta-blocking agents

Beta-blocking agents are used *prophylactically* in angina pectoris and may be considered to be beneficial by the following actions:

1 Decreasing sympathetic action on exertion (in 'angina of effort') or excitement (in 'angina at rest'). The bradycardia allows better coronary perfusion while the decrease in force of contraction lowers the myocardial oxygen requirement.

2 Increasing the endocardial: epicardial flow ratio during the prolonged diastole. This can be best understood by a realisation of the actions of isoprenaline under similar conditions. This drug, by massive, general dilation of coronary vessels diverts blood to the epicardial half of the myocardium during diastole (this is termed 'coronary steal') and the accompanying precipitate tachycardia (Table 10.4) radically curtails diastole: both represent counter-productive mechanisms in the selective perfusion of the endocardial half of the myocardium during diastole. Blockade of similar maleficent actions generated via endogenous sympathetic mechanisms is therefore helpful.

These agents also appear to be protective in patients who have survived acute myocardial infarctions.

Side-effects of β-adrenoceptor agonists are detailed in 3.5. Caution is necessary in incipient heart failure (especially if verapamil is also being given—*see* below).

The α- and β-blocker, labetalol, will additionally relieve any α-adrenoceptor-mediated coronary spasm.

Calcium channel blocking agents (4.11)
As shown in Table 4.8, all groups are used *prophylactically* in angina pectoris and the relevant beneficial actions (varying with each group) can involve
1 Resistance (and, to a lesser extent, capacitance) vessel dilation thus decreasing cardiac afterload (and preload).
2 Coronary artery dilation (if healthy) and especially if in spasm: therefore, particularly indicated in 'variant angina'.
3 Negative inotropy means less cardiac work with decreased oxygen requirement.
4 Bradycardia (*not* nifedipine) results in augmented coronary perfusion.

Side-effects of calcium channel blocking agents—see 4.11. *Note*: The combination of verapamil and a β-blocker is potentially very dangerous by the production of heart failure—exercise extreme caution.

10.11 The treatment of congestive heart failure
There are a number of different types of heart failure but one of the commonest involves inadequate contraction of either the right and/or the left ventricle with consequent systemic venous congestion, pulmonary oedema or a mixture of both. Modern treatment involves
• a *diuretic*. This is mandatory and frusemide which is potent and rapidly-acting (given i.v. if necessary) is used. This removes sodium chloride and water from the extracellular fluid, thus relieving the oedema and taking excessive strain off the heart by decreasing the circulating blood volume. In addition its venodilator effect is valuable in acute pulmonary oedema. *See* Table 12.4 and accompanying text

- a *vasodilator* is commonly added to lessen heart work by resistance and/or capacitance vessel dilation
- a *positive inotropic agent* may additionally be required to strengthen the cardiac contraction. The classical medicament for stimulation of cardiac contraction is *digoxin*. The complex cardiac actions of this drug (arranged numerically, 1 → 4 to indicate low → high dose effects), which is the type substance of the cardiac glycosides, are shown in Table 10.5.

It is agreed that the positive inotropic effect is caused by an increase in activator (free, intracellular) Ca^{2+} ions. A likely genesis is shown in Fig. 10.12. Digoxin competes for the attachment site of potassium ions on the outer surface of the Na^+, K^+-activated ATPase so that the 'pump' is blocked. This leads to a significant increase in sodium ion concentration within the cell which activates a sodium–calcium exchange mechanism (this operates in either direction depending on intra- and extracellular concentrations of the relevant cations) to bring calcium ions into the cell. Thus, there is more excitation–contraction coupling at the same end-diastolic volume, i.e. a positive inotropic effect. This hypothesis is supported by much of the available evidence. The objection that *at low concentrations* (which, however, are sufficient to produce some positive inotropy) digoxin *stimulates* the 'sodium pump' (4.8) may be valid and would require an alternative explanation. Suggestions are: increased slow inward current (Fig. 10.14), enhanced trigger calcium release (Fig. 10.9) and decreased calcium sequestration (Fig. 10.9). Digoxin is only useful therapeutically at relatively high concentrations where the major mechanism is probably the one shown in Fig. 10.12. In the same diagram note that, *because of the much higher intracellular concentration of K^+* than Na^+ ions, a significant decrease in internal potassium ions, will only occur (as a 'late' effect, Fig. 10.12) when digoxin is used in high dosage (Table 10.5, toxic effect 4b and *see* p. 283). *See also* cumulation, p. 434.

As just stated, to be effective in uncomplicated heart failure, *digoxin* has to be given to near-toxic levels. These are recognised clinically (Table 10.5) by excessive slowing (pulse below 55 beats per minute) and *occasional* ventricular extrasystoles (a coupled beat is a normal beat followed by an extrasystole) with anorexia, nausea and vomiting (Fig. 13.1), diarrhoea and visual disturbances (18.4) often prominent. Thus, this drug has been replaced by frusemide ± a vasodilator as an initial measure. However, it is valuable when *atrial flutter or fibrillation* complicates the heart failure. Then the chief beneficial effect is to protect the ventricles from the erratic atrial beat by conduction blockade (Table 10.5, actions 3a and 3b, shown by increased PR interval) and the contraction is also strengthened (action 1); however, the atrial situation is worsened (flutter can progress to fibrillation, by action 4a which is accordingly given a minus sign in the table) and

Table 10.5 Comparison of the effects of digoxin, acetylcholine, isoprenaline and lignocaine on the four main facets of heart action, with the important relevant ionic changes *on their right*. How these responses contribute to their major cardiac indications and toxic effects. Numbers indicate usual order of appearance as drug concentration is increased

Heart action	Digoxin		Acetylcholine		Isoprenaline		Lignocaine (US: lidocaine)	
inotropic effect	1. Positive	$Ca_i^{2+}\uparrow$	2. Negative	$\downarrow i_{Ca}$	1. Positive	$\uparrow i_{Ca}$	3. Negative	$\downarrow i_{Na}$
chronotropic effect	2. Negative†		1. Negative	$\downarrow i_{Ca}$	2. Positive‡	$\uparrow i_{Ca}$		
conduction	3a. Slows at atrio-ventricular node* 3b. Slows in His–Purkinje system		3. Slows at atrio-ventricular node	$\uparrow i_K$	4. Quickens—only if greatly depressed	$\uparrow i_K$	2. Slows particularly in His–Purkinje system	$\downarrow i_{Na}$
automaticity	4a. Increases atrial† 4b. Increases ventricular	$Ca_i^{2+}\uparrow\uparrow$ $K_i^+\downarrow$	4. Increases atrial	$\uparrow i_K$	3. Increases in His–Purkinje fibres, especially if dominant (sinus) pacemaker of heart is concomitantly slowed (*see* text)		1. Depresses in ectopic ventricular foci more than in sinu-atrial node	
Indications	Atrial flutter or fibrillation: 3a + 3b + 1 − 4a Cardiac failure: 1 ± 2				Stokes–Adams attacks: 4		Ventricular tachycardia or ectopic beats: 1	
Toxic effects on the heart	Excessive slowing: 2 + 3 Ventricular extrasystoles (coupled beats): 4b		Excessive slowing, even stoppage: 1		Ventricular tachycardia or extrasystoles: 3		Atrioventricular block	

↑↑, increased excessively; ↑, increased: ↓, decreased. For each current (i), *see* 10.12. Subscript 'i' indicates *internal* ionic concentration (as in Fig. 10.12). For digoxin:

* Indicates reflex or direct central effect acting via the efferent vagus.

† Ditto but possible additional action directly on the heart.

‡ *See* footnote to Table 10.4.

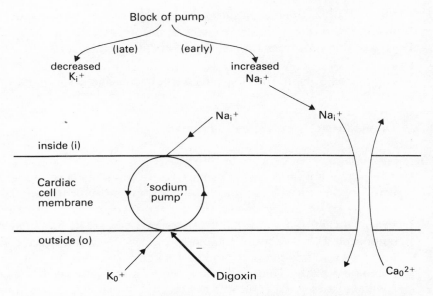

Fig. 10.12 A mechanism whereby digoxin could produce a positive inotropic effect (*see* text). Exact ratios of cations exchanged are not indicated. $-$, inhibition.

requires subsequent treatment. In uncomplicated heart failure, the positive inotropic effect is the major action but it may be accompanied by slowing (± 2 in Table 10.5, Indications), especially if the beat is initially rapid. This bradycardia is probably mainly reflex by removal of capacitance volume reflexes (Table 10.1) as the venous congestion is relieved.

The poor therapeutic range of digoxin has encouraged attempts to find a better positive inotropic agent. Many of these drugs (some in the latest stages of their clinical trials) are inhibitors of phosphodiesterase III but with an additional property which can be
- *either* vasodilation (which might be their main mechanism in the relief of congestive heart failure), e.g. milrinone
- *or* enhanced response of the myofibrils to the combination of calcium ions with troponin C (p. 262): 'calcium sensitisers', e.g. pimobendan.

Adrenoceptors involved in the human positive inotropic response
In pathological myocardia excised from heart transplant patients, the ratio of $\beta_1 : \beta_2$ receptors in different cardiac areas is at least $2:1$ with even fewer α-receptors. But all these mediate positive inotropy (Fig. 10.13): β_1- and β_2- via increased cAMP; α- by phosphatidylinositol disphosphate hydrolysis. In chronic heart failure there is down-regulation of β_1-receptors (due to increased sympathetic outflow, Table 10.1) and less response to phosphodiesterase inhibitors. This suggests

the use of α_1-adrenoceptor agonists, e.g. phenylephrine but their maximum positive inotropic effect is, unfortunately, very small (only 10% of that of isoprenaline on human papillary muscle).

A synopsis of major mechanisms of inotropic changes is given in Fig. 10.13.

10.12 Drugs affecting cardiac rate and rhythm

Physiological basis

The cardiac action potential in 'pacemaker' tissues (shown in Fig. 10.8) is redrawn in Fig. 10.14 with the major ionic movements expressed as currents (i) occurring during the defined phases 0, 1–4, Table 10.6. First, consult 8.2 for ionic currents in nerve. The heart is more complicated as it requires the plateau (phase 2) to introduce calcium ions for excitation-coupling and also requires rhythmicity ('pacemaker potential', phase 4). In addition the voltage-operated K^+ channel characteristics (1–3, Table 4.9) are much more complex than in nerve.

The major ionic currents activated and inactivated during the various stages of cardiac action are shown in Table 10.6 and the resultant effects as manifested in Fig. 10.14 will now be particularised.

Resting potential

This is maintained by the background current, i_{K_1} ('inward rectifier', Table 4.9, 3).

Phase 0. The rising phase of the action potential in the *His–Purkinje* fibre tracing (Fig. 10.14, left) is, for an initial depolarisation of about 40–50 mV, dependent upon i_{Na}, and this determines the speed of conduction because, the more rapid the rate of rise, the greater (and more extensive) the local circuit activation external to the fibre and, therefore, the faster the impulse conduction rate. Inactivation of i_{K_1} also occurs on depolarisation. The 'slow inward current' (i_{si}) also termed i_{Ca} as it is mainly carried by calcium ions (via L channels, 4.10) is present during the later stages of the His–Purkinje rising phase. *This current is the predominant phase 0 mechanism in sinu-atrial and atrioventricular nodal tissues* (Fig. 10.14, right).

Phase 1. The 'overshoot' (A, Fig 10.14) is followed by a slight repolarisation due to a *t*ransient *o*utward potassium current (i_{to}, Table 4.9, 2). At the same time i_{Na} has inactivated (Table 10.6).

Phase 2. The plateau is maintained by the i_{si} (i_{Ca}) which is now opposed by the delayed rectifier i_K (Table 4.9, 1) which is *inwardly* rectifying. This means that it is relatively weak at less negative (i.e. plateau)

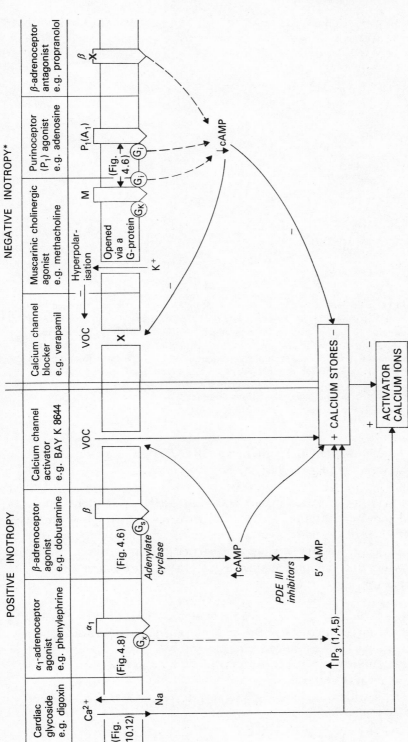

Fig. 10.13 Inotropic mechanisms. VOC, voltage-operated (calcium) channels; PDE III, phosphodiesterase III. For routes connected with guanine nucleotide-binding regulatory proteins: G_s and G_i, see Fig. 4.6; G_x, see Fig. 4.8. ↑, +, increased; ↓, −, decreased. Interrupted lines indicate multiple stage processes; all lines indicate excitatory actions unless accompanied by a minus sign (inhibitory). **X**, sites of blocking effects. * in whole preparations: in isolated preparations will only be significant if either i_{Ca} or cAMP is increased first. *See also* negative inotropy produced by potassium channel openers (p. 259)

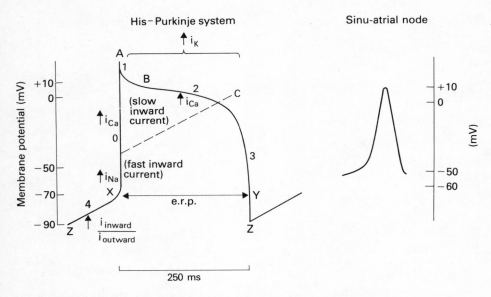

Fig. 10.14 Important ionic movements in relation to the cardiac action potential in 'pacemaker' tissues. i, ionic current across the tissue membrane. Sodium (Na^+) and calcium (Ca^{2+}) ions are passing inwards; potassium (K^+) ions are going outwards. At the sinu-atrial node (*and atrioventricular node*) the action potential is much more dependent on i_{Ca} (i_{si}, period of importance delineated by interrupted line) than on i_{Na}. ↑, increased; Z, maximum diastolic potential; X, threshold; X ↔ Y, effective refractory period (e.r.p.); ZX, pacemaker potential (phase 4); XA, rising phase (phase O); A, overshoot; AB, slight immediate repolarisation (phase 1); BC, plateau (phase 2); CZ, repolarisation (phase 3).

potentials and, therefore, provides a safety margin as less i_{si} is necessary to maintain the plateau (*see* Fig. 10.15).

Phase 3. Repolarisation occurs because i_{si} inactivates about ten times more rapidly (footnote, Table 10.6) than i_K—which, also, decreases relatively little (initially) as more negative potentials are reached (due to inward rectification). This phase is carried to completion to reach the maximum diastolic potential (Z, Fig. 10.14) by the activation of i_{K_1} as this point is approached.

Phase 4. The slow diastolic depolarisation (as indicated in Fig. 10.14) results from an increase in the ratio inward current/outward current. Over the pacemaker range (-90 to -50 mV) there are a number of background currents (e.g. i_{K_1}, Table 4.9, 3) but the main currents which are significantly varying are
- inactivation of i_K (and i_{K_1}), giving a decrease in outward current
- activation of i_{si}

Table 10.6 Ionic currents (i; Na^+ and Ca^{2+} inwards, K^+ outwards) present during the resting potential and the various phases of the cardiac action potential

Phase number		i_{K1}	i_{Na}	$i_{si}(i_{Ca,L})^*$	$i_{to}(K^+)^\dagger$	i_K
	Resting potential‡	+				
0	Rising phase					
	early ('fast inward current')	−	+			
	later ('slow inward current')			+	+	
1	Slight immediate repolarisation		−	+	+	
2	Plateau			+		+‖
3	Repolarisation					
	early			−§		+‖
	late	+				
4	Pacemaker potential ('slow diastolic depolarisation')	at more negative potentials (−)				−§
		at less negative potentials		+		

+, activation; −, inactivation; (−), inactivation but significance doubtful.

* i_{si} mainly consists of current via calcium L(ong) channels—4.10, which are activated by BAY K 8644 or β-adrenoceptor agonists and closed by calcium channel blockers or β-adrenoceptor antagonists (as shown in Fig. 10.13).

† i_{to} is a *t*ransient *o*utward current carried by potassium ions (Table 4.9, 2).

‡ Resting potential in non-pacemaker tissues: usually termed maximum diastolic potential (Z, Fig. 10.14) in pacemaker tissues.

§ Time constants of inactivation (vary with tissue and voltage): i_{si}, *c.* 20–100 ms; i_K, *c.* 200–1000 ms.

‖ *See* Fig. 10.15.

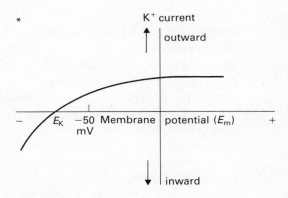

Fig. 10.15 Current–voltage relationship for a potassium current (E_K − 70 mV) showing inward (-going) rectification. The channels act as rectifiers passing inward better than outward current. Therefore, as E_m becomes less negative, there is relatively less increase in i_K.

- activation of i_f (see later).

Both these latter activations give an increase in inward current.

Inactivation of the delayed rectifier current (i_K) *generated by the immediately preceding action potential* has a time constant *c.* 500 ms in Fig. 10.14 and, therefore, is certainly occurring over the pacemaker potential time range.

Activation of i_{si} (mainly $i_{Ca,L}$) is most marked over the less negative part of the pacemaker potential range.

The inactivation of the potassium current predominates in *His–Purkinje tissue*. At the *sinu-atrial and atrioventricular nodes* it also produces the early part of the pacemaker potential but i_{si} becomes important in the later stages ($i_{Ca, T(ransient)}$ can link these two stages but is not essential: activated *c.* -65mV and rapidly inactivated—4.10). The so-called 'calcium' (slow inward current-mediated) action potential (Fig. 10.14, right) has a slower rising phase and, thus, a slower conduction rate across nodal tissues.

An inward current i_f (carried by both Na^+ and K^+ ions) is activated over the whole pacemaker range (-50 to -90 mV) and is considered by some workers to modulate the i_K and $i_{Ca,L}$ effects on the slow diastolic depolarisation.

Sympathomimetic and parasympathomimetic agents

Let us now compare the effects of sympathomimetic and parasympath-omimetic agents on the heart, especially in relation to the underlying mechanisms involved. It must be stressed that some of the effects obtained at higher concentrations are produced by exogenous applica-tion of the drugs and cannot occur following relevant nerve stimulation. Table 10.5 shows actions of isoprenaline (preferred to adrenaline here because of its cardiac indication) and of acetylcholine (because many of the actions of digoxin are vagally mediated, *see* Table 10.5, footnotes). The influx of calcium ions induced by the catecholamines (10.7) satisfactorily accounts for their positive inotropic effect (Fig. 10.13) and positive chronotropic effect (increased i_{Ca} at sinu-atrial node): the dysrhythmic action will be discussed in 10.13. Acetylcholine elicits its characteristic bradycardia by decreasing i_{Ca} at the sinu-atrial node: it also decreases i_f. When perfused through a Langendorff heart prepara-tion, acetylcholine produces a negative inotropic effect (due to decreased i_{Ca}) at a lower concentration than the slowing, but this is less significant on vagal stimulation in the whole animal (therefore designat-ed 2, in Table 10.5). (For conduction and dysrhythmic changes, *see* next section.)

A pathological note. Infarction, inflammation or other damage to the heart often results in some myocardial fibres (e.g. those adjoining an infarcted area) becoming partially depolarised (probably for several reasons—loss of intracellular potassium ions by hypoxic 'sodium pump' failure is a manifest possibility) so that they become more dependent on 'calcium' action potentials with a resultant loss in conduction velocity and a greater liability to develop dysrhythmias (*see* next section, under refractory period protractors). Release of and increased sensitivity to noradrenaline is also reported, together with pH fall (CO_2 and lactic acid accumulation)—these are further dysrhythmogenic factors.

10.13 Dysrhythmic and antidysrhythmic actions produced by drugs

Automaticity may be defined as the ability to generate an impulse spontaneously. For this to occur, the tissue must be at (or close to) threshold (X, Fig. 10.14) at a time outside its refractory period. There are a number of differently measured refractory periods but a convenient one is the 'effective refractory period' shown in Fig. 10.14. One important point to remember is that, *provided the shape of the action potential does not change markedly* (e.g. develop a slow repolarisation phase, Fig. 10.16b) the width of the action potential (say at 75%

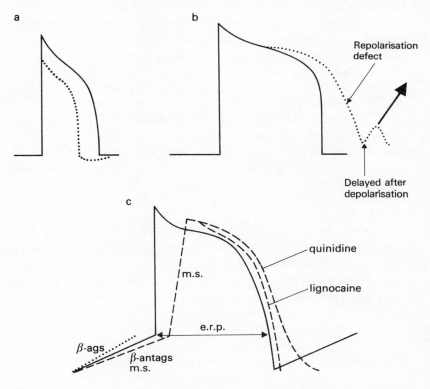

Fig. 10.16 The effects of dysrhythmic (dotted lines) and antidysrhythmic drugs (interrupted lines) on various cardiac action potentials (continuous lines show control responses). a, atrial muscle: effect of acetylcholine or digoxin; b, ventricular muscle: effect of digoxin: for significance of large arrow, *see* text.; c, Purkinje fibre: effects of β-agonists (β-ags) and β-antagonists (β-antags) compared with those of membrane stabilisers (m.s.). Lignocaine marginally shortens the the action potential duration (APD). Quinidine increases APD and the effective refractory period.

repolarisation) can usually be taken as an appropriate measure of refractory period (more refined techniques are used by specialists). Further, it must be appreciated that the refractory period is only *one* factor in automaticity and not necessarily the major one. For example, the very important antidysrhythmic agent, lignocaine, in fact slightly decreases the action potential duration (Fig.10.16c) but this apparent disadvantage is overshadowed by its beneficial actions.

A classification of antidysrhythmic and dysrhythmic effects produced by different drugs is shown in Table 10.7 and will be discussed under the *antidysrhythmic class headings. Most antidysrhythmic drugs have effects in more than one category* but are mentioned here under their major property.

Class I: sodium channel blockers
Their action results in a slower rising phase of the action potential but they also slow the rate of rise of the pacemaker potential in the His–Purkinje system. The subtypes 1A, 1B (lignocaine) and 1C (the latter not shown in Table 10.7) represent groups in which, additionally, the action potential duration is increased, decreased or negligibly altered.

Now, go through the actions of lignocaine shown in Table 10.5.
1   The major action of this drug is to decrease i_{Na} (local anaesthetic effect, 8.2): it slows the rate of rise both of the pacemaker potential and the rising phase of the action potential in *ventricular* foci (Fig. 10.16c). As the sinu-atrial node mainly depends upon a 'calcium' action potential, lignocaine has a preferential effect upon the ectopic focus which allows the predominance of sinus rhythm to be reinstated.
2   Slowing of conduction from atria to ventricles only occurs with high doses of the drug unless the system is already depressed. It may, therefore, exacerbate atrioventricular block and is not used in atrial dysrhythmias.
3   The negative inotropic effect is extremely weak and could only occur therapeutically if an overdose was given intravenously. Care is necessary because lignocaine (when used as an antidysrhythmic) *is* given by this route (taken orally, it has a high, 'first pass' hepatic inactivation)— as a bolus injection followed by continuous infusion—which could also lead to CNS effects (excitement first, depression later).

Class II: β-adrenoceptor antagonists
Beta-agonists increase the rate of rise of the pacemaker potential in the His–Purkinje system (Fig. 10.16c) which generates *ventricular* extrasystoles (isoprenaline, action 3, Table 10.5) and in excessive dosage can lead to ventricular tachycardia and fibrillation.

Such ectopic beats are particularly likely to occur if the sinu-atrial node is simultaneously depressed, as it is (reflexly) with noradrenaline in the whole animal (Table 10.4). However, all these substances can

Table 10.7 A classification of antidysrhythmic and dysrhythmogenic mechanisms.

	Antidysrhythmic					Dysrhythmogenic	
Class	Description	Drug example(s)	Reference	Parameter		Drug example(s)	Reference(s)
I	Membrane stabilisers			i_{Na}	→		
A	Also ↑APD	Quinidine*	Fig. 10.16c				
B	Also ↓APD	Lignocaine Phenytoin†	Fig. 10.16c				
II	β-Adrenoceptor antagonists	Propranolol	Fig. 10.16c	Rate of rise of pacemaker potential	↓ →	β-Adrenoceptor agonist, e.g. isoprenaline on His–Purkinje system ↑	Table 10.5 (action 3); Fig. 10.16c
III	Refractory period protractors	Amiodarone Quinidine		Effective refractory period	↑ →	Digoxin } on atrial muscle Acetylcholine }	Table 10.5, 4a Fig. 10.16a Table 10.5, 4
IV	Calcium channel blocking agents	Verapamil		Calcium ion entry	↓ →	Digoxin on ventricular muscle ↑	Table 10.5, 4b; Fig. 10.16b
	Digoxin (in atrial flutter or fibrillation)			Conduction in AV node and bundle of His	→		

↑, increased; ↓, decreased. APD, action potential duration.
* Quinidine was the original antidysrhythmic drug. It has some dangerous cardiac side-effects (e.g. myocardial depression; paradoxically, ventricular tachycardia) but is still, carefully, used.
† Main use in digoxin toxicity (*see* text)

induce ventricular dysrhythmias, therefore avoid intravenous use. Halothane (Table 8.7) also slows the dominant pacemaker and can potentiate dysrhythmogenic effects of circulating catecholamines.

The β-agonists increase the rate of rise of the pacemaker potential by enhancing the appropriate events described on pp. 276–8 viz. inactivation of i_K and activation of $i_{Ca,L}$ (and/or i_f): these effects are opposed by β-adrenoceptor antagonists. Many β-blockers also have 'membrane stabilising' activity (Table 3.4) but *see* p. 86.

Class III: refractory period protractors

Dysrhythmias in this category are usually *re-entrant* phenomena. Re-entry circuits (Fig. 10.17) become common under pathological conditions and are exacerbated by shortening of the refractory period and/or slowing of conduction. The increased atrial automaticity caused by acetylcholine is, like that of digoxin (action 4a, Table 10.5), due to increased i_K which produces the action potential change illustrated in Fig. 10.16a, namely attenuated rising phase (resulting in lower conduction velocity) and more rapid repolarisation (with slight hyperpolarisation), resulting in decreased refractory period. These are good conditions for re-entry which is also helped by the concomitant negative chronotropic effect of both agents, which lessens pacemaker predominance.

There are many antidysrhythmic drugs which increase the refractory period (e.g. all Class 1A) but the type substance is usually taken to be *amiodarone*. This is not a good choice as it also has Class 1 properties and can act as a non-competitive α and β-adrenoceptor blocker (Class II). It has some unusual side-effects. The molecule contains an iodine atom which results in multiple interactions with thyroxine function such that either hypo-or hyperthyroidism can ensue. Amiodarone antagonises the action of phospholipase A_2 which, clinically, can cause

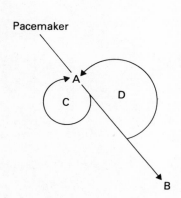

Pacemaker

Fig. 10.17 Re-entry processes in cardiac muscle. The arrow AB represents the pacemaker-generated impulse taking its orderly course. C and D show possible re-entry circuits (normally ineffectual because A is refractory) which can reactivate A prematurely if its refractory period is less than the time taken to pass via either C or D to A, i.e. if refractory period < (length of circuit/velocity of conduction) and if the next pacemaker-generated impulse has not yet reached A.

phospholipid accumulation (*see* Fig. 4.7) in nerve, lung tissue, liver, skin or eye (the corneal microdeposits, which may partly contain the drug or a metabolite, are harmless and disappear on cessation of therapy). *See also* surfactant (p. 296) and phototoxicity (Table 18.3).

Class IV: calcium channel blocking agents
Verapamil is the type substance. These drugs are obviously most useful in the treatment of dysrhythmias involving overaction of calcium channels, e.g. sinu-atrial or atrioventricular nodal tachycardias, e.g. pathological situations (p. 278) which have resulted in depolarisation of heart muscle so that ectopic foci are mainly dependent on the 'slow inward' current (*see also* digoxin toxicity, next).

Ventricular toxicity caused by digoxin (action 4b, Table 10.5) has been extensively studied. Two major factors are involved, namely
• *calcium 'overload'.* The positive inotropic effect of digoxin is due to Ca^{2+} ion entry into the cell (Fig. 10.12) which directly or via release from intracellular stores (Fig. 10.13) increases activator calcium which is subsequently sequestered (returned to the stores). However, excess of the drug—and, remember, the therapeutic range is narrow—will result in a calcium 'overload' and the exaggeration of the above effects. Specifically there ensues an oscillatory Ca^{2+} ion release from intracellular stores which produces *both* a direct stimulatory action on the contractile actin–myosin system which causes additional 'after contractions' *and* a transient inward current across the myocardial cell membrane resulting in a delayed after depolarisation (Fig. 10.16b) which can produce a propagated action potential (with associated subsequent cardiac muscle contraction) if the threshold potential is attained (large arrow in figure)
• *a fall in potassium ion concentration.* If this occurs generally in the body, the toxic effects of digoxin on the ventricular muscle are enhanced (e.g. frusemide *plus* digoxin, p. 434). However, the fall in K^+ ion concentration, produced at high cardiac glycoside concentrations *by the drug itself,* is *in*side the myocardial cell (Fig. 10.12) so that the K^+ ion gradient across the membrane falls and, therefore, less i_K will pass on opening the channel gates. Thus, a '*repolarisation defect*' occurs (Fig. 10.16b) which means that there is an increased likelihood of the delayed after depolarisation reaching the threshold potential (*see* above) *outside the refractory period.* Additionally, there is recent evidence that a decrease in internal K^+ ion concentration can increase the transient inward current induced by calcium overload.

Antidysrhythmic therapy in digoxin toxicity involves
1 The passage of more potassium ions into the cell by the administration of
• potassium chloride (Table 12.6): also competes with digoxin for attachment to the 'sodium pump' (Fig. 10.12)

- phenytoin: stimulates the 'sodium pump' (more potassium passes inwards) and exerts a positive inotropic effect—*see* low doses of digoxin (10.11). It is also a membrane stabililiser
- glucagon produces a hyperglycaemia which releases insulin; this, in turn, causes potassium ions to enter cells (p. 345). Glucagon is also positively inotropic (p. 112).

2 The prevention of calcium ion entry into the cell with, e.g., verapamil.

3 In severe poisoning, purified Fab fragments of digoxin-specific antibodies are available: expensive and only available in a few centres as yet.

Note the *anti*dysrhythmic action of digoxin in atrial flutter or fibrillation by blocking atrioventricular conduction (Tables 10.5 and 10.7).

Envoi
Nowadays electrical stimulation (electroversion) is commonly used in *hospital* practice to procure normal (sinus) rhythm but even so antidysrhythmic drugs are still useful prophylactically or subsequently to maintain the eurhythmic state.

11 Respiratory System

11.1 Pharmacokinetic considerations

Route of administration
Inhalation is limited to gases, vapours or finely suspended particles (p. 14), which all produce *rapid* effects
• locally, e.g. inhalations for bronchial asthma—salbutamol, sodium cromoglycate or beclomethasone. With the latter low concentrations are effective and, even if some of the drug is swallowed, it is not absorbed (Table 14.2) so that systemic side-effects are minimised although husky voice is common and local opportunistic infections (e.g. candidosis) may be precipitated
• systemically. The maintenance of general anaesthesia (8.6).
For intranasal absorption of a peptide *see* desmopressin (p. 310).

Metabolism
Pulmonary changes may produce (5.6)
• activation, e.g. the conversion of angiotensin I to angiotensin II
• inactivation, e.g. the breakdown of prostaglandins, 5-hydroxytryptamine, or bradykinin.

Excretion
The respiratory tract is an extremely important route for excretion of gaseous or volatile general anaesthetics (1.8) but it can also be significant for other drugs (e.g. iodide expectorants, 11.9).

11.2 Effects of drugs upon the tracheobronchial smooth muscle
While, therapeutically, the emphasis relates to the *terminal* bronchioles (bronchial asthma), methods are available to examine drug actions upon any part of the system, e.g. perfused tracheal smooth muscle. In practice the major pharmacological techniques determine the *overall* resistance of the respiratory pathways (Table 11.1). Using the unanaesthetised *guinea-pig* preparation, it can be shown that propranolol increases pulmonary airway resistance, implying that sympathetic bronchodilator tone is normally present and acting via β-adrenoceptors; whereas atropine does not affect the resistance, indicating a lack of parasympathetic, bronchoconstrictor tone. In *human* airways smooth

Table 11.1   Methods used to measure changes in bronchial calibre

$$\frac{1}{Calibre} \propto Resistance = \frac{Pressure\ (recorded\ at\ inflow\ site)}{Flow}$$

Experimental preparation	Pressure divided by	Flow equals	Resistance
Frog lung perfused with isotonic saline from reservoir at constant height*	Constant	Measure	Calculated
Konzett–Rössler method: anaesthetised guinea-pig on artificial respiration which is giving constant inflow to the lungs	Measure	Constant	Calculated
Unanaesthetised guinea-pig breathing spontaneously	Measure†	Measure†	Calculated

* This preparation, with scissor cuts in the dependent parts of the lungs to allow outflow of fluid (which is measured) may appear to be a crude variation of normal airway function but it is, nevertheless, capable of detecting acetylcholine (causing bronchoconstriction) down to 10^{-12} molar: compare with contraction of guinea-pig ileum, which is sensitive to a lower limit of 10^{-9} molar.
† At equal volumes during inspiration and expiration when the elastic elements are stretched to equal lengths.

muscle, the situation shown in Fig. 11.1 applies—i.e. the vagi co-release acetylcholine which is bronchoconstrictor via muscarinic receptors and a non-adrenergic non-cholinergic transmitter (? vasoactive intestinal peptide, VIP) which is bronchodilator—*except that there is little direct sympathetic innervation to the smaller airways.* However, like animal preparations, the human tissues dilate in response to circulating catecholamines and β_2-adrenoceptor agonists.

The direct effects of other bronchoactive agents—which are broadly similar in animals and humans—are shown in Fig. 11.1. The additional effects (1–3) mentioned in the figure legend have not been confirmed in the human but could explain

• the well known dangers of β-adrenoceptor antagonists in asthmatic patients (3.5)
• the use of atropine-like drugs in bronchial asthma treatment.

11.3 Bronchoconstrictor substances
These are important in

Experimental pharmacology
As just stated, in *guinea-pigs* the bronchodilator is stronger than the bronchoconstrictor tone, i.e. the pathways are normally relatively relaxed. Under such conditions, to show significant bronchodilation, it is necessary first to decrease the calibre of the airways with a

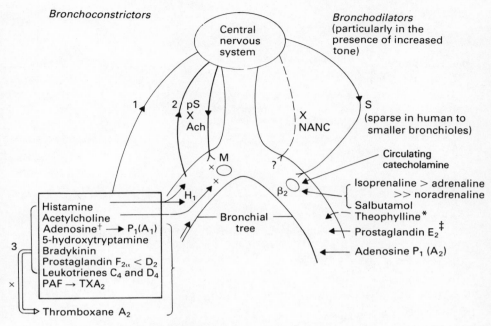

Bronchoconstrictors

Bronchodilators
(particularly in the
presence of increased
tone)

Fig. 11.1 Bronchoconstrictors (left) and bronchodilators (right). All agents shown probably act via specific receptors (not all indicated), e.g. M, muscarinic; H_1, histamine; β_2, adrenergic; *see* p. 290 for possible mechanism(s) of action; †contraction only significant in asthmatic patients, bronchodilator effect via P_1 (A_2)-purinoceptors — *also see* Table 5.8 — predominates in most animal experiments. ‡can produce bronchoconstriction in low tone preparations (*see* p. 290). pS, parasympathetic (X, vagus; ACh, acetylcholine); NANC, non-adrenergic non-cholinergic transmitter; ?, unknown receptor; S, sympathetic innervation; TX, thromboxane. Additional effects, *shown in animal preparations*, are as follows. 1. All bronchoconstrictor agents tested so far, reflexly produce some compensatory bronchodilation via β_2-adrenoceptors. 2. Histamine activates lung irritant ('cough') receptors situated in the epithelia of the larger passages and the intrapulmonary bronchioles which, reflexly, cause hyperpnoea and cholinergic bronchoconstriction (? in an attempt to expel the irritant substance by a strong current of air through narowed channels). 3. Histamine and the leukotrienes C_4 and D_4 can liberate thromboxane A_2 by a process blocked by atropine. x, atropine-sensitive mechanisms, PAF, platelet activating factor, and bradykinin also liberate TXA_2.

bronchoconstrictor. Commonly employed drugs are methacholine (which has the disadvantage of hypotension with bradycardia, 2.4), histamine or 5-hydroxytryptamine (both of which show different changes in blood pressure depending on the species, 5.5).

Pathological situations
These include malignant carcinoid syndrome (liberation of 5-hydroxytryptamine and bradykinin, 5.6) and bronchial asthma (Fig. 11.2).

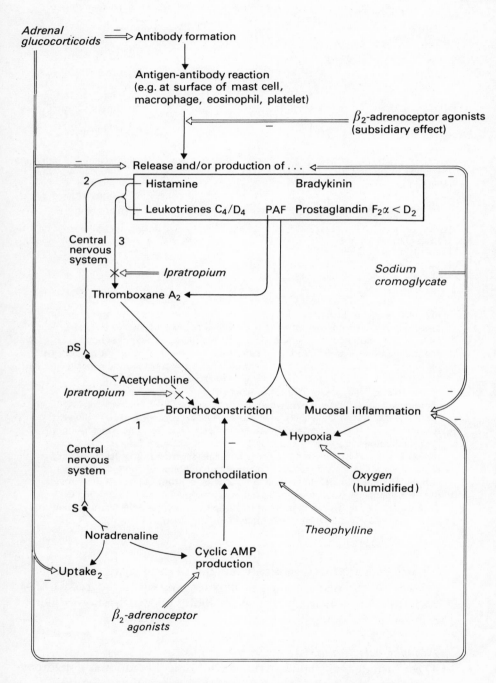

Fig. 11.2 Major sites of action of drugs (italicised) useful in the treatment of bronchial asthma. −, inhibition. Figures and symbols as Fig. 11.1.

Toxicology/pathology

In anticholinesterase poisoning (2.6) the lethal bronchial actions of cholinergic constriction accompanied by an increase in secretions are reversed by atropine. This bronchodilator drug is less useful in asthma as it tends to *thicken* bronchial mucus but it also blocks constrictor effects mediated via lung irritant receptors and thromboxane A_2 generation (2 and 3, Fig. 11.1 legend). Ipratropium is presently the preferred antimuscarinic drug (11.5).

11.4 Bronchodilator drugs

These are of paramount value in bronchial asthma and in bronchospasm (commonly associated with chronic bronchitis).

The main group is the β_2-sympathomimetic agonists so that isoprenaline > adrenaline ≫ noradrenaline. The latter is, therefore, insignificant therapeutically as a bronchodilator, although it is the transmitter activating the innervated β_2-adrenoceptors shown in Fig. 11.1. The major disadvantage of isoprenaline and adrenaline is that, by simultaneous activation of β_1-adrenoceptors, they cause a quickening and more forcible action of the heart which is undesirable. Thus, their use has been replaced by that of selective β_2-agonists, type substance, salbutamol (Ventolin®; US: albuterol). A further advantage of the latter lies in its longer duration of effect. Isoprenaline (Table 3.2) is not removed by uptake₁ and, following extraneuronal uptake (uptake₂), it is resistant to monoamine oxidase but susceptible to catechol-O-methyl transferase. As salbutamol is neither a substrate for monoamine oxidase nor a catecholamine, it is more persistent. The relevant properties of similar drugs used in the treatment of bronchial asthma are shown in Table 11.2. It is important to appreciate that substances such as salbutamol are β_2-*selective not* β_2-specific; in other words higher

Table 11.2 Beta-sympathomimetic substances which have been used in the treatment of bronchial asthma

Drug	β_2-Adrenoceptor selectivity	Breakdown by catechol-O-methyl transferase	Relative duration of action
Isoprenaline	0	+	Short
Orciprenaline (US: metaproterenol)	0	0	Long
Salbutamol (US: albuterol)	+	0	Long
Terbutaline	+	0	Long
Rimiterol	+	+	Short

+, present; 0, absent.

concentrations will affect the heart. This side-effect is obviously minimised if the drug is administered locally by inhalation.

Theophylline (as the compound, aminophylline) is a useful broncho-dilator. Beta$_2$-adrenoceptor-activated bronchodilation (like β_1-adreno-ceptor-activated cardiac actions) is mediated via cyclic AMP. A characteristic effect of theophylline is to prevent the breakdown of this second messenger by phosphodiesterase III but at therapeutic plasma concentrations this effect is minimal. Alternative suggestions (compare p. 235) include antagonism of adenosine on P$_1$ (A$_1$) receptors (Fig. 11.1) and *de*crease in activator Ca^{2+} ions.

The effects of bronchoactive substances depend on the initial tone present in the system. Therefore, *bronchodilators* are more effective in the presence of a higher tone: in fact, PGE$_2$ can *contract* airways smooth muscle if the initial tone is low (Fig. 11.1). Conversely, *bronchoconstric-tors* (e.g. methacholine, histamine, 5-hydroxytryptamine) produce increased responses
• in low tone preparations (? natural tonic influence absent)
• after epithelial removal (? due to loss of epithelium-derived relaxing factor(s))
• after indomethacin pretreatment (effect reversible by PGE$_2$).

The latter observations have led to the suggestion that PGE$_2$ could be one endothelium derived factor regulating airways smooth muscle tone.

11.5   The treatment of bronchial asthma (Fig. 11.2)
This condition is characterised by spasmodic attacks of bronchocon-striction which result in hypoxic hypoxia (11.6) and are usually exacerbated by concomitant local vasodilation and inflammation. It often has an immunological basis but anti-(H$_1$) histamines are not normally useful because of the involvement of other autacoids. Clinic-ally important drugs act under one or more of the following headings.

Functional antagonists
Beta$_2$-adrenoceptor agonists (Table 11.2). These are the most important agents used therapeutically, i.e. to abort or treat an asthmatic attack. They produce marked bronchodilation via increased cyclic AMP—an effect which (5.3) also *subsidiarily* results in decreased release of substances important in the genesis of bronchial asthma: also decreased capillary permeability (Table 5.4). Salbutamol—given by inhalation (preferably), orally, s.c., i.m. or i.v.—is a most valuable agent producing minimal cardiac stimulation and, rarely, muscle tremor (β_2, Table 2.3).

Theophylline. This is particularly indicated in
• nocturnal asthma (as a sustained release preparation, orally)

• status asthmaticus. While waiting for the adrenal glucocorticoid to produce its relief (see later), the bronchodilator effect of theophylline (given i.v. as aminophylline) is useful.

Muscarinic antagonists. Herbal preparations containing atropine and related substances have a long history in the treatment of asthma but fell into disrepute because they tend to thicken bronchial secretions. A more recent drug, ipratropium (isopropyl atropine, given as an aerosol) is mainly indicated in chronic bronchitis.

Adrenal glucocorticoids, e.g. beclomethasone

As shown in Fig. 11.2, these have multiple sites of action. They decrease

• antibody formation (longer term)
• release of asthmatic mediators
• bradykinin, eicosanoid and PAF formation, i.e. are anti-inflammatory (5.17)
• uptake$_2$: thereby potentiating the effects of naturally released adrenaline and noradrenaline.

They are indicated specifically in

• status asthmaticus (acute severe asthma) e.g. attacks unrelieved by maximal β_2-adrenoceptor therapy. They take a few hours to be effective, during which time the patient must be sustained with aminophylline and oxygen therapy
• severe repeated episodes. Beclomethasone (by inhalation—thus minimising systemic side-effects) is the treatment of choice but can lead to candidal superinfection of the respiratory tract. If systemic usage is necessary, the dose of glucocorticoid must be rapidly reduced to below that producing significant side-effects (14.2).

Prophylaxis

Sodium cromoglycate (Intal®; US: cromolyn). This is useful prophylactically not only in allergic asthma but also against other types (e.g. exercise-induced asthma). It is inhaled as a dispersed powder which may activate lung irritant receptors (2, Figs. 11.1, 11.2) to cause bronchoconstriction: in this case precede with a salbutamol inhalation to induce functional bronchodilation. Sodium cromoglycate is an important preventive agent (especially for children) and in severe, chronic cases allows the dosage of adrenal glucocorticosteroids to be reduced to a level producing insignificant side-effects.

The original 'mast cell stabilisation theory' for cromoglycate action is now untenable but the drug is 'anti-inflammatory' in asthma probably by several effects including lessened generation of inflammatory agents and antagonism of inflammatory responses especially the prevention of increased 'capillary' permeability.

Symptomatic relief

The paramount deficiency is hypoxic hypoxia and the provision of oxygen—humidified, to keep secretions fluid—is essential in severe acute asthma.

A note for the future

Many of the processes involved in bronchial asthma, e.g. mast cell degranulation, smooth muscle contraction and inflammation, require calcium ions as intermediate messengers. *Calcium channel-blocking drugs*, e.g. nifedipine or *potassium channel openers*, e.g. cromakalim (p. 259) can antagonise histamine-induced bronchospasm.

11.6   Oxygen therapy

Lack of oxygen (hypoxia) is divisible into:

1 Hypoxic hypoxia: insufficient oxygen enters the blood, e.g. by prevention of air passage into the alveoli, as in bronchial asthma.

2 Hypoxaemic hypoxia: lack of oxygen contained in the blood. The two main categories are

• anaemia. Treat as such (17.1)

• carbon monoxide poisoning. This gas is produced by incomplete combustion of carbonaceous compounds, e.g. petrol (exhaust fumes) or household contents (buildings on fire). It combines avidly (*c.* 200 times more than O_2) with haemoglobin—thus displacing oxygen—a process which must be reversed, once the victim has been removed from the scene of the catastrophe, by the provision of maximum oxygen.

3 Ischaemic (stagnant) hypoxia: although the blood contains sufficient oxygen, there is a tissue deficiency of the gas because the blood supply to the tissue is inadequate, e.g. myocardial infarction.

4 Histotoxic hypoxia: oxygen is available to the tissues but cannot be used because of, e.g., cyanide poisoning of the cytochrome oxidase system: give hydroxocobalamin or dicobalt edetate (Table 20.5).

Normally, inspiring air (*c.* 21% O_2), the oxygen content of arterial blood (19–20 cm^3 per 100 ml fluid, 19–20 vol %) is predominantly in the form of oxyhaemoglobin (over 95% saturated) with only about 0.3 vol % in simple solution. Therefore, when the oxygen concentration in the inspired air is increased, the amount of oxyhaemoglobin will only be marginally raised and the main gain will be in the dissolved element—to the extent of 2.2 vol % per atmosphere of pressure (i.e. the solubility of O_2 in blood at 37 °C). There are *three* types of oxygen therapy.

1 *High-pressure* (hyperbaric) use necessitates special chambers within which the patient is subjected to 2–3 atmospheres pressure, thus increasing the dissolved arterial oxygen to 4.4–6.6 vol %. This method is not commonly used but may be life-saving in a severe anaerobic infection (e.g. gas gangrene) to inhibit organismal growth.

2 *High-concentration* (high-level) administration is the usual tech-

nique. It involves oxygen delivery via a face-mask or nasal catheters (more comfortable) to bring the inspired concentration to 35–60%, a satisfactory level in bronchial asthma, barbiturate poisoning (9.6), or myocardial infarction. Downward adjustment may be made as improvement occurs.

3 *Low-concentration* (low-level) oxygen. In chronic bronchitis, prolonged hypoxia leads to a situation where arterial PO_2 is low and arterial PCO_2 high; the chemoreceptors become acclimatised to the raised CO_2 tension so that respiration is dependent on the hypoxic drive via the *peripheral* chemoreceptors (Fig. 11.3). To provide adequate tissue oxygenation, especially during acute exacerbations of the disease, additional oxygen is required but its use must be tempered to allow spontaneous respiration to continue and to avoid carbon dioxide narcosis (11.7). This is satisfactorily achieved by the prolonged inhalation of 24–28% oxygen in air by means of a special mask. Due to the *steepness* of the oxygen dissociation curves at low arterial PO_2 a small rise in alveolar PO_2 and hence arterial PO_2 (insufficient to remove the hypoxic drive) will result in a substantial increase in arterial oxygen content (for tissue usage).

Deleterious effects of oxygen therapy are infrequent. They can be systematised as follows
• prolonged 40% usage in premature babies (suffering from a lack of surfactant) can result in retrolental fibroplasia
• over 60% for more than 12 hours. Respiratory irritation and infection; pulmonary atelectasis (due to absorption of oxygen distal to an obstruction); 'popping' of the ears (Eustachian tube occlusion); headache (nasal sinus blockage)
• two atmospheres for greater than 6 hours or three atmospheres for longer than 2 hours may produce the effects described above, often accompanied by central nervous system manifestations varying from twitching of limbs and paraesthesiae (in milder cases) to convulsions.
In poisoning with hyperbaric oxygen, there is inhibition of some of the enzymes which break down glutamate so that this transmitter collects, producing fits and a concomitant increase in the blood ammonia (Fig. 6.3). Experimentally, lithium salts antagonise the convulsions, possibly by combination with ammonium ions.

Similar effects can occur during deep-sea diving and must be avoided by diluting the oxygen content of the inspired air. The obvious choice, nitrogen, is dangerous because it is relatively soluble in body fluids and, on too rapid decompression, causes gaseous emboli ('the bends' if into joints; 'the chokes' if into the respiratory tract or its control systems). A preferable diluent is *helium*, which has a low aqueous solubility: it is also of low density so that it can be used in some types of upper respiratory obstruction as a helium-oxygen mixture is easier to breathe than either air or pure oxygen.

11.7   Respiratory stimulants
Carbon dioxide is the natural agent (via both central and peripheral chemoreceptors) and, as such, is already acting in many cases of respiratory depression (an important exception is chronic bronchitis, 11.6). Given as carbogen (5–7% CO_2—air contains *c*. 0.04%—in oxygen) it will

- increase respiratory depth and rate. It was once used in carbon monoxide poisoning to increase ventilation and thus allow (by simultaneously administered oxygen) quicker dissociation of the carboxyhaemoglobin. This is now achieved by the use of respiratory pumps without the production of respiratory acidosis (*see* below)
- produce an ambivalent effect upon the blood pressure—the CNS stimulant effects on the cardiovascular centres being opposed by a negative inotropic effect and overall (direct) peripheral vasodilation. So, it is hypotensive in patients with CNS depression.

The administration of higher (10% or greater) concentrations of carbon dioxide or the retention of this gas by respiratory depression causes a respiratory acidosis and, if prolonged, can result in CO_2 narcosis, characterised by headache, dizziness and mental confusion. Carbon dioxide still has a few specialised uses in anaesthesiology and to produce acidosis (by rebreathing) in alkalotic tetany (p. 372).

Other respiratory stimulants. Respiratory depression caused by poisoning is most efficiently reversed by the use of specific antagonists (e.g. naloxone in the treatment of opiate overdosage, 7.12). Functional antagonists (e.g. picrotoxin which stimulates the respiratory centres) were once used in barbiturate poisoning (for modern treatment, *see* p. 237). Uncommonly, respiratory stimulants (e.g. doxapram, p. 234) are useful as temporary measures in the chronic bronchitic to allow occasional relief from continuous oxygen therapy.

11.8   Effects of drugs on CNS respiratory control
These are illustrated in Fig. 11.3 and allow the student to revise many of the actions mentioned previously.

11.9   Effects of drugs on tracheobronchial secretions
A cough may be unproductive or productive.

Unproductive: the cough is an irritant nuisance causing, for example, loss of sleep: suppression is indicated. Opiate receptor agonists act in the L-configuration both as analgesics and antitussives (anti-cough agents). If they are converted to the D-isomers, they lose their pain-relieving effect but retain their antitussive action. Thus, *dextro*methorphan is a potent agent in this connection. Other useful antitussives are codeine and diamorphine. The latter is a very effective agent but must

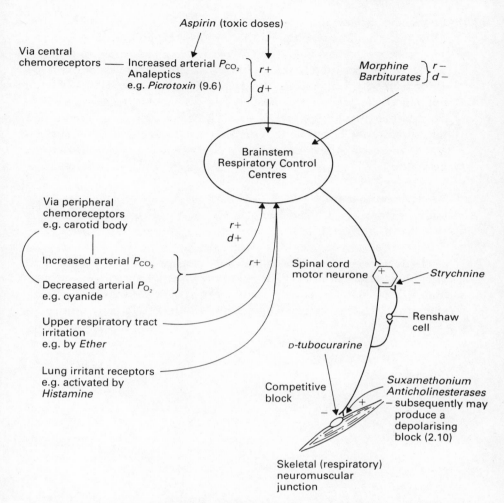

Fig. 11.3 Some drug actions (italicised) modifying (+, increasing; −, decreasing) the rate (*r*) and/or depth (*d*) of breathing.

be prescribed with care because of its severe dependence-producing liability.

Productive, i.e. the cough results in the expulsion of phlegm from the system. This beneficial event may be improved by the use of an *expectorant* such as potassium iodide which is excreted by the bronchial mucosa and simultaneously increases its secretions. In a tenacious situation, *mucolytics* decrease sputum viscosity by cleaving mucopolysaccharides (bromhexine) or mucoproteins (acetylcysteine). Inhalations of steam containing menthol or eucalyptus are valuable both to encourage cough and to aid in the liquefaction of sinusitic accretions.

11.10 Pulmonary surfactant

This fluid contains a complex mixture of phospholipids and proteins which are synthesised in alveolar Type II cells and secreted in response to an increased tidal volume or sympathetic stimulation (via β_2-adrenoceptors). Amiodarone by decreasing phospholipase A_2 activity not only causes pulmonary phospholipidosis but also interferes with the synthesis of dipalmitoyl phosphatidylcholine which is a major surface tension-lowering constituent of surfactant. Thus a less effective surfactant is secreted which can cause respiratory distress syndrome in neonates.

11.11 Nasal decongestants

Sodium cromoglycate and beclomethasone (11.5) are used in allergic rhinitis. In 'stuffy nose', sympathomimetic agents, e.g. ephedrine (Table 3.2) can be applied locally to constrict the mucosal vessels by an α-adrenoceptor effect. Repeated use can produce tolerance and 'rebound' vasodilation. (?β_2-adrenoceptor-mediated, as with adrenaline, 10.2). The latter is uncommon with *systemic* agents, e.g. *pseudo*-ephedrine (a stereoisomer of ephedrine with less CNS penetration).

12 Drugs and Renal Function

12.1 Pharmacokinetic considerations

Metabolism. A specific function occurring in the kidney is the activation of vitamin D (16.2). The juxtaglomerular apparatus is the source of renin which produces angiotensin I by enzymatic breakdown of a plasma α_2-globulin derivative (Fig. 5.5).

Excretion. The renal tract is the major route of removal of drugs and their metabolites from the plasma. The principles involved are explained in 1.1 and some variations indicated in 1.10.

12.2 Ions, body fluids: control of composition

A *labile* ion (Table 12.1) is a charged particle which can be converted to a negligibly charged form in the body, e.g.

$$H^+ + HCO_3^- \rightleftharpoons H_2CO_3 \rightleftharpoons H_2O + CO_2$$

Because of the availability of such mechanisms both in intracellular and in extracellular compartments:
1 Almost immediate stabilisation of pH ('buffering') is possible.
2 The buffer capacity can be restored
• rapidly via the lungs (variations in CO_2 removal)
• more slowly via the kidney (all ions shown in Table 12.1) An important corollary is the use of these processes to alter the pH of the urine (12.10).

A *fixed* ion is always present in the fully dissociated form and so its ionic content in the body cannot be adjusted by any metabolic manipulation. Accordingly, control of deficient or plethoric states *ultimately* depends on the appropriate modifications in input and/or output—as classified in Table 12.6.

Fixed ion contents of potassium and sodium are intimately involved with intra- and extracellular fluid volumes, respectively, and are of vital importance for the maintenance of corporeal isotonic conditions, membrane charges and passage (co-transport) of important metabolites (e.g. glucose) across cellular barriers. Adequate control of these 'internal environments' is essential to life. Intracellular changes are usually reflected in extracellular fluid variations which are constantly being monitored with respect to

Table 12.1 Fixed and labile ions. Labile ions can be converted to molecules which are insignificantly ionised, thereby allowing buffering in the body tissues and restoration of buffer capacity by the appropriate excretion of salts in the urine (lower table)

	Fixed	Labile	
		Fully ionised form	Weakly ionised form
Cation	Na^+	NH_4^+	Urea (via ornithine cycle)
	K^+	H^+	H_2O
Anion	Cl^-	HCO_3^-	CO_2
		PO_4^{3-}*	Organically combined, e.g. with glucose, adenosine

* Alters body buffer capacity by changes in the ratio NaH_2PO_4/Na_2HPO_4 in the urine (*see* below).

Buffer content of urine

	Under alkalotic conditions	Under acidotic conditions
Sodium bicarbonate	High	Low*
Sodium dihydrogen phosphate / Disodium hydrogen phosphate	Lower (e.g. 10:1)	Higher (e.g. 50:1)
Ammonium chloride†	Negligible	High

* Achieved (in stages) by Na^+ ion absorption in exchange for an H^+ ion, which, then (by the reaction shown in 12.2) forms CO_2 in the tubular lumen. The CO_2 is next absorbed to form HCO_3^- in the plasma, i.e. (overall) $NaHCO_3$ has been absorbed.
† Ammonia (produced from L-glutamic acid, Fig. 6.3, or glutamine) is secreted by the distal tubule and combines with H^+ ions in the lumen to produce ammonium ions, thus sparing the excretion of fixed cations with the chloride anion.

- volume
- pressure (blood; hydrostatic or osmotic)
- sodium and/or potassium ion concentration(s).
  Subsequent major executive processes (*which are closely integrated*) to correct imbalances are
- the renin–angiotensin–aldosterone system
- vasopressin (antidiuretic hormone, ADH)
- atrial natriuretic peptides (also diuretic).

12.3 Removal of water and ions via the kidney

A *diuretic* is a substance which produces an increased flow of urine. This is useful to flush out injurious agents (e.g. forced diuresis with mannitol, 20.8; e.g. extra water intake during cyclophosphamide therapy to dilute irritant metabolites, p. 411) or to prevent crystallisation of a naturally excreted compound in the urinary tract (e.g. drink plenty of water during treatment of gout with uricosurics, 12.8).

A *saluretic* is a type of diuretic which, in addition to water, results in significant loss of 'salts' (in particular sodium, usually combined with chloride) from the body; this is a prerequisite in the major use of 'diuretics', namely the treatment of oedema (cardiac, renal or hepatic).

Action
Primary sites of action are divisible into extrarenal and renal.

Extrarenal diuretics. Water taken orally is absorbed from the gut and lowers the osmotic pressure of the plasma. This, via the hypothalamo-pituitary axis, inhibits the release of ADH—thus resulting in less reabsorption of water from the fluid in the distal tubules and collecting ducts of the kidney (Fig. 12.1). Ethanol-containing liquors, in addition to their aqueous content, also inhibit vasopressin secretion directly.

Extrarenal saluretics. Digoxin, in heart failure associated with atrial fibrillation (10.11), raises cardiac output thereby relieving venous congestion in the renal circulation and, possibly, increasing glomerular filtration rate, so that less retention of salts (particularly sodium chloride) and water takes place.

Renal
Glomerular. Methylxanthines (e.g. theophylline) can increase renal blood flow and hence the glomerular filtration rate (determined by an inulin clearance test); however, even here, the weak diuretic effect is mainly tubular in origin (*see* Table 12.2, footnote).

Tubular. All the important diuretics act by tubular mechanisms. The physiological background is depicted in Fig. 12.1.
• *Tubular diuretics.* Mannitol is the type substance for the *osmotic diuretics*. It is filtered freely at the glomerulus and not reabsorbed to any appreciable degree by the renal tubular cells. It therefore retains an isosmotic equivalent of water at all sites of passive reabsorption of the latter (namely proximal convoluted tubule, descending loop of Henle and collecting duct). Due to this disturbance of renal function, secondary changes produce an increase in electrolyte loss but this is not enough in most forms of oedema fluid. Mannitol can be given (by i.v. infusion) to produce a forced diuresis (p. 445) and in acute cerebral oedema.
• *Tubular saluretics.* These are the prime agents used to achieve the appreciable *salt* and water loss which is essential in the treatment of the common types of oedema. They all act by increasing the total amount of fixed ions in the tubular fluid which, in turn, osmotically raises urinary

water output. Analysis of the urine produced at maximum diuresis (Table 12.2) shows that saluretics differ in the volume, ionic spectrum and pH of excreted fluid which they produce—making them apposite in particular circumstances. Some important means whereby these variations are achieved are discussed in the next section but it must be emphasised that *overall effects are commonly multifactorial and, in many cases, still not fully elucidated.*

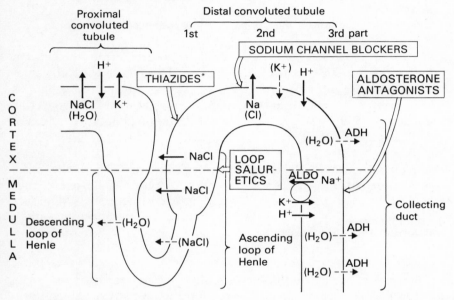

Fig. 12.1 Major ionic and water exchanges along the renal tubule. Active, e.g. Na ──▶ ; passive, e.g. (Na) --▶ : hormonal control (ALDO = aldosterone; ADH = antidiuretic hormone). Clinically used drugs act at sites shown.* *See* footnote, Table 12.3.

	Movements *in relation to tubular fluid*				
	Outward			Inward	Outward/inward
Site	Na^+	Cl^-	Water	H^{+*}	K^+
Proximal convoluted tubule	+	+	(+)	+	+ (out)
Descending loop of Henle			(+)		
Ascending loop of Henle					
thin segment	(+)	(+)			
thick segment	+	+			
Distal convoluted tubule	+	(+)		+	(+)(in)
Collecting duct	+†		(+)§	+	+(in)‡

+, present, active; (+) if passive. * Dependent upon (*see* text) acid–base balance of body fluids and carbonic anhydrase function. Under the control of † aldosterone; ‡ possibly aldosterone; § antidiuretic hormone (vasopressin). Carbon dioxide and ammonia exchanges (mentioned in footnotes to Table 12.1, lower) are not shown.

Table 12.2　Some properties of saluretics (schematic)

Group	Representative drug(s)	Relative potency*	Urinary concentration of ion at maximum diuresis†				pH of urine‡	Main site(s) of action
			Na^+	Cl^-	K^+	HCO_3^-		
Potassium-losing								
'High-ceiling' ('loop')	Frusemide, Bumetanide, Ethacrynic acid	+++	+++	+++	0	0	6	Medullary and cortical segments of thick, ascending loop of Henle (TAL)
Thiazides§	Chlorothiazide, Bendrofluzide	++	+++	+++	+	+	7.5	Cortical segment of TAL ‖ / Early distal convoluted tubule ‖
Carbonic anhydrase inhibitors¶	Acetazolamide	+	+	0	++	+++	8	Proximal and distal convoluted tubule
Potassium-sparing								
Sodium channel blockers	Amiloride, Triamterene	+	+++	++	−	+	7	*Later* distal convoluted tubule
Aldosterone antagonists	Spironolactone	+	+++	++	−	+	7	Collecting duct

* Relative potency (maximum rate of urine production possible); +++, strong; ++, moderate: +, weak.

† Urinary ion concentrations (compared to control values): +++, large increase; ++, moderate increase; +, small increase; 0, negligible change; −, decrease.

‡ To nearest 0.5 unit.

§ Strictly, benzothiodiazides.

‖ *See* footnote*, Table 12.3.

¶ Never used as saluretics (*see* text). Neither is theophylline: potency, weak; pH and ionic content of urine similar to frusemide.

12.4   Mechanisms of tubular saluretic action

The main sites are shown in Fig. 12.1.

Effects upon the thick, ascending loop of Henle

These are shown by changes in 'free-water production' as illustrated in Fig. 12.2. This relates the total clearances of all osmotically active molecules in the urine to the corresponding urine volumes in the presence of the saluretic under two different experimental conditions of the subject—dehydrated and highly hydrated. The 'free-water production' is defined as the amount of distilled water which must be added to (dehydrated subject: negative 'free water production', $T^c_{H_2O}$) or subtracted from (hydrated subject: positive free water production, C_{H_2O}) the

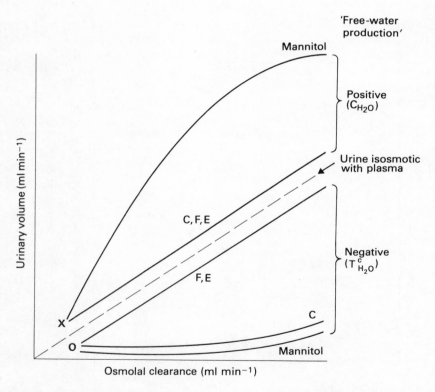

Fig. 12.2 Effects of representative diuretics on 'free-water production'. Lines— origin O—*below* the isosmotic (interrupted) line were obtained when the subject's water intake had been restricted and indicate the ability to *concentrate* urine (negative 'free-water production'; old terminology, $T^c_{H_2O}$). Lines—origin X—*above* the isosmotic line were obtained when the subject's water intake had been large and are indicative of the ability to *dilute* urine (positive 'free-water production'; old terminology, C_{H_2O}). C, chlorothiazide; E, ethacrynic acid; F, frusemide. For conclusions *see* Table 12.3.

Table 12.3   Interpretation of 'free-water production' data

Inability to	Shown by inhibition of	Indicates action on thick, ascending loop of Henle	By mannitol	By frusemide, ethacrynic acid	By chlorothiazide
Concentrate urine	Negative 'free-water production'	Medullary segment	0	+	0
Dilute urine	Positive 'free-water production'	Cortical segment*	0	+	+

+, present; 0, absent.
* Functionally it is difficult to separate this cortical segment from the *first* part of the distal tubule. Therefore, many workers consider that thiazides *mainly act on the early distal tubule.*

urine to render it isosmotic with plasma. Inhibitions of these processes (Table 12.3) are considered to represent actions upon the thick, ascending loop of Henle—medullary and cortical segments, respectively. The 'high-ceiling' ('loop') diuretics (frusemide, ethacrynic acid) are carboxylic acids and, accordingly, secreted into the proximal convoluted tubular fluid (*see* Fig. 1.5,c). They exert their major actions upon both segments of the thick, ascending loop. Thiazides are amphoteric and similarly secreted but have to pass further along before they are capable of effective action upon the cortical segment (*see* footnote, Table 12.3). Due to their proximal tubular secretion, all these drugs can interfere with uric acid excretion and precipitate an attack of gout (12.8).

Effects upon the distal convoluted tubule and the thick, ascending loop of Henle
Might be analogous to those which occur in the toad bladder or frog skin. These amphibians lack distal renal tubules, so that essential salts are reabsorbed from (toad) the bladder lumen or (frog) the external environment (e.g. pond). If amphibian results can be transferred to mammalian renal pharmacology—a bold assumption—the situation might be as envisaged in Fig. 12.3. From the lumen, sodium ions (either via an NaCl symport* or alone, passively) cross a sodium-permselective membrane along a concentration gradient which is maintained by the presence of an active sodium–potassium exchange pump, located on the non-luminal side of the cell. In the frog-skin preparation, the pores on

*In co-transport systems, the transport of one substance must be accompanied by the simultaneous or sequential transport of one or more other substances. The mechanism is termed a *symport* if all are passing in the same direction across the membrane: an *antiport* if substances are crossing in opposite directions.

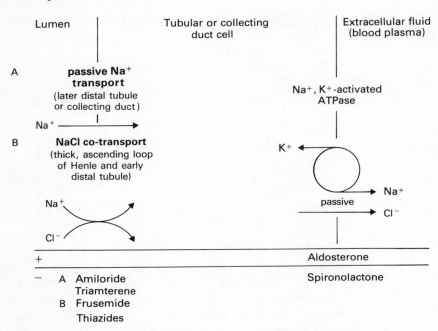

Fig. 12.3 One simplified model for sodium ion reabsorption in the distal convoluted tubule, collecting duct or thick, ascending loop of Henle of the mammalian kidney. Putative agonists $(+)$ and antagonists $(-)$ of the passive and active components of the system are shown.

the external surface of the membrane (equivalent to mammalian renal luminal surface) are closed by amiloride and triamterence (both contain 'guanidine moieties', like tetrodotoxin which also blocks Na^+ ion channels, p. 216). Recent evidence suggests that the 'loop' diuretics and thiazides are only effective when applied to the luminal surface of the appropriate tubular membrane, i.e. they inhibit the NaCl symport.

Aldosterone induces synthesis of 'sodium pump' protein—a process which takes several hours—so that its actions and those of its antagonist, spironolactone, are not immediate. The active process on the non-luminal side of the cell also appears to be dependent upon the intermediation of cyclic AMP. It has been shown *in vitro* that this is inhibited by saluretics acting as analogues of cyclic AMP (frusemide, thiazides) or antagonists of adenylate cyclase (ethacrynic acid). However, there is no correlation between the diuretic effects of these agents and their inhibition of either the 'sodium pump' or cyclic AMP activity.

A specific effect upon such widely distributed mechanisms as those shown in Fig. 12.3 could be due to the renal concentration of these drugs. This is vividly exemplified by the fact that digoxin—a potent blocker of the 'sodium pump' at higher concentrations (4.8)—exerts its diuretic action by circulatory improvements (12.3). But following injection into the renal artery in experimental animals, it has a direct diuretic effect on the kidney tubules.

Carbonic anhydrase inhibition
The reaction sequence

$$H_2O + CO_2 \overset{\textcircled{1}}{\rightleftharpoons} H_2CO_3 \rightleftharpoons H^+ + HCO_3^-$$

is catalysed (at the molecular stage, ①) by the enzyme, carbonic anhydrase, to produce hydrogen ions. In acidotic conditions these are exchanged for sodium ions and thus allow the changes in buffer content of urine which are specified in Table 12.1 (lower). Enzyme inhibition particularly results in increased sodium bicarbonate content of the incipient urine entering the distal tubule. Here, where normally Na^+ ion reabsorption is balanced by cationic H^+ plus K^+ ion secretion (Fig. 12.1), the lack of hydrogen ions results in a greater loss of potassium. Thus, the characteristic urinary ion spectrum of a carbonic anhydrase inhibitor (type substance, acetazolamide, Table 12.2) is a large increase in bicarbonate ion excretion associated mainly with extra K^+ loss. This might account in part for the enhanced potassium bicarbonate content of the urine produced by thiazides, as they have some carbonic anhydrase inhibitory activity.

It is instructive to consider why acetazolamide is no longer used as a saluretic. It is too weak, it has the wrong ionic spectrum (K^+ rather than Na^+ is excreted) and it is self-limiting. Excretion of such an alkaline urine causes a systemic acidosis which results in the series of reactions depicted above, proceeding in the *absence* of enzyme function. Therefore, sodium bicarbonate is reabsorbed and the saluretic effect lost. Acetazolamide is used in glaucoma (18.1).

12.5 Saluretics used in clinical practice
These are most conveniently divided (Table 12.2) into
- potassium-losing ('high-ceiling', thiazides)
- potassium-sparing (sodium channel blockers, aldosterone antagonists).

'High-ceiling' ('loop') and thiazide saluretics
Salient properties are compared in Table 12.4. The additional action of 'loop' saluretics on the medullary segment of the thick, ascending loop of Henle (Table 12.3) increases their relative potency (by diminishing the counter current osmotic gradient which is further depleted by an increase in medullary blood flow) and makes them indispensable in many conditions (e.g. heart failure, p. 270; forced diuresis, p. 445). They are even effective in chronic renal failure, when the glomerular

Table 12.4 Comparison of the pharmacological properties of chlorothiazide with those of frusemide

	Chlorothiazide	Frusemide (US: furosemide)*	
Saluretic action	Moderate	'High-ceiling'	
Route of administration	Oral	Oral	i.v.
Time of onset (minutes)	60	30–peak 60	10–peak 30
Side-effects:			
hypokalaemia (Table 12.5)	+	+	As oral *plus*
hyponatraemia (Table 12.5)	+†	+†	dehydration,
precipitation of gout (12.8)	+	+	urinary
hyperglycaemia (p. 350)	+	(+)	(prostatic)
allergic manifestations	(+)	(+)	retention,
(most common, rash)			deafness (rare)
Other uses		Congestive heart failure	
	Hypertension (10.5)	Hypertension associated with chronic renal failure; acute pulmonary oedema	
	Nephrogenic diabetes insipidus (12.7)	Forced diuresis	
		Hyperkalaemia (12.6)	
	Hypercalciuria (16.4)	Hypercalcaemia (Table 16.3)	

Side-effects: +, can occur; (+), uncommon.
* Bumetanide: similar to frusemide *plus* can cause myalgia.
† Especially in elderly patients.

filtration rate is greatly diminished. If a milder action is required, frusemide is preferable to ethacrynic acid as its less steep dose–response curve (Fig. 12.4) makes it easier to select an appropriate dose. This is important because a torrential saluresis may result in hypovolaemia, hyponatraemia (Table 12.5) or other effects shown in Table 12.4.

When thiazides are employed as saluretics, *potassium supplements* may be required—given as the chloride (in slow-release or effervescent form as too rapid, local release gives ileal ulceration). While the 'high-ceiling' diuretics produce less excretion of K^+ ions *per ml* of urine than the thiazides (Table 12.2), they may also necessitate potassium supplements (12.6), especially if used in higher dosage or with digoxin (p. 283), for two reasons:

1 The much larger volume of urine.

2 Greater sodium and water depletion will activate the renin–angiotensin–aldosterone system more and enhance K^+ ion loss into the collecting ducts; this is not limitless however as angiotensin II 'feeds back' to decrease renin release (p. 137). Additionally, frusemide (but not bumetanide in equi-diuretic dose) releases renin.

To reinforce the point that frusemide causes urinary potassium loss, remember that this drug is useful in hyperkalaemia (12.6).

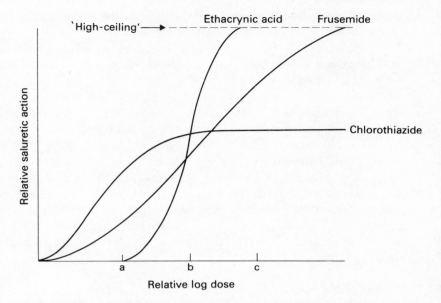

Fig. 12.4 Dose–response curves for ethacrynic acid, frusemide and chlorothiazide (diagrammatic). Relative doses: a, low; b, medium; c, high.

Saluretics can modify the excretion of elemental cations other than those already mentioned. Calcium ion excretion is increased by frusemide and decreased by thiazides: thus indicating subsidiary uses shown in Table 12.4. Magnesium depletion can occur with frusemide or thiazides.

In the treatment of mild-to-moderate essential hypertension (10.5) thiazides are first-line drugs and achieve their action by a combination of saluretic and direct vasodilator properties. Frusemide appears to have less vasodilator activity in relation to saluretic effect but is extremely useful when an antihypertensive action is required in chronic renal failure, or in acute pulmonary oedema where its vasodilation has been shown to produce relief even in the absence of a diuresis (e.g. in patients undergoing dialysis).

Finally, it must be stressed that all these saluretics are most valuable drugs with minimal side-effects.

Potassium-sparing saluretics
Sodium channel blockers. Their main site of action is the distal tubule where they close sodium channels on the luminal surface of the membrane (Figs. 12.1 and 12.3). They are weaker than the 'high-ceiling' diuretics and thiazides with which they are often given in combination because:

1   Their actions tend to be compensated by the activation of more

proximal physiological mechanisms which will be prevented by drugs acting on the thick, ascending loop of Henle.

2   They balance the potassium-losing effects of the latter agents.

Their main side-effect is potassium retention. Amiloride or triamterene is usually given.

Aldosterone antagonists (type substance, spironolactone—a structural analogue of the hormone) are specifically indicated when there are excessive aldosterone plasma levels for example Conn's syndrome (primary hyperaldosteronism) or hepatic cirrhosis (lack of breakdown of the hormone due to decreased liver function). They also potentiate the saluretic actions of frusemide and thiazides by blockade of aldosterone-mediated compensatory mechanisms (*see* earlier). Side-effects are uncommon but, due to a chemical similarity to sex hormones, include imbalances such as (male) gynaecomastia and (female) hirsutism.

12.6   Control of Na^+ and K^+ ion concentrations in body fluids

Illustrative drugs and other important factors which alter the plasma concentrations of these ions are shown in Table 12.5. As explained in 12.2, control must finally be achieved by alterations in input or output. Available methods are shown in Table 12.6. Most of the drug actions

Table 12.5   Some important factors modifying plasma concentrations of sodium or potassium ions

Genesis	Hyponatraemia	Hypernatraemia	Hypokalaemia	Hyperkalaemia
Gastrointestinal	Purgation (13.6)		Purgation (13.6)	
Metabolic			Alkalosis Glucose (14.4)*, insulin (14.4) β_2-Adrenoceptor stimulation (e.g. circulating adrenaline)†	Acidosis (e.g. diabetic ketoacidosis, 14.4)
Renal	Saluretics		Potassium-losing saluretics	Potassium-sparing saluretics, including aldosterone antagonists
		Mineralocorticoids (Table 14.1)	Mineralocorticoids	
		Carbenoxolone (13.5)	Carbenoxolone	Captopril (p. 256)
		Renal insufficiency		Renal insufficiency

* Via insulin release.

† By stimulation of Na^+, K^+ - activated ATPase.

Table 12.6 Methods for correcting sodium and potassium ion imbalances in the body fluids.*

	Defect in extracellular fluid		Defect in extracellular fluid	
	Na⁺ lack	K⁺ lack	Na⁺ excess	K⁺ excess
Alteration of INPUT by changing:				
Gastrointestinal absorption	Oral NaCl	Oral KCl†	Oral —'low salt' diet	Oral —'low K⁺' diet —cation-exchange resin (*see* text)
Plasma concentration	i.v. NaCl	i.v. KCl†		NaHCO₃‡ Insulin plus glucose‡
Alteration of OUTPUT by changing:				
Plasma concentration				Dialysis
Renal excretion	Mineralocorticoid (e.g. fludrocortisone, 14.2)	Potassium-sparing saluretics§	Thiazide or frusemide plus an aldosterone antagonist (e.g. spironolactone)	Frusemide

* Treatment also requires correction of cause.
† Passes into cellular fluid by normal mechanisms.
‡ Causes passage of K⁺ ions into the cells.
§ If K⁺ lack due to potassium-losing saluretics.

indicated have already been discussed in this chapter; some used in the treatment of hyperkalaemia will now be specified.

The appropriate *cation-exchange resin* (e.g. Resonium A®) contains a polystyrene sulphonate which has a higher affinity for potassium than for sodium ions. Therefore, given orally as the sodium salt, it retains within the gut potassium in the diet as well as enhancing its normal excretion into the large intestine; it can, however, produce nausea and vomiting. Given as a retention enema, this side-effect is avoided and the colonic action still occurs.

Passage of potassium ions from the extracellular fluid into the cells is enhanced (Table 12.5) by insulin, alkalosis, or β_2-adrenoceptor activation (which acts by stimulating the 'sodium' pump', Table 2.3, p. 47). In severe, acute *hyper*kalaemia, i.v. calcium gluconate (with monitoring of plasma Ca^{2+} concentration) may be necessary to oppose the toxic effects of potassium (particularly on the heart).

12.7   Vasopressin action on the kidney: diabetes insipidus treatment

The antidiuretic action of vasopressin is mediated via a specific adenylate cyclase (Table 4.5) which renders the collecting ducts permeable to water, resulting in passive water reabsorption due to the counter-current osmotic gradient (Fig. 12.1). Diabetes insipidus may be caused by

1   Hypothalamopituitary inadequacy. Treatment is by:
•   replacement therapy. The oral route is unsatisfactory for a peptide and, unusally, nasal insufflation is an alternative to s.c/i.m. injection in milder cases and for short-term maintenance therapy. The preferred compound is 1-desamino-8-D-arginine vasopressin, *desmopressin*, which has a prolonged action (p. 138)—up to a day—with negligible smooth muscle contraction
•   chlorpropamide (an oral hypoglycaemic agent, 14.4) or carbamazepine (an antiepileptic, 7.1) which sensitises the renal collecting ducts to the action of any residual pituitary vasopressin secretion and may be useful if this is still present.
2   A renal defect (nephrogenic diabetes insipidus). Here, paradoxically, a thiazide can lessen the flow of urine. The mechanism(s) involved are unclear but the drug only works *if given with a low salt diet*. Overall, under these forced conditions of sodium lack, more sodium ions (and therefore, osmotically, more water molecules) are reabsorbed from the renal tubular fluid.

12.8   Gout

This extremely painful condition is due to an excess of uric acid in the body fluids. Deposition—as (mono) sodium urate (large concentrations are termed 'tophi')—at various sites classically involves the joints of the great toe, where periodically it sets up an inflammatory reaction manifested as an acute attack. Also, renal calculi may form. Therapy is accordingly directed towards the control of three factors.

Inflammation

See the note on aspirin at the end of this section.

Indomethacin is usually preferred (naproxen is an alternative). Colchicine (the traditional remedy) stabilises lysosomal membranes and depolymerises microtubules (4.11) in leucocytes thus reducing their enzymatic and phagocytic activities, respectively, which are creating the acid milieu favourable to the precipitation of sodium urate. Further, it inhibits urate-stimulated production of leukotriene B_4 which is a potent chemotactic agent (footnote, Table 5.12). Colchicine can be used *diagnostically* because it only has a significant anti-inflammatory action in gout. However, in effective dosage to relieve *an acute attack* it often produces intolerable nausea, vomiting and diarrhoea—probably due to antimitotic effects on gastrointestinal epithelial cells (Table 19.2); it is rarely used. In lower dosage, it is an alternative to indomethacin as a suppressant, prophylactically (*see* next paragraphs).

Uric acid formation

The major pathways are outlined in Fig. 12.5. The hypoxanthine analogue, allopurinol—which is an *inhibitor* of hepatic microsomal enzymes (1.9)—also depresses xanthine oxidase activity. As a result, any small amount of uric acid which is formed, together with its more soluble precursors (hypoxanthine and xanthine), is usually readily excreted without precipitation in the urinary tract. This is the treatment of choice for maintenance therapy as it is effective even in cases where uricosurics—*see* below—fail (e.g. renal insufficiency, urate stones). Paradoxically, the drug may bring on an acute attack (probably by mobilisation from tophi producing a temporary hyperuricaemia),

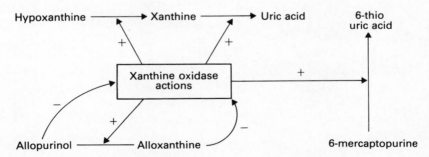

Fig. 12.5 Xanthine oxidase functions. Both allopurinol and its metabolite, alloxanthine, are enzyme inhibitors which prevent the formation of uric acid and the breakdown of 6-mercaptopurine (*see* text). +, stimulation; −, inhibition.

which should be covered by simultaneous use of a suppressant. Allopurinol has few side-effects but can produce allergic skin reactions.

During antileukaemic therapy, massive breakdown of leucocytes results in a secondary hyperuricaemia. Allopurinol should be given but in lower dosage if azathioprine (Fig. 19.7) is used, as the xanthine oxidase inhibitor will prevent catabolism of the active agent, 6-mercaptopurine (Fig. 12.5), and result in an increased incidence of side-effects (*see* Table 19.2).

Uric acid excretion

Two opposing mechanisms present in the renal tubules are shown in Fig. 12.6. The effects of drugs can be rationalised by assuming that the reabsorptive process has the greater capacity but a higher threshold.

Uricosuric agents increase the output of uric acid in the urine. The type substance—*probenecid* (Fig. 1.5,c)—is considered to bind to a carrier necessary both for secretion and for absorption and, as the drug itself is only slowly excreted, daily doses are adequate. Acute gout can be precipitated by inadequate dosage or early in treatment (as with allopurinol). Uricosurics are only alternative drugs, e.g. in patients allergic to allopurinol. To avoid urate stone formation, increase the dose of the drug gradually, maintain a high fluid intake and make the urine alkaline. Side-effects are not marked: rashes more common than gastrointestinal upsets.

Note. Aspirin, except in high doses, makes gout worse and also antagonises uricosuric actions: *so avoid its use.* 'High-ceiling' saluretics and thiazides can precipitate a gout attack (Table 12.4).

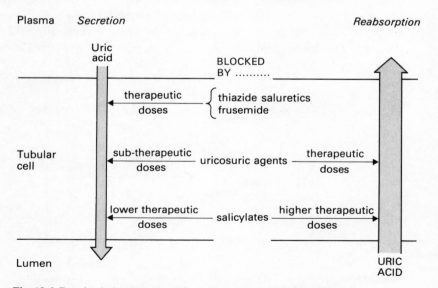

Fig. 12.6 Renal tubular transport of uric acid and its *inhibition* by drugs.

12.9   Renal side-effects and toxicity (add further examples yourself)
1   *Side-effects* by interference with specific processes
• water and/or ionic imbalances with saluretics
• lithium inhibits the action of vasopressin on the collecting ducts to produce diabetes insipidus (7.5).
2   *Allergic responses* in the kidney are often type III, i.e. microprecipitates in or around small blood vessels. Drugs with such a proclivity include warfarin (p. 384). Nephrotic syndrome can result from an autoimmune reaction induced by gold salts or penicillamine (Table 5.13).
3   *Toxic effects*. The kidney is particularly vulnerable because many drugs or their metabolites become highly concentrated within the tubules as in 'analgesic nephropathy' (7.9), or nephrotoxicity (necrosis, e.g. particularly of the proximal convoluted tubules, with aminoglycosides, 19.6). Cyclophosphamide metabolites can cause bladder irritation (cystitis, p. 411).

12.10   Alteration of urinary pH
This is achieved (within the range 4.5–8.5) by changing the alkali reserve in the appropriate direction, when the normally functioning kidney will respond accordingly. Thus, to make the urine
• *alkaline*, administer a salt which consists of fixed cation with a labile anion (Table 12.1), e.g. sodium bicarbonate or potassium citrate (the citrate ion enters the tricarboxylic acid cycle, Fig. 14.5)
• *acid*, give a salt of a labile cation with a fixed anion (e.g. ammonium chloride) or an organic acid which is non-toxic and significantly excreted in the urine (e.g. ascorbic acid).
   Some major indications are
• to prevent stone formation, e.g. with uricosuric drugs in gout, 12.8
• to facilitate excretion, e.g. make alkaline in aspirin poisoning or acid in gentamicin toxicity, e.g. alkalinise with sulphonamides (p. 408).
• to prevent excretion, e.g. make alkaline in gentamicin therapy of renal parenchymal infections.
• to create a hostile environment, e.g. make alkaline in coliform urinary tract infections.

13 Digestive Tract and Liver

13.1 Route of administration

General principles in respect of oral administration are discussed in 1.2. For a *local* effect (e.g. purgatives, 13.6, anthelmintics, 19.8), this route is obligatory. For a *systemic* effect, this is the most convenient method provided that the drug is non-irritant, not inactivated and neither required urgently (the sublingual route is an exception) nor in extremely accurate dosage. Lipid solubility is the prerequisite for absorption by simple diffusion although a few drugs (e.g. α-methyldopa and lithium), due to their similarity to natural dietary constituents (phenylalanine and sodium, respectively), are actively transported. However, ion-trapping can occur if lipid solubility is grossly diminished at intracellular pH (e.g. aspirin in the gastric mucosa, *see* Fig. 1.3). An additional complication is the extent of hepatic 'first pass' metabolism. This may be vital in drug activation but, much more commonly, it results in inactivation.

Rectal administration (by suppository or enema) is useful for local effects. For systemic actions, this route may be used if the patient is vomiting or unconscious and results in a relatively low hepatic first pass metabolism. However, drugs can irritate the rectal mucosa, absorption is not always reliable and rather slow.

13.2 Metabolism

This can occur at the following sites.

Lumen of the alimentary canal. Digestive enzymes naturally break down carbohydrates, fats (to some extent) and proteins prior to absorption. The latter (including simpler peptides) are commonly used therapeutic agents which cannot be given orally, e.g. insulin.

Epithelial cells of the gastrointestinal tract. The presence of monoamine oxidase here means that adrenaline is ineffective when swallowed. Conversely, tyramine and some other sympathomimetic substances contained in foods are normally inactivated in the gut wall and liver but can become troublesome during monoamine oxidase inhibitor therapy (p. 184).

314

Hepatocytes. These are the major site of metabolism in the body (1.9) with vital implications regarding
- route of administration (1.2)
- caution when using drugs in combination(s) (20.5) or in patients with inadequate liver function.

13.3 Excretion

Salivary. Uncommon but can be useful as a non-invasive method to estimate plasma concentrations, e.g. for paracetamol, p. 32.

Small intestinal. Hepatic cells pass drugs and/or their metabolites into the bile canaliculi, reabsorptive or secretory processes occur in the gall bladder and the resultant bile is passed into the gut, where its constituents may become involved in an enterohepatic circulation (1.10).

13.4 Emetics and anti-emetics (Fig. 13.1)
Emetic drugs can act on:

Stomach wall. Irritation produces a reflex stimulation of the vomiting centre either directly or via the chemoreceptor trigger zone. Sodium chloride and mustard are readily available household materials which can be mixed with water and given orally in the emergency situation.

Chemoreceptor trigger zone. Most of the centrally acting emetics exert their action here. It is situated in the area postrema at the posterior end of the floor and roof of the fourth ventricle and *is not protected by the blood–brain barrier,* so that it can be affected by drugs which do not normally enter the brain from the circulation. The major receptor in the chemoreceptor trigger zone is dopaminergic (D_2) and it is stimulated by dopamine (Table 7.2), ergometrine and ergotamine (Table 15.5) and apomorphine (Table 6.4). For the latter, and less selective opioids such as morphine, specific opiate receptors may also be involved. Digoxin (10.11) also acts on the chemoreceptor trigger zone.

Both sites. For example ipecacuanha (or one of its active constituents, emetine). Other emetics may also have this dual action, e.g. digoxin can irritate the gastric mucosa; e.g. copper sulphate—the classical experimental agent for the production of reflex emesis—can, *after section of the vagi,* produce delayed retching movements which are abolished by bilateral ablation of the chemoreceptor trigger zone.

Final coordination is provided by the vomiting centres in the medullary reticular formation which are also activated in motion

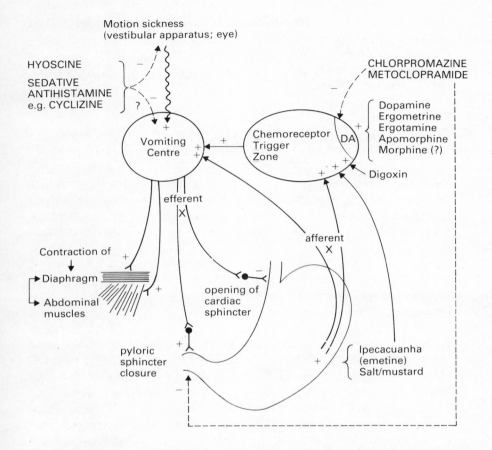

Fig. 13.1 Sites of actions of emetics and anti-emetics (in capitals). DA, dopamine receptor (mainly D_2); +, activation; −, antagonism; ?, possible site; X, vagus.

sickness by signals from the organs of balance, particularly vestibular apparatus, and eye. Efferent pathways produce
- (via the vagi) opening of the cardiac and closure of the pyloric sphincter
- (via the phrenic and thoracic nerves) contraction of the diaphragmatic and abdominal musculature (retching) which increases intra-abdominal pressure and expels gastric contents orally.

Therapeutic emesis is valuable in the treatment of poisoning provided the patient is conscious (20.8). Oral ipecacuanha preparations are the most suitable.

Anti-emetics

First, as all drugs used produce significant side-effects, do not prescribe them unless absolutely necessary. A specific indication is often cancer chemotherapy which commonly produces vomiting (Table 19.2). Cisplatin (p. 412) is particularly liable to cause this and is, therefore, the drug against which anti-emetic actions are often measured.

Secondly, the route of administration can pose a problem. Obviously, oral therapy is most satisfactory for prophylactic use, e.g. in motion sickness, but in acute vomiting drug treatment must be parenteral (the rectal route is too slow).

Anti-emetics acting in relation to the chemoreceptor trigger zone
These are dopamine (D_2) antagonists. The type-substance, *chlorpromazine* (or a related phenothiazine) is useful in drug-induced vomiting—additionally, in terminal cancer patients, it potentiates the analgesic action of morphine (p. 203). *Metoclopramide*—as indicated in Fig. 13.1—not only depresses the chemoreceptor trigger zone, but also relaxes the pyloric sphincter, so that it promotes gastric emptying. This dual action is particularly indicated in patients whose nausea is associated with pylorospasm, and in migraine (p. 260). Both chlorpromazine and metoclopramide cross the blood–brain barrier and, so, are liable to cause extrapyramidal syndromes (p. 178) especially on chronic usage. *Domperidone* is an alternative D_2-receptor antagonist which negligibly crosses the blood–brain barrier but can block effects on the chemoreceptor trigger zone (which is outside the barrier). However, it has been reported to cause cardiac dysrhythmias following *intravenous* injection. In cancer chemotherapy patients, domperidone or metoclopramide is usually combined with dexamethasone (a synthetic glucocorticosteroid introduced after patients receiving similar agents as part of their treatment were found to suffer less severe nausea and vomiting) or nabilone (a synthetic anti-emetic cannabinoid). Recently $5-HT_3$ antagonists (Table 5.3) have been used against (cisplatin-induced) vomiting, suggesting that the latter might be caused by 5-HT mechanisms related to the gut.

Anti-emetics acting in relation to the vomiting centre. Muscarinic and/or H_1-histamine receptors have been identified in the vestibular nuclei, in the vomiting centre itself and at functionally associated sites. These findings conveniently explain the two major groups of drugs used prophylactically in the prevention of *motion sickness*
• antimuscarinic drugs, especially those with a marked central sedative effect, e.g. hyoscine, 2.7. This is satisfactory for a short journey (up to 4 hours) but can produce peripheral antimuscarinic side-effects, namely blurring of vision and dry mouth, in addition to drowsiness
• sedative anti-(H_1) histamines (e.g. promethazine, Table 5.5). These are longer-lasting with similar side-effects to the first group, due to their strong antimuscarinic activities. Cyclizine (Fig. 13.1) and cinnarizine are less sedative.

Sickness associated with pregnancy. The particular danger here is teratogenicity (20.7). If absolutely indicated (e.g. hyperemesis gravid-arum) give a well-tried agent, e.g. promethazine.

13.5   Peptic ulceration

The physiological background is shown in Fig. 13.2. Increase in the hydrochloric acid to mucus ratio results in ulcer formation accompan-ied by pain (due to irritation by the acid) in the stomach, duodenum or oesophagus (by reflux). Ulcerogenic drugs are obvious from Fig. 13.2: nicotine (Table 2.5) and those which decrease prostaglandin concentra-tions (Table 5.10, e.g. aspirin, adrenal glucocorticoids); also ethanol.

Therapy of peptic ulcer involves pain relief, healing of the lesion, and the prevention of recurrence.

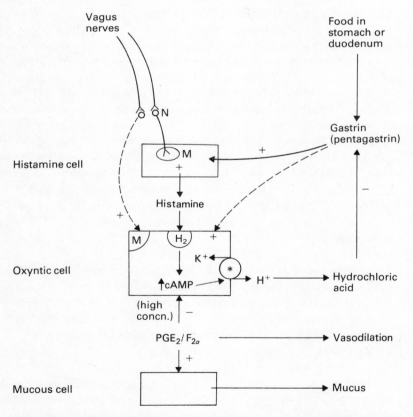

Fig. 13.2 Physiological control of gastric hydrochloric acid and mucus productions. Identified receptors (for acetylcholine): N, nicotinic; M, muscarinic; (for histamine) H_2. +, activation, −, antagonism. Interrupted lines indicate possible additional pathways. *H^+, K^+-ATPase. Concn., concentration.

Pain relief

Pain relief can be achieved by an increase of stomach pH (normally 1.5) to about 3.5 which will dilute the acid approximately a hundredfold. Such a change will not result in *significant* 'rebound' increase in secretion due to lessened negative feed-back of hydrochloric acid upon gastrin production. Acid dilution will also accelerate healing, especially in duodenal ulceration (where the gastric acid secretion is particularly high). Methods available are:

Histamine (H_2)-antagonists (type substances cimetidine, ranitidine)
These diminish hydrochloric acid secretion from the oxyntic cells. Figure 13.2 shows the major mechanisms involved. The cephalic phase of the gastric acid secretion via the vagi is not completely prevented by all H_2-antagonists and may be acting partly directly on oxyntic cells. The gastric and intestinal phases (possibly through postganglionic parasympathetic links) mainly use gastrin as an intermediate which primarily acts by local release of histamine. *In parenthesis*, pentagastrin (a polypeptide which consists of the five amino acids essential for the gastrointestinal actions of the seventeen amino acids in gastrin) can be given s.c. as a test for achlorhydria; the *functional* type will respond to the extra stimulus.

Therapeutically, cimetidine or ranitidine is used *as first-line treatment* in peptic ulceration, reflux oesophagitis and the Zollinger–Ellison syndrome (gastrin-secreting adenoma of the pancreas or gut). Side-effects (uncommon) include gastrointestinal upsets, mental confusion (in the elderly), gynaecomastia (weak anti-androgenic action—cimetidine) and galactorrhoea (increased prolactin secretion). Cimetidine inhibits hepatic microsomal enzymes and therefore can potentiate the action of drugs such as phenytoin or propranolol.

Antimuscarinic drugs
These are seldom sufficient treatment alone but may be useful adjuncts to decrease the acid secretory responses to vagal stimulation. The preferred drug is *pirenzepine*, which is an M_1-selective agent so that it is most likely acting at postsynaptic M_1-muscarinic receptors in the gastric parasympathetic ganglia (*see* p. 61). Due to its selectivity and only slight passage of the blood–brain barrier, it has a relatively low incidence of 'atropinic' side-effects (Table 2.7).

Antacids
These common, inexpensive remedies are bases which lessen the acidity by:
1 *Neutralisation*, i.e. chemical reaction. Examples are sodium bicarbonate and magnesium hydroxide. They have a rapid effect with duration dependent both upon gastric emptying time and degree of

absorption from the small intestine (*see* later). Sodium bicarbonate (rarely) can produce too much carbon dioxide with excessive, unsocial eructation.

2   *Adsorption* (also weak chemical neutralisation). These agents have a slower but more prolonged action and include

• aluminium hydroxide gel
• magnesium trisilicate. This adsorptive antacid reacts slowly with gastric hydrochloric acid to form magnesium chloride (neutralising salt) and silicic acid (silica gel) which adsorbs further acid.

Other relevant properties of gastric antacids are

1   The extent of their absorption into the systemic circulation. This is greatest with sodium bicarbonate which has, accordingly, a brief local action and can produce a systemic alkalosis. Negligible amounts of magnesium and aluminium ions are absorbed.

2   Their direct actions upon the gut. Overall, magnesium salts produce purgation (13.6) and aluminium compounds are constipating; but, usually, these effects are not noteworthy.

Gastric proton pump inhibitors

Omeprazole inhibits the H^+, K^+-ATPase (Fig. 13.2) by forming an intermediate compound which binds to the thiol (.SH) groups of the enzyme. This drug conversion only occurs in conditions of strongly acid pH and, therefore, is effectively limited to the secretory canaliculi of the oxyntic cell. Its action is long-lasting (> 12 hours) and powerful (but this can stimulate excessive gastrin release by decreasing the negative feedback of HCl, Fig. 13.2). Prolonged hypergastrinaemia produced by repeated very high (experimental) doses of omeprazole resulted in oxyntic mucosal hyperplasia (mouse/dog) or carcinoid tumours (enterochromaffin cell overgrowth, in rats). Omeprazole can inhibit microsomal enzymes in the liver.

Recently, a drug SCH 28080 has been shown to inhibit the proton pump by combination at the *luminal* K^+-binding site of the enzyme.

Healing of the ulcer

This is encouraged by decreasing gastroduodenal acidity: *the anti-(H_2)-histamines are most satisfactory* in this connection. Other measures (if necessary) include:

Stop smoking. Nicotine (Table 2.5) increases gastric acid and adrenal glucocorticoid secretions, and (swallowed) tobacco smoke constituents are irritant.

Bismuth chelate. This is a colloidal preparation which protects the ulcer base and allows healing. Often a satisfactory alternative, although prolonged usage can precipitate an encephalopathy. Recently it has been suggested that its beneficial effects are partly due to an antibacterial action which leads to the removal of *Campylobacter pylori*, an organism found in the gastric mucosae of peptic ulcer patients.

Sucralfate. This complex compound of aluminium hydroxide and sulphated sucrose is converted by gastric acid into a protective gel which preferentially adheres to the ulcer site. It may also increase the production of prostaglandins and mucus. The main side-effect is constipation.

Carbenoxolone. A preparation from liquorice (glycyrrhiza) root which promotes healing by increasing the life-span of the gastric epithelial cells and enhancing mucus production. This may partly be due to decreased breakdown of mucosal prostaglandins. Side-effects are sodium and water retention with potassium ion loss (? weak mineralocorticoid action—structural similarity to aldosterone). Carbenoxolone is largely absorbed in the stomach and mainly excreted in the bile. Treatment of duodenal ulceration therefore necessitates the formulation of a delayed-release preparation avoiding gastric digestion. Its use has largely been superseded by cimetidine/ranitidine treatment.

Prostaglandins. Synthetic $E_{1/2}$ analogues, which improve mucosal protection by increased blood flow and mucus production, and (in high doses) inhibit acid secretion (Fig. 13.2) are available clinically e.g. misoprostol.

Prevention of recurrence
This has to be separately assessed in each case. Commonly involved factors are stress, bad eating habits such as infrequent or irregular meals and ingestion of substances which are irritant (e.g. spices) or those which tend to increase gastric acid secretions (e.g. excessive coffee drinking, p. 234).

13.6 Purgatives
Alternative titles are laxatives or aperients (for mild agents) or cathartics (for strong drugs—which are never used nowadays). These substances are commonly self-prescribed.

Uses
Rational indications are for
• bedridden patients, especially where straining at stool might be dangerous (e.g. myocardial infarction, *see* Table 7.15)
• persons on low-residue diets
• the removal of orally taken poisons or with anthelmintics (19.8)
• an easier defaecation in the presence of painful anorectal lesions (e.g. haemorrhoids)

- evacuation of the gut contents prior to childbirth, bowel surgery or examination.

They are *absolutely contraindicated* in undiagnosed obstruction of the gastrointestinal tract when they can produce, for example, perforation of an infected appendix.

Properties

The relevant properties of clinically useful purgatives are collated in Table 13.1.

Bulk purgatives

These increase the volume of the bowel contents which activates sensory elements in the gut wall to enhance peristaltic (propulsive) intestinal movements.

Polysaccharides, such as bran and methylcellulose, are not digested (except in ruminants) and absorb water, resulting in a gentle, satisfactory evacuaton.

Salines are not significantly absorbed and retain an isosmotic volume of fluid within the alimentary tract (osmotic purgatives). A dose of Epsom salts (magnesium sulphate) is taken in a tumblerful of water. More concentrated solutions are either emetic or elicit a pre-emetic action namely closure of the pyloric sphincter (Fig. 13.1), which delays the purgative effect. Normally, the response is fairly rapid so that they are useful, for example, in poisoning, but the watery, diarrhoeic nature of the stool renders them unpopular for general use. However, magne-

Table 13.1 Purgatives

Type	Drug example	Site of action in intestine	Time to produce effect*	Consistency of stool
Bulk				
polysaccharides	Bran, methylcellulose	Entire length	Long	Well-formed
salines	Magnesium sulphate	Entire length	Short	Aqueous ('loose')
	Magnesium hydroxide	Entire length	Short	Moderately formed
Emollient (faecal softeners)	Liquid paraffin	Entire length	Long	Well-formed
	Docusate sodium	Entire length	Long†	
Stimulant				
anthraquinones	Senna, cascara	Colon	Long	Moderately formed
diphenylmethanes	Bisacodyl	Mainly colon	Long‡	Well-formed
	Phenolphthalein		Long	Moderately formed

* Time of action: long (greater than 6 h)—give at night; short (1–6 h)—give in the morning; ultra-short (less than 1 hour) when given by retention enema (†) or suppository (‡).

sium hydroxide (taken as an aqueous suspension, milk of magnesia) acts first as an antacid to form magnesium chloride which itself is a mild purgative especially useful for children.

Emollient purgatives
Emollients (L: *mollis*, soft) soften the faeces—a marginal action of polysaccharide bulk purgatives.

Liquid paraffin is incorporated into the bowel contents and also acts as a lubricant during the evacuation. The main disadvantage is that, by solution in the paraffin, vital fat-soluble substances—particularly vitamins A, D and K—may be prevented from absorption. This interdicts its use habitually, especially in children (vitamin D) or patients on warfarin therapy which is potentiated by vitamin K deficiency (*see* Table 17.2).

Docusate (dioctyl sulphosuccinate) *sodium* lowers surface tension which allows water to enter scybalous masses. It is also given by retention enema in faecal impaction.

Stimulant purgatives
A heterogeneous group chemically, which may act by direct stimulation of the gut wall or by inhibition of salt and water absorption (like saline bulk purgatives) so that in either case they increase intestinal propulsion.

Anthraquinones (senna, cascara) are converted to the active agents (emodins) in the colon (by bacterial action). They sometimes cause griping pains. Active derivatives can be secreted in the milk (15.5).

Diphenylmethanes. Phenolphthalein partly undergoes enterohepatic circulation and acts mainly on the colon. It may produce griping or an allergic rash. It is still contained in some proprietary formulations. A more satisfactory agent is bisacodyl which is effective both orally and as a suppository.

Summary
Do not rush to drugs. Improvements in diet and evacuative habits, and general retraining are most successful in the long term. If help is temporarily required, a short course of a bulk polysaccharide or an anthraquinone is probably best: specific indications for other agents have been mentioned. Remember that purgation is naturally followed by a period of constipation, as there is little to excrete. Habitual users of purgatives may also suffer water and electrolyte depletion (*see* Table 12.5).

A note on lactulose
This is used in hepatic encephalopathy. It is a disaccharide which is broken down by bacterial action in the colon to form (mainly) lactic and acetic acids. These reduce ammonia and amine passage into the blood

(the aim of treatment) by lessening their production by inhibition of ammonia-producing bacteria and decreasing their absorption by protonation (p. 6), and by causing an osmotic diarrhoea.

13.7   Prophylaxis and treatment of some intestinal conditions

Specific

Bacillary dysentery
Only severe cases (usually due to *Shigella dysenteriae*) require antibiotic therapy. At one time poorly absorbed sulphonamides were used but these have been replaced by those which act systemically now that it is realised that the infection has to be attacked *within* the gut wall. Co-trimoxazole is probably the treatment of first choice (19.3).

Typhoid fever
This is one of the few indications for chloramphenicol (19.6). Carriers respond well to amoxycillin.

Amoebic dysentery (see 19.8)

Worms (see Table 19.6).

Non-specific

Traveller's diarrhoea
Fluid replacement is the prime necessity. 'Oral rehydration salts' (dissolved in water prior to use) which contain glucose and NaCl (these help each other's absorption from the gut), sodium citrate or $NaHCO_3$ (to combat any acidosis) and KCl (to replace potassium loss) are used. Otherwise, as the condition is almost always self-limiting, symptomatic treatment is usually all that is necessary. Anti-diarrhoeal agents act by thickening the gut contents (e.g. kaolin, chalk); or decreasing intestinal hurry, with *either* opioids, e.g. morphine, codeine (mechanisms of these explained on p. 202), e.g. diphenoxylate, loperamide—two constipant compounds related to pethidine (7.12)—or antimuscarinic drugs, e.g. atropine.

Tablets of codeine phosphate are most convenient. Mixed preparations are sometimes used such as kaolin and morphine mixture ('mixture', pharmaceutically, indicates a *bottle* of medicine), or diphenoxylate with atropine (Lomotil®). Poisoning by the latter, especially in children, manifests (up to 3 hours after ingestion) central atropinic effects (*see* Table 2.7) and, subsequently, morphine-like overdose actions (respiratory depression, 7.11): treat accordingly. Loperamide is preferable because there is less systemic absorption.

Pre-operative preparation for bowel surgery: use metronidazole (p. 413) and magnesium sulphate.

Ulcerative colitis

This condition may be auto-immune in origin. In acute exacerbations of the condition, adrenal glucocorticosteroids are valuable, such as *prednisolone* (i.v., orally or by retention enema—p. 13—for severe, moderate or mild attacks, respectively). *Sulphasalazine* is useful in the prevention of relapses. Its use represents an interesting delivery problem. The drug is a diazo compound of a sulphonamide (sulphapyridine) with 5-aminosalicylic acid (mesalazine) which is the active agent liberated in the colon by bacterial action—if it were given alone orally it would be absorbed in the small intestine. Side-effects are mainly caused by the sulphonamide so, if they occur, give mesalazine *orally* as an enteric-coated tablet or as a diazo compound which is split to form two molecules of mesalazine or *rectally*.

13.8 Treatment of hyper-β-lipoproteinaemias

Plasma lipoproteins consist of specific globulins (apoproteins) combined with fatty acid esters of glycerol (triglycerides) and of cholesterol plus phospholipids. *As lipids have a greater density than proteins*, it is possible to separate the lipoproteins by ultracentrifugation into the broad classes shown in Table 13.2. Additionally, the fatty acids contained in low-density lipoproteins (LDLs) are largely saturated whereas those in high-density lipoproteins (HDLs) are mainly unsaturated. Excessive levels of plasma LDLs and cholesterol are definitely related to the production of vascular atheromatosis.

LDLs are being found to have an increasing number of functions but, essentially, in the present connection they may be considered to be transporting lipids from the liver to other tissues for cellular oxidation and membrane synthesis, for example. Figure 13.3 shows a broad outline of lipoprotein metabolism. Lipoprotein lipases are important in the synthesis and breakdown of lipoproteins in the liver and tissues, but

Table 13.2 Compositions of different lipoproteins

Lipoprotein	Contents (%)*			
	Triglycerides	Cholesterol	Phospholipids	Apoproteins†
VLDL	*60*	20	10	10 (B, C, E)
LDL	5	*45*	20	30 (B)
HDL	10	20	20	50 (A, C, E)

VL, very low; L, low; H, high; DL, density lipoproteins.
* Average values (to nearest 5%). Figures in italics indicate major contents.
† Sub-groups present indicated within brackets.

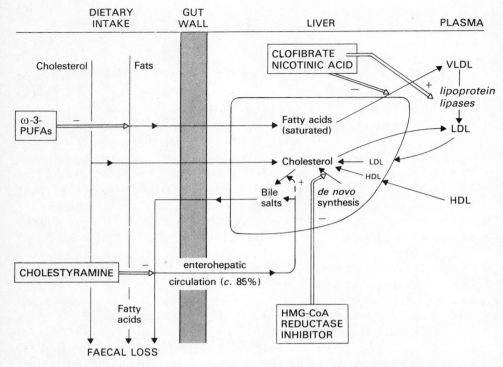

Fig. 13.3 Lipoprotein metabolism and its modification by antihyperlipidaemic drugs. Only major pathways are shown. Antagonistic drugs (in rectangles) act at sites indicated by thick, open arrows. Hepatic receptors are in small capitals; HDL, LDL. ω-3-PUFAs, omega-3-*p*oly*u*nsaturated *f*atty *a*cids. +, activation; −, inhibition.

in the plasma they also hydrolyse the core triglycerides of VLDLs thus converting them to LDLs which are then cleared from the plasma via hepatic LDL receptors. ('Up-regulation' of these receptors by some drugs—Table 13.3—increases LDL plasma clearance.) Conversely, HDLs are functionally transporting cholesterol back to the liver for elimination in the bile and they appear to have a 'protective' effect against atheroma formation.

Current methods available for the treatment of hyper-β-lipoproteinaemias—which probably prevent further lipid deposition rather than significantly 'dissolving' existing plaques—are:

General
Eliminate risk factors—hypertension, obesity, smoking.

Dietary changes
In addition to a low calorie intake (if overweight); decrease fat intake (especially of cholesterol and saturated fatty acids), lower sugar and ethanol content (decreases triglyceride levels) and introduce a high fibre element (lowers triglyceride and cholesterol levels) into the diet.

Table 13.3 Major effects of representative lipid-lowering drugs on plasma lipid levels

| Drug | Lowering the plasma concentrations of | | Main mechanism of action |
	Triglycerides	Cholesterol	
Cholestyramine		+	Adsorption of bile salts in the gut†
Clofibrate	+	> +*	Decreased synthesis and more breakdown of VLDLs†
Nicotinic acid	+	> +	Decreased synthesis and release of VLDLs
Omega-3-marine triglycerides	+		Lowered saturated fat intake
HMG-CoA reductase inhibitor		+	Decreased synthesis of cholesterol†

+, present.
* More marked with bezafibrate and gemfibrozil (*see* text).
† Additionally, 'up regulates' the hepatic LDL receptor number.

The above measures are usually sufficient in most cases. For those with familial hyper-β-lipoproteinaemias or otherwise at high risk, drugs may be necessary. Their major sites of action are indicated in Fig. 13.3 and summarised together their main effects on plasma lipids in Table 13.3.

Cholestyramine
An anion-exchange resin which—taken orally—remains in the gut and interchanges its chloride ion for a bile acid or bile salt anion. This lowers the enterohepatic circulation of the latter so that more cholesterol is converted to bile acids in the liver. Also, the lack of functional bile salts in the intestine diminishes fat and cholesterol absorption. It also 'up' regulates hepatic LDL receptors. The main effect is a decrease in the plasma cholesterol concentration. Side-effects include abdominal discomfort and constipation. Also, lipid-soluble substances (e.g. vitamins, A, D and K) may not be absorbed, and orally administered drugs may bind to the resin (e.g. warfarin, Table 17.2).

Clofibrate
An ethyl ester which is well absorbed from the gut and hydrolysed to the active agent, chlorphenoxyisobutyric acid, in the liver. Its major effects are: decreased synthesis and release of VLDLs, increased conversion of VLDLs to LDLs with a resultant greater biliary excretion of cholesterol (see side-effects) and 'up regulation' of hepatic LDL receptors. The drug reduces triglyceride, and to a lesser extent, cholesterol plasma levels.

Side-effects (usually mild, gastrointestinal upsets in a small percentage of patients) can, however, be dangerous and include increased incidence of cholesterol gallstones (indicative of enhanced biliary excretion of cholesterol). The related compounds bezafibrate and gemfibrozil are reported to have a greater effect on plasma cholesterol reduction and a lower incidence of gall bladder problems in the long term.

Nicotinic acid (US: niacin)
This decreases triglyceride more than cholesterol plasma levels. Its main action appears to be by decreasing the synthesis and release of VLDLs. To be effective the drug has to be given in high dosage, so that side-effects are common: especially flushing (vasodilation); also pruritus, gastrointestinal upsets and (rarely) depression of liver function.

Omega-3-marine triglycerides
As explained on p. 381, the 'Eskimo' diet containing eicosapentaenoic acid (which has an additional double bond in the ω-3 position, compared with arachidonic acid, p. 143) forms PGI_3 and TXA_3 with a resultant low degree of platelet aggregation. Eskimo plasma contains (relative to 'Western' plasma) low triglyceride and 'total cholesterol' levels and high HDL concentrations. In 'Western' patients, the major effect of a fish oil concentrate containing ω-3 polyunsaturated fatty acids is a sustained fall in plasma triglycerides. The use of the diet revolves round the questions of whether reduction of triglycerides is important in the *prevention* of atheroma and/or whether the diet lowers cholesterol levels consistently in non-Eskimos.

HMG-CoA reductase inhibitors
A number of drugs can decrease the synthesis of cholesterol (e.g. clofibrate) but the rate-limiting step is the synthesis of mevalonic acid from 3-*h*ydroxy-3-*m*ethyl*g*lutaryl-*co*enzyme *A* (HMG-CoA) by the appropriate reductase. Selective inhibitors of this enzyme, are becoming available. These drugs also 'up regulate' hepatic LDL receptors.

Summary
Methods which are successful in the treatment of hyper-β-lipoprotein-aemias are available, but primary preventive drugs for use by the (symptomless) general population are still very much at the experimental stage.

13.9   Sites of side- or toxic effects

Digestive tract
The following list is not exhaustive but merely indicative of some of the drugs which affect or effect

Appetite: alimentary upsets
Bowel activity
Changes in microorganismal content and activity
Damage.

Anorexia, nausea, vomiting, colic and diarrhoea may all occur with digoxin (10.11). Vomiting (associated with premonitory nausea) is common with many other drugs—examples in 13.4.

Bowel activity changes such as *diarrhoea* can be caused by purgatives (13.6), excessive parasympathetic activity (e.g. anticholinesterase poisoning, cholinergic crisis in myasthenia gravis), or block of sympathetic tone (e.g. reserpine, guanethidine, 3.2). It may be haemorrhagic (e.g. ferrous sulphate poisoning, 17.1; 'antimitotic drugs', Table 19.2). *Constipation* results from loss of parasympathetic tone (e.g. ganglionblocking agents, 2.8) or loss of parasympathetic tone plus contraction of gut musculature (e.g. morphine, p. 202).

Changes in gut flora are induced by orally administered broad-spectrum antibiotics (e.g. tetracyclines, 19.6) which can result in opportunistic infections (p. 414)

Damage. Any part of the digestive tract can participate in general allergic reactions but this is unusual. Ulceration may be
• gastric: prostaglandin cyclo-oxygenase inhibitors, e.g. aspirin
• gastrointestinal, e.g. oral iron poisoning (17.1).

Liver
The liver, like the kidney, is a vulnerable organ insofar as it often receives high concentrations of drugs or their metabolites, and it also has a large number of enzymatic processes which may be deranged. Specific hepatic toxic responses may be classified as:
1 *Allergic*
• hepatocellular, e.g. monoamine oxidase inhibitors, 7.5; possibly halothane, Table 8.7
• cholestatic, e.g. chlorpromazine, Table 7.6; imipramine, 7.5.
2 *Dose-related*
• hepatocellular, e.g. paracetamol metabolites, 1.9; ferrous sulphate poisoning, 17.1
• cholestatic, e.g. 17-methyltestosterone, p. 358.

The most obvious manifestation of all the above hepatic toxic effects is jaundice.

14 Endocrine Pharmacology

Hormonal action can involve extra- or intracellular receptors (Fig. 4.5) and a variety of intermediate messengers (Table 4.5, Figs 4.6, 4.8 and 14.6). Control of most body functions is secured by nervous and/or hormonal factors. The prime site at which these two systems are integrated is the hypothalamo-pituitary complex. Major exceptions to this generalisation are discussed elsewhere, namely calcium homeostasis (16.3), insulin release (*see* Table 14.6) and the renin–angiotensin system (5.9, for aldosterone *see also* 14.2).

14.1 Hypothalamo-pituitary axis (Fig. 14.1)
Posterior pituitary hormones are released following stimulation of the appropriate hypothalamic neurones: vasopressin (5.9), oxytocin (15.3).

Intermediate lobe hormones: α- and β-melanocyte-stimulating hormones (18.5).

Anterior pituitary hormones are liberated in response to releasing hormones (RH) secreted into the blood draining the hypothalamus (hypophysial portal system). There are some release-*inhibiting* hormones (RIH), e.g. somatostatin (growth hormone RIH), e.g. prolactin RIH, which is activated via a dopamine receptor, *see* Fig. 14.7 (accounting for the galactorrhoea as a *side-effect* of chlorpromazine, *see* Table 7.6 and the *use* of bromocriptine to terminate lactation, 15.1). The pharmacology of the anterior pituitary (and their target organ) hormones will now be discussed in detail, with those primarily involved with reproduction deferred to Chapter 15.

14.2 Drugs acting in relation to the adrenal cortex
Table 14.1 shows the major actions of the three types of hormone released by adrenal cortical cells and the resultant side-effects (when used as indicated in Table 14.4). Effects of multifactorial or uncertain provenance are included under the (known) main or (unknown) most likely cause(s).

The type substance, prednisolone, has mainly glucocorticoid but some mineralocorticoid action (Table 14.2). Its effects are most readily remembered under the headings 'organic constituents' i.e. carbohydrate, fat, protein (*see* Fig. 14.3), 'inorganic elements' (i.e. calcium, sodium and potassium) and anti-inflammatory. With regard to side-

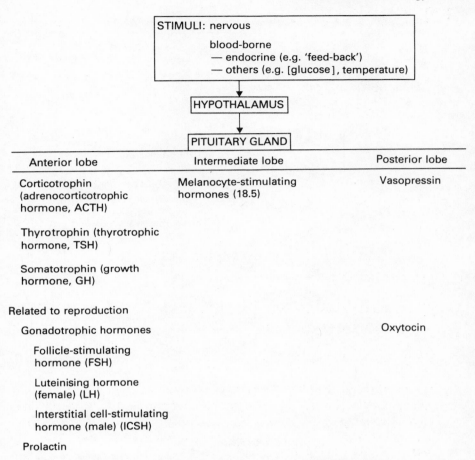

Fig. 14.1 Hypothalamo-pituitary control of endocrine functions. In American terminology, the '*h*' of trophin is elided resulting in the corresponding 'tropins'.

effects, a useful *aide-mémoire* is to consider the simple measurements (italicised in Table 14.1) which can be used to monitor them during prolonged therapy, namely

• *blood sugar level*—the hyperglycaemic action is predominantly due to glucocorticoid effects (as specified in Tables 14.1 and 14.5) but also involves a mineralocorticoid element, as potassium ion loss from the body results in a decrease in insulin release

• *height*—decreases due to vertebral osteoporosis and osteomalacia

• *weight*—increases due to sodium and water retention

• *blood pressure*—hypertension is probably mainly due to elevated extracellular fluid volume (mineralocorticoid action), and increased sensitivity of blood vessels to catecholamines—possibly partly resulting from blockage of uptake$_2$ in the peripheral vasculature (3.1).

Other adrenal corticoid-like substances are shown in Table 14.2.

Table 14.1   Actions and side-effects of the three types of adrenal corticoid hormones

Type	Actions	Side-effects*
Glucocorticoid (hydrocortisone; US: cortisol)	Carbohydrate glyconeogenesis; less peripheral usage of glucose	Raised *blood sugar level*[†]
	Fat lipolysis/ redistribution	'Buffalo' obesity—hump on neck and shoulders; 'moon face'— roundness of features
	Protein catabolism	Stunting of body growth (children); muscle wasting; delay in wound and peptic ulcer healing; thinning of skin (striae); osteoporosis—loss of *height*[†‡]
	Ca^{2+} decreased gut absorption (results in increased release of parathyroid hormone);	Osteomalacia—loss of *height*[†‡]
	increased renal excretion	Kidney stones
	Lessened inflammatory responses (p. 147)	Reactivation or spread of infection, e.g. in skin; increased liability to infection
	Immunosuppression Anti-'stress' Cardiovascular system lymphocytopenia; eosinopenia; increased capillary fragility	Bruising
	Central nervous system negative feed-back on adrenocorticotrophin secretion;	Adrenal cortical atrophy: danger of acute adrenocortical insufficiency if therapy suddenly stopped
	mood changes	Neurosis or psychosis
	Eye	Glaucoma: cataract (following prolonged high dosage)
Mineralocorticoid (aldosterone)	Sodium and water retention	Oedema—increased *body weight* Raised *blood pressure*[†]
	Potassium loss	Hypokalaemia: results in decreased insulin release → raised *blood sugar level*[†]
Sex hormones (mainly androgenic corticoid)	Protein anabolism Secondary male characteristics	Hirsutism (in the female)
	Increased sebum secretion	Acne

* All are chronic effects—iatrogenic Cushing's syndrome (Table 14.4 and *see* text).
† May be of multiple causation (*see* text).
‡ Osteoporosis usually predominates.

Table 14.2   Natural (N) and synthetic adrenal corticoids

Drug	Glucocorticoid action	Mineralo-corticoid action	Indication(s)
Hydrocortisone (N) (US: cortisol)	+	±	Emergency i.v.
Prednisolone	+ +	±	General glucocorticoid
Betamethasone	+ + +	0	General glucocorticoid
Beclomethasone	+ + +	0	Bronchial asthma (11.1 and 11.5)*
Fludrocortisone	+ +	+ + +	Mineralocorticoid
Aldosterone (N)	±	+ + + +	Nil* (*see* text)

Strength of action: + + + +, very strong; + + +, strong; + +, moderate; +, present; ±, weak; 0, negligible.
* Inactive orally.

Tetracosactrin

The rate-limiting step in the synthesis of adrenal gluco-, mineralo- and sex corticoids is the conversion of cholesterol to pregnenolone which is stimulated by corticotrophin and inhibited by aminoglutethimide, p. 425). Corticotrophin is a peptide which consists of the first 39 amino acids of opiocorticotropin (Table 6.8): the active moiety lies in the initial 24 amino acids and this preparation—tetracosactrin (Gk: *tetra*, four; *eicosi*, twenty), Table 14.3—is preferred in therapy as it produces fewer allergic responses. It has the following actions

• (main): facilitates the synthesis of adrenal glucocorticoids (hydrocortisone is the chief constituent) and androgens. Release ensues as there is little storage of hormones in the gland. The plasma glucocorticoid concentration provides a negative feed-back on the hypothalamo-pituitary axis

• (subsidiary): produces growth of the adrenal cortex

• (slight): there is usually a negligible action upon aldosterone production and release, which is mainly dependent upon angiotensin II/III stimulation (5.9).

The main advantage of tetracosactrin is that it causes less retardation of growth in children because the protein anabolic effect of the androgens opposes the protein catabolism associated with glucocorticoid action. However, it has the major disadvantages of parenteral administration (even if only bi-weekly) and relatively low glucocorticoid selectivity and production, and is not often used.

Glucocorticoids

General medical indications are shown in Table 14.4.

Appreciate that while acute adrenal glucocorticoid *lack* can be lethal, side-effects of excess only develop in the longer term. Therefore:

Table 14.3 Pharmacology of a corticotrophin compared with that of a glucocorticoid

	Corticotrophin (e.g. tetracosactrin; US: cosyntropin)	Adrenal glucocorticoid (e.g. prednisolone)
Pharmacokinetics		
Route of administration	s.c./i.m. (depot preparation)	Any route
Plasma protein binding	Small	*c.* 90%
Plasma half-life	*c.* 15 min	2–4 h
Pharmacodynamics		
Presence of adrenal cortex	Necessary	Unnecessary
Plasma concentration of adrenal glucocorticoids obtainable	Up to four times the resting level*	Limited only by side-effects
Other adrenal corticoids released	Androgens mainly	Nil
Side-effects (for same glucocorticoids activity)	As Table 14.1 but more sodium retention,* hypertension,* hirsutism, acne	Table 14.1
Advantages	Less growth inhibition (children), no adrenal cortical atrophy	

* Mainly hydrocortisone (therefore, less glucocorticoid selectivity, Table 14.2); normal resting level shows diurnal variations (so give two-thirds daily dose a.m., one-third p.m.— in replacement therapy).

1 *Acute* therapy presents no problems: give the appropriate drugs in acute adrenal insufficiency or life-threatening situations, e.g. Gram-negative septicaemia (plus antibacterial chemotherapy).

2 *Chronic* therapy will in many cases produce iatrogenic Cushing's syndrome; if so, first decide whether this is preferable to the diseased state. If the decision is made to administer adrenal glucocorticoids chronically, i.e. for more than a few weeks

• lower the dose as soon as possible to one which will maintain the control of the pathological situation but produce minimal side-effects

• make sure that the patient does not miss taking a dose (or increasing it in a stressful situation such as infection). When in doubt, advise to take the drug and contact the doctor

• at the end of a course of treatment, taper off the dosage slowly so that the hypothalamo–pituitary–adrenal cortical balance gradually returns to normality. Exogenous adrenal glucocorticosteroids (by the negative feed-back mechanism mentioned earlier) inhibit corticotrophin release:

Table 14.4 Uses of glucocorticoids

Use(s)	Side-effects*
Ophthalmological/dermatological (*see* caveats 18.3 and 18.6)	Absent
Replacement therapy (plus mineralocorticoid): acute or chronic (Addison's disease) adrenal insufficiency	
Suppression of adrenocorticotrophic hormone due to pituitary overactivity or adrenogenital syndrome, for example	Only if excessive doses required
Hypercalcaemia associated with sarcoidosis or vitamin D overdosage (by virtue of anti-vitamin D action, Table 16.3) Bronchial asthma (11.5)	
Anti-inflammatory indications (excluding most dermatological)	Often inevitable (iatrogenic) Cushing's syndrome, i.e. side-effects shown in Table 14.1
Immunosuppressant, e.g. in auto-immune conditions and transplantation reactions (19.11)	
Life-threatening situations, e.g. lymphatic leukaemia	

* Side-effects only develop during chronic therapy.

the resultant atrophy of the adrenal cortical cells begins within a few days but only achieves significance after a few weeks. Fortunately, it is reversible on (gradual) cessation of therapy, though this may take months (or even years).

Mineralocorticoids

Aldosterone is mainly concerned with the maintenance of the extracellular fluid volume which it procures primarily by renal actions (*see* Fig. 12.1). Like the naturally produced adrenal glucocorticoids, aldosterone is inactivated in the liver but to such an extent that it is ineffective orally. In conditions of mineralocorticoid insufficiency, therefore, fludrocortisone (Table 14.2) is used. Conversely, in hepatic cirrhosis (and in some other conditions where hyperaldosteronism is present), the aldosterone antagonist, spironolactone, is indicated as a saluretic (p. 308).

14.3 **Drugs acting in relation to the thyroid gland (excluding calcitonin, 16.3)**
The physiological background is shown in Fig. 14.2.

Circulating iodide anions are actively transported into the gland. In the epithelial cells, an oxidised form of the element is produced which iodinates tyrosine to form its mono- and di-iodo derivatives (attached to thyroglobulin) which, in turn, are converted into liothyronine (L-triiodothyronine, T_3) and L-thyroxine (T_4): the first and third of these reactions (labelled a and b in Fig. 14.2) are catalysed by a peroxidase.

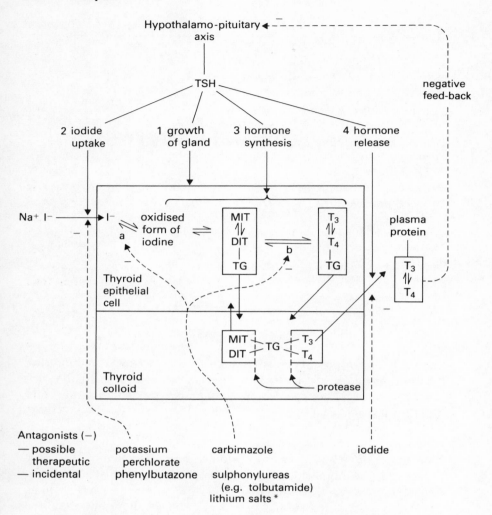

Fig. 14.2 (*Above*) actions of thyrotrophic hormone upon the thyroid gland and (*below*) its antagonists at specific sites (*see* text). TSH, thyrotrophin; TG, thyroglobulin; MIT, mono-iodotyrosine; DIT, di-iodotyrosine; T_3, tri-iodothyronine; T_4, thyroxine. a and b indicate sites of peroxidase action. −, inhibition. *See p. 185.

All the iodinated compounds are stored with thyroglobulin in the colloid vesicles of the gland. This cache of available hormones means that changes produced by drugs acting on thyroid function only manifest themselves slowly (over weeks). T_3 and T_4 release involves protease activity, which may take place within vesicles contained in the epithelial cells (not illustrated in Fig. 14.2).

In the bloodstream, the hormones are heavily plasma protein bound and their free forms pass into the tissues to elicit *control of normal growth and development, and metabolic stimulation.* Characteristic signs of thyroxine overdosage are increased basal metabolic rate with raised body temperature (*see* Table 7.10) and cardiac stimulation, particularly tachycardia and dysrhythmias. In this connection the following observations are pharmacologically interesting. Hearts taken from hypothyroid animals show a prolongation of action potential duration (and effective refractory period) similar to that produced by the antidysrhythmic agent, amiodarone (10.13), and a decrease in β-adrenoceptor number (increase of latter in hyperthyroidism).

Overall, however, there is sufficient similarity between these effects and those of the appropriate sympathetic stimulation to justify the use of adrenergic β-blocking agents in the relief of some hyperthyroid symptoms, e.g. tachycardia, muscle tremor; e.g. lid retraction (guanethidine, p. 392). Another suggestion is that β-adrenoceptor antagonists also prevent the conversion of T_4 to T_3 (*see* next paragraph). Despite this there are some discrepancies; for example, diarrhoea is a good indicator of thyroxine excess yet is usually produced by sympathetic block (e.g. reserpine, guanethidine, 3.2).

T_4 is partly converted to T_3 in the tissues. Their overall effects are similar because, although T_3 is roughly three times as potent as T_4, its duration of effect is only about one-third of the latter (plasma half-lives: T_3 about 2 days; T_4, about 6 days). T_4 (L-thyroxine) is the usual form of therapy.

The other major effect exerted by the hormones is a *negative feedback* (via the hypothalamo-pituitary system) *on thyrotrophin release.* Thyrotrophin acts on its target organ (Fig. 14.2) to increase

1 Glandular size *and vascularity.*
2 Uptake of iodide.
3 Synthesis of iodinated compounds.
4 Release of T_3 and T_4.

These effects are mainly mediated via cyclic AMP production.

Therapy

Iodide is required in the prophylaxis of *simple goitre*

Hypothyroid conditions

L-thyroxine (US: levothyroxine) is used. Indications are:
• *cretinism.* Give the *highest* dose possible without producing hyperthyroid symptoms (e.g. tachycardia, diarrhoea). The prognosis is better the earlier the treatment is commenced
• *adult myxoedema.* Give the *lowest* dose which relieves the hypothyroidism. These patients often have hyper-β-lipoproteinaemia (thyroxine increases conversion of cholesterol to bile acids) and cardiac stimulation can precipitate angina pectoris
• *drug-induced hypothyroidism.* In conjunction with carbimazole, to

prevent thyroid enlargement (see later). Fig. 14.2 shows other drugs which can produce thyroid hypofunction (and goitre) as a side-effect: this is uncommon

• *post-operative or post-radiation hypothyroidism, see* later.

Hyperthyroid conditions

A common type—usually occurring in young adults—is *exophthalmic goitre* (Graves' disease). This presents two difficulties. First, the paradox that there is an increased activity of thyroid hormones associated with the goitre yet decreased thyrotrophin concentration (due to negative feed-back). Long-*a*cting *t*hyroid *s*timulator (LATS) is an immunoglobulin present in the plasma of many thyrotoxic patients which appears to act like thyrotrophin (though for longer, as its name implies), but it is produced in lymphoid tissue and is, therefore, not susceptible to the negative feed-back mechanism. The second difficulty is that the exophthalmos (mainly due to an increase in the retro-orbital fat) cannot be produced experimentally by an increase in circulating thyroid hormones: despite a number of theories (e.g. exophthalmos-stimulating factors) its genesis remains unknown. From middle-age onwards, thyroid *neoplasms* are relatively common; these are mostly adenomata and, rarely, carcinomata.

Supportive therapy includes β-adrenoceptor blocking agents and guanethidine (as described earlier), and oral anticoalgulants (p. 382) if it is considered that an atrial thrombus is likely to result in embolism.

Definitive treatment consists of the following alternatives.

Surgery

There are specific indications for this such as pressure effects on the trachea (e.g. most neoplasms). Preliminary carbimazole with or without iodine therapy (*see* later) is usually given. Any patients who become hypothyroid post-operatively are placed on L-thyroxine therapy.

Radioactive [131]I

This is taken up by the thyroid gland which it then irradiates mainly with β-rays of little penetration (*c*. 2 mm) but also with a small amount of γ-rays (of greater penetration), which give the uptake count. The inhibitory effects on thyroid glandular activity begin to manifest themselves within a month and reach a maximum at about 3 months. This treatment often finally results in hypothyroidism but this is effectively controlled with L-thyroxine. Radioactive iodine must not be used in either sex before reproductive life is finished because of the possibility of germ cell mutagenicity. In carcinomatous conditions, the radioactive compound might reasonably be expected to be particularly effective by concentration in secondary growths but sometimes, unfortunately, the metastatic growths are so anaplastic that they lack a functional iodine uptake mechanism.

Antithyroid drugs (see Fig. 14.2)

Potassium perchlorate prevents iodide ion uptake into the gland. However, its potential to produce blood disorders (agranulocytosis, aplastic anaemia) is so great that it has become obsolete.

Thiourea derivatives. These inhibit the synthesis of T_3 and T_4 by antagonism of the peroxidase enzyme (at sites a and b in Fig. 14.2).
    Carbimazole is the currently preferred agent because it has minimal side-effects which may be categorised as
• *a*granulocytosis: rare and never fatal (can be with phenylbutazone, Fig. 14.2)
• *a*llergy (most commonly a rash)
• *a*lopecia
• *a*thropathy. Both these latter are rare.
It is usually given initially for a few months when, according to the response, it is either continued for 1–2 years as the sole therapy or surgery is performed.
    This drug, by decreasing the negative feed-back of thyroid hormones on the hypothalamo-pituitary axis, increases the secretion of thyrotrophin and, thus, can result in a hypervascular, enlarged gland. This effect can be mitigated by the concomitant administration of a *small* dose of L-thyroxine. Carbimazole also crosses the placental barrier and is excreted in the milk, to produce (by the same mechanism) either a fetal or a puerperal goitre. Thus, in these circumstances, it should be used in lower dosage, and breast feeding avoided.

Iodide. As shown in Fig. 14.2, this ion prevents the release of active thyroid hormones into the blood (though it can marginally oppose the other actions of thyrotrophin). However, the beneficial effects only persist for up to a fortnight so that it can be used pre-operatively when, over 10 days, it reduces the thyrotoxic symptoms as well as the gland's vascularity (rendering surgery less hazardous). It is given orally (as aqueous iodine solution) which consists of molecular iodine disssolved in potassium iodide solution: occasionally patients are allergic to this.

14.4   Blood glucose concentration

Hormonal control
A constant supply of this energy substrate is vital for most tissues and organs, particularly the brain, so that hypoglycaemia usually presents

with mental confusion, ('light-headedness'), often with signs of compensatory sympathetic activation (sweating, tachycardia, tremor).

To allow for a variety of physiological contingencies, the control mechanism consists of one hypoglycaemic hormone—insulin (released from the β-cells of the pancreatic islets, and with the actions shown in Fig. 14.3)—opposed by a number of hyperglycaemic hormones (major effects shown in Fig. 14.3 and Table 14.5) which can be preferentially activated under any requisite circumstance, e.g. exercise, starvation.

Many factors influence insulin release; some of those which are important pharmacologically are shown in Table 14.6. Glucose is the natural stimulus in most animal species (including man) and it releases insulin in two phases: a rapid initial surge of preformed hormone; and a

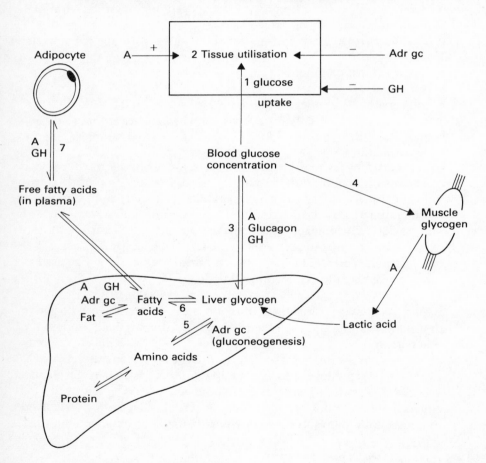

Fig. 14.3 Hormonal control of blood sugar level. 1–7 indicate actions of insulin (Table 14.5): action 1 is not necessary in certain tissues, e.g. the brain—except for the satiety centres, 9.5. For many of the chemical interconversions involved *see* Fig. 14.5. +, increase; −, decrease. A, adrenaline; Adr gc, adrenal glucocorticoid; GH, somatotrophin.

Table 14.5 Insulin actions (1–7, Fig. 14.3) compared with those of its major hormonal antagonists; and insulin release produced by the same antagonists, directly or indirectly

	Tissue glucose uptake* 1	Tissue glucose utilisation 2	Glycogenesis Liver 3	Glycogenesis Muscle 4	Gluconeogenesis 5	Lipogenesis 6	Free fatty acid release into the circulation 7	Insulin release Directly	Insulin release Indirectly (due to hyperglycaemia)
Insulin	+	+	+	+	−	+	−		
Adrenaline	+	+	−	−†	(+)	−	+	−	+
Glucagon‡			−		(+)	(−)	(+)	+	+
Somatotrophin	−	−	−			−	+	0	+
Adrenal glucocorticoids		−			+	−	(+)	0	+

+, Increase; −, decrease; 0, negligible action: bracketed signs show marginal or permissive effects (not illustrated in Fig. 14.3).
* Also promotes entry of K^+ ions and amino acids into cells. Not necessary for glucose uptake in brain (except satiety centres) or liver cells.
† Strictly, muscle glycogenolysis (see Fig. 14.3).
‡ Produced by the α-cells of the pancreatic islets.

Table 14.6 Important factors/drugs involved in the control of insulin release

Increased release	Decreased release
Hexoses, particularly glucose absorbed from the gut (*see* gastric inhibitory peptide below) or otherwise increased in concentration in the blood, e.g. by all the hormones antagonising the actions of insulin (Table 14.5) producing a hyperglycaemic effect	Hypoglycaemia; exercise;* starvation*
	Somatostatin
Glucagon (direct)†	Adrenaline (direct via α-adrenoceptors)
Vagal stimulation	Sympathetic stimulation (via α-adrenoceptors)
Secretin, GIP	
Amino acids, e.g. leucine	Hypokalaemia
Fatty acids (especially in cattle)	
Sulphonylureas, e.g. tolbutamide	Diazoxide; thiazide saluretics (possibly); streptozotocin

* In these situations, preference is given to production of energy requirements by fat, rather than carbohydrate, catabolism (effectuated, e.g. by somatotrophin, Table 14.5).

† Overall effect of glucagon is *hyper*glycaemia. GIP, gastric inhibitory peptide.

slowly developing, more prolonged output which is prevented by puromycin (a blocker of protein synthesis, Table 19.4)—probably newly synthesised hormone. It is interesting that glucose by mouth produces more insulin than when given intravenously: this is due to the fact that local gut hormones activated by the first but not the second route (particularly gastric inhibitory peptide, GIP and secretin) enhance the release of insulin.

The molecular mechanisms involved in glucose-induced insulin release are shown in Fig. 14.4. Glucose enters the β-cell and is metabolised which increases the ATP level. This results in closure ($\ominus$) of the ATP-dependent K^+ ion channels (*see* Table 4.9) with consequent depolarisation of the cell surface. Voltage-operated Ca^{2+} ion channels are thus opened, allowing calcium to enter the cell and bring about insulin release. A sulphonylurea hypoglycaemic agent, e.g. tolbutamide, inactivates ($\ominus$) the potassium channels, therefore leading (via the stages mentioned above, interrupted line) to insulin release. Conversely diazoxide produces the opposite effect by activation of the potassium channels.

Insulin and glucagon actions

The molecular mechanisms of these (Table 14.7) illustrates some important pharmacological principles (Chapter 4). The experiments have mainly been performed on adipocytes, lymphocytes and liver cell

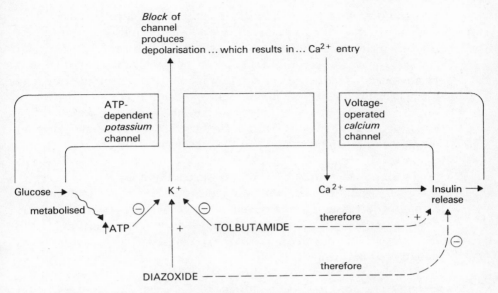

Fig. 14.4 Glucose-induced insulin release from a pancreatic β-cell and its modification by drugs. For explanation *see* text. All actions are excitatory unless denoted by $\ominus$.

Table 14.7 Molecular mechanisms of insulin action compared with those of glucagon

	Insulin	Glucagon
Molecular structure	Globular: rigid	Linear: flexible
Site of receptors on cell membrane	External surface	External surface
Binding type	Lock-and-key	Zipper model
Binding characteristic	Negative cooperativity	
Number of receptors	Down regulation	Down regulation
Intermediate messenger process(es)	Decrease in cyclic AMP-mediated effects via tyrosine kinase (Fig. 14.6) Decrease in cyclic AMP*	Increased cyclic AMP
Resultant effect on hepatic carbohydrate metabolism (Fig. 14.5)		
phosphorylase a activity	Decreased	Increased
glycogen synthase activity	Increased	Decreased

* Only if raised beforehand (*see* text).

preparations. Attachment of either hormone to a large polysaccharide (sepharose) molecule prevents entry into the cell but potentiates their actions, by maintaining the concentration in contact with the outer surface, where the receptors are situated. While insulin combination is immediately effective (like a key in a lock) at triggering intermediate messenger mechanisms, the glucagon molecule needs to adhere at a number of sites which require too much total energy to be possible all at once but are achieved in a *series of steps* each of which is (energetically) feasible—in a similar manner to the closure of a zip-fastener—hence the term 'zipper model'.

As the concentration of insulin is raised, there is

• down regulation, i.e. with time the number of available insulin receptors decreases. Normally, on combination with insulin, receptors group together and the complexes move to the inner surface of the membrane: later the receptors are externalised. This cycle becomes unbalanced in down regulation

• negative cooperativity, i.e. the binding of insulin molecules to their receptor sites diminishes, resulting in decreased sensitivity of target cells to the hormonal action.

These two processes may be considered to ensure maximum sensitivity at low concentrations of insulin and to prevent overstimulation by the hormone at higher concentrations.

Glucagon acts in the liver to increase cyclic AMP concentrations (compare its similar action on the myocardium, p. 112) which—by phosphorylation—results in activation of phosphorylase kinase kinase (producing more phosphorylase a) and inactivation of glycogen synthase (Fig. 14.5). Insulin opposes these effects (to produce glycogenesis) but in a less straightforward manner. For example, lowering of cyclic AMP concentrations can usually only be shown after tissue levels of the intermediate messenger have first been raised (e.g. with glucagon). Conversely, insulin given alone can exert its glycogenetic action without lowering the cyclic AMP level.

These findings could be explained by the scheme shown in Fig. 14.6. The insulin receptor is undoubtedly a ligand-dependent protein tyrosine kinase. Combination of insulin with the α-subunit activates protein tyrosine kinase activity in the β-subunit and this is essential for insulin action. Subsequent stages are still problematical but it is probable that the tyrosine kinase will act:

a via cAMP-independent mechanisms to modify relevant enzyme activity (only two major enzymes shown)

b via phospholiphase C hydrolysis of rather unusual phosphatidyl inositol glycans (*see* Fig. 4.7a with a glycan—polymer of a monosaccharide or glucosamine—in place of the terminal diphosphate) to produce

• inositolphosphate glycans which by actions 1–3 lower a raised cAMP

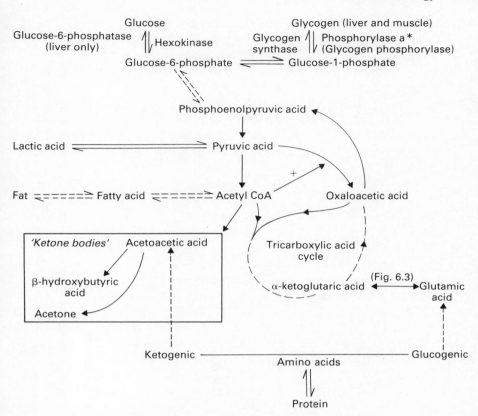

Fig. 14.5 Glucose metabolism—anaerobic to pyruvate, aerobic via tricarboxylic acid (Krebs') cycle—and important interactions with fat and protein catabolism. *Cyclic AMP activates this enzyme through a series of actions which are initiated by phosphorylation of inactive phosphorylase kinase kinase. +, activation. Interrupted lines indicate multiple stages.

- diacylglycerol, which is membrane bound (? important in membrane actions of insulin)

Finally, a summary of the multifarious actions of insulin:

1 Metabolic effects (Fig. 14.3, actions 2–7).

2 Membrane actions: increased cellular uptake of glucose, amino acids and potassium ions (*see* Table 14.5).

3 Stimulation of cell growth. It is interesting that receptors for several growth factors (the most studied is EGF, epidermal growth factor) like insulin respond to ligand attachment by generating protein *tyrosine* kinase activity.

Drug effects

Idiopathic diabetes mellitus is a common condition. It arises from a genetically determined or acquired defect at one or more stages from the synthesis of insulin to its final effector mechanisms. The aim of

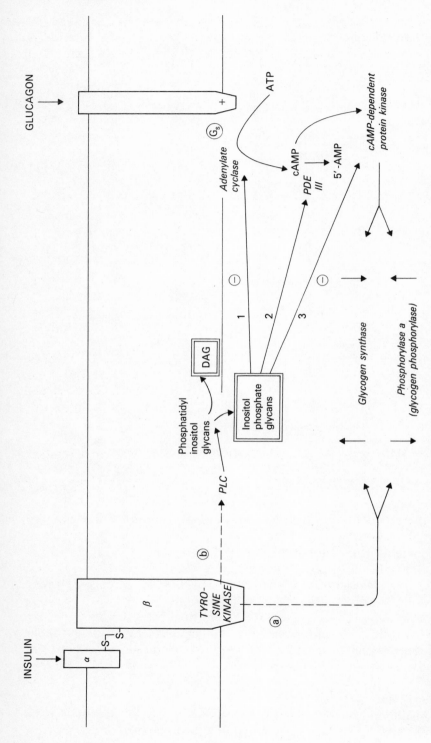

Fig. 14.6 Subcellular mechanisms for glucagon and insulin (probably) effects following their separate attachments to specific extracellular receptors (schematic). For explanation *see* text. The insulin receptor consists of two *α*- and two *β*- subunits; only one of each type connected by a disulphide bridge is shown. Interrupted lines indicate unknown pathways. Clustering and internalisation of receptors (explained in text) not shown here. ⊝, inhibitory action.

treatment is to control the blood sugar level within normal limits and thus prevent (acutely) hypo- or hyperglycaemic crises and (chronically) serious complications due to degenerative lesions in blood vessels and nerve demyelination.

Treatment (for life) is with *either*
• insulin (usually given s.c.): *insulin dependent diabetics*
or
• an oral hypoglycaemic agent: *non-insulin dependent diabetics*
plus
• dietary changes. These are particularly necessary if insulin is being taken and involve adjustment of carbohydrate intake to the type of insulin used and its time of administration, avoidance of rapidly absorbed sugars, high fibre content and low fats mainly polyunsaturated. Also, obesity must be corrected if it is present (*see* p. 93).

Insulin
The preparations available are divisible into short-, medium-, and long-acting (Table 14.8). Possible adverse effects are:
1 *Local reactions* and/or *atrophy of fat* at the repeatedly used injection sites. Rotation is advisable as absorption can be erratic from such sites.
2 *Hypoglycaemia.* This can be intensified by *ethanol* (which increases endogenous insulin release by glucose) or by *β-blockers* (3.5) which prevent the mitigating liver and muscle glycogenolysis and also mask the tachycardia and tremor of hypoglycaemia so that the diabetic is less aware of this developing danger. Treatment is with glucose orally (or i.v. in severe cases), or glucagon (s.c. or i.m.).

Hyperglycaemia. Hyperglycaemia in the controlled diabetic can occur when there is
• additional depression of pancreatic β-cell function (*see* diazoxide, under iatrogenic hyperglycaemia, p. 350)
• an increase in insulin requirements (e.g. infections). Here, the patient commonly eats less and imagines that the insulin requirement is correspondingly diminished, whereas it is in fact greater
• a decrease in glucose tolerance (e.g. oestrogens, Table 15.2), possibly by an anti-insulin action peripherally.
Hyperglycaemic ketoacidosis occurs in uncontrolled insulin-dependent diabetics. The reduced glucose metabolism produces insufficient oxaloacetate to cope with the increased acetyl CoA consequent upon the greater fat catabolism necessary for calorie requirements (Fig. 14.5). Thus ketone bodies collect with resultant acidosis and hyperventilation. Meanwhile, the glycosuria has effected an osmotic diuresis with consequent dehydration.
Treatment of this condition (which can be precipitated by an infection) consists of

Table 14.8 Preparations of insulin with relevant temporal characteristics (when given subcutaneously)

Type of insulin*	Approximate time (in hours) when given s.c., of			Notes
	Onset	Maximum effect	Total duration	
Short-acting				
Soluble insulin	2/3	2	6	Crystalline insulin in aqueous solution (pH 7). Acid insulin is a similar preparation at pH 3
Intermediate-acting				
IZS (amorphous)				Suspensions of insulin zinc (IZS). Smaller particles (amorphous) act more rapidly; larger particles (crystalline) have a slower onset but more prolonged effect. IZS is a mixture of 30% amorphous with 70% crystalline.
IZS				
IZS (crystalline)	2	6	18	
Isophane				Suspension of insulin with a protamine zinc complex (Fig. 1.4,d)
Long-acting				
Protamine zinc	4	12	36	Suspension of an insulin-protamine zinc complex (Fig. 1.4,d)

* All were originally prepared from pig or ox (beef) pancreas. Nowadays highly-purified preparations are still used but are being gradually superseded by human insulins (only one amino acid different from the porcine) produced either by modification of pig insulin (designated 'emp') or biosynthetically (designated 'crb' or 'prb'). Very rare cases of allergy to animal protein contaminants are the only *absolute* indication for human insulin.

• neutral insulin therapy by i.v. *infusion* (due to its short half-life—under 10 minutes): average rate 0.1 unit $kg^{-1} h^{-1}$
• correction of dehydration, and acid–base imbalance (if pH<7)
• initially there is a deficit of *total* body potassium with either hypokalaemia (due to predominance of urinary loss) or hyperkalaemia (due to acidosis and lack of insulin, Table 12.5). As the latter two conditions are ameliorated, hypokalaemia will occur unless potassium supplements (which also correct the intracellular K^+ deficit) are given. Therefore, repeated estimations and control of plasma potassium are necessary
• treat any causative condition and warn the patient accordingly, to prevent future episodes.

Oral hypoglycaemic agents
There are two groups: sulphonylureas and biguanides.

Sulphonylureas (type substance, tolbutamide) act by
• increasing insulin release (Fig. 14.4). Unlike glucose (*see* earlier) these drugs only pass *pre*formed hormone into the blood and do not encourage *de novo* synthesis and extrusion (glibenclamide may do these latter: it *is* more potent)
• increasing tissue sensitivity to insulin by 'up regulation' of receptors in body tissues

A comparison of the pharmacological properties of three representative compounds is presented in Table 14.9.

Tolbutamide has the shortest half-life due mainly to catabolism in the liver microsomes. It can mutually potentiate warfarin by competition for hepatic enzymes (Table 17.2).

Chlorpropamide is 20% excreted unchanged in the urine and has a prolonged action. It has rather more side-effects than its congeners, but even so the total incidence is low (*c.* 5%). It may occasionally produce a transient, cholestatic jaundice. It is contra-indicated in patients with obesity problems as it tends to increase appetite; and in those to whom alcohol is a way of life, due to a disufiram-like action (and *see* footnote to Table 14.9). Its use in pituitary diabetes insipidus is described in 12.7.

Glibenclamide is a potent agent which can work when the others fail but is, correspondingly, more likely to produce hypoglycaemia.

Biguanides (type substance, metformin) lower the blood sugar *in diabetics* but mechanisms are uncertain. Suggestions include decreased glucose absorption from the gut, decreased gluconeogenesis, and increased peripheral glucose utilisation. These are different to those of the sulphonylureas, to which they are sometimes added. Metformin also lessens appetite which is useful in obese patients. High doses can result in lactic acidosis (due to a block in pyruvate metabolism, Fig. 14.5) which is extremely serious and has resulted in the obsolescence of phenformin—the original biguanide.

A large-scale, but controversial, study reported a higher incidence of cardiovascular mortality in non-insulin-dependent diabetics treated with diet plus tolbutamide or phenformin than in those treated with diet alone. Accordingly, stress is laid on achieving the control of hyperglycaemia *by diet alone* before resorting to oral hypoglycaemic agents.

Iatrogenic hyperglycaemia
Corticotrophin and adrenal glucocorticoids (Table 14.1) raise blood sugar levels.

Table 14.9 Pharmacology of three important sulphonylurea oral hypoglycaemic agents

	Tolbutamide	Chlorpropamide	Glibenclamide (US: glyburide)
Pharmacokinetics			
Plasma protein binding	+++	+++	+++
Hepatic metabolism	+++	++	+++
Renal excretion (unchanged)	0	+	0
Plasma half-life (average, in hours)	5	35	7
Pharmacodynamics			
Action			
potency	+	++	+++
duration	+	+++	++
Side-effects (uncommon)			
hypoglycaemia	±	++*	++
gastrointestinal	++	++	+
increased appetite	0	++	0
leucopenia	+	+	
cholestatic jaundice		+	
porphyria (in susceptible individuals)	+	+	+
Interactions			
warfarin (mutual potentiation)	+	0	
alcohol intolerance	+	++†	±
Use in pituitary diabetes insipidus	+	+	

+++, marked/higher; ++, present/intermediate; +, some/lower; ±, slight; 0, negligible.
* Especially in renal impairment and the elderly.
† There is a familial variety of this condition.

Thiazide saluretics can also cause hyperglycaemia (Table 12.4) probably by decreasing insulin release. This effect is much stronger with *diazoxide* and one of the prime factors preventing its *chronic* use against hypertension (Table 10.3). The major mechanism involves lessened insulin release (Fig. 14.4) which can be put to practical use in diazoxide treatment of

• leucine-sensitive children who release insulin excessively in response to this amino acid (Table 14.6).

• inoperable islet-cell carcinoma. An alternative drug is streptozotocin, an alkylating agent (Fig. 19.8) which destroys islet β-cells, including those in metastases.

14.5 Growth hormone

The physiological background is shown in Fig. 14.7.

Somatotrophin (growth hormone, GH) has two main functions :

1 To encourage fat rather than carbohydrate catabolism in conditions such as starvation (Table 14.6, footnote).

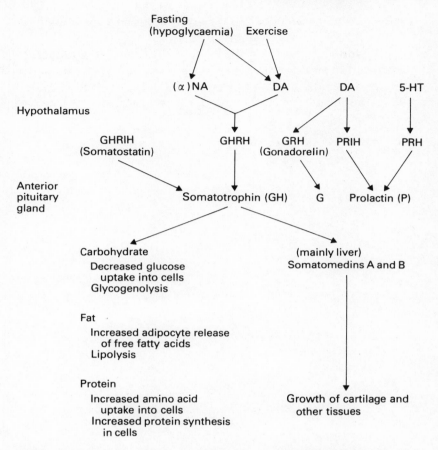

Fig. 14.7 Somatotrophin formation and function. (*Upper right*) gonadotrophin (G) and prolactin production (*see also* Fig. 15.1). NA, noradrenaline; DA, dopamine; 5-HT, 5-hydroxytryptamine; RH, releasing hormone; RIH, release-inhibiting hormone.

2   Growth of body tissues: mediated directly or via somatomedins.

In dwarfism *due to GH lack*, human replacement therapy is given. In acromegaly or gigantism (due to a rare acidophil tumour of the pituitary), pressure symptoms demand surgery or radiotherapy. Medical treatment uses bromocriptine—a dopamine agonist which, paradoxically, *de*creases GH production and release in *these* patients. It also lessens prolactin production from similar acidophil, anterior pituitary cells and, thereby alleviates any gynaecomastia and galactorrhoea which may be present.

Depression of GH overactivity with somatostatin is unsatisfactory because this peptide has

• a short half-life (minutes)

• very widespread effects. In addition to its hypothalamic existence, it occurs in other parts of the central nervous system and in the gastrointestinal tract (including α_2-cells in the pancreatic islets); actions have also been reported at other sites.

Bovine somatotrophin (BST) is injected into cattle to increase milk yield and to produce more lean meat in relation to fat. Some BST does occur in the final product (milk or meat) but it is stated to be destroyed in the human gut when such products are ingested.

15 Reproductive Pharmacology

The relevant hormonal factors are schematised in Fig. 15.1

15.1 Anterior pituitary (and similarly acting) agents and their antagonists

Gonadotrophic hormones
These induce (in the primary sex organs—ovary and testis) gametogenesis (other factors are also involved), and sex hormone formation and release. In the fertile female during the reproductive ages sex hormones produce, by their *differential* feed-back (not shown in Fig. 15.1), the correct sequences of the menstrual cycle. This system becomes unbalanced by two major events: pregnancy and the menopause.

In pregnancy, human chorionic gonadotrophin (HCG) is produced by the syncytiotrophoblast (following implantation of the fertilised ovum) to maintain the corpus luteum: the latter provides sufficient oestrogens and progestogens (to exert adequate feed-back on the hypothalamo-pituitary axis to prevent menstruation and further ovulation) until the requisite production of placental oestrogens and progestogens is established. HCG is excreted in the urine to provide a 'pregnancy test' and, on extraction, to be available as a natural replacement hormone with primarily luteinising hormone activity.

Following the menopause, diminished ovarian function results in less negative feed-back on to the hypothalamo-pituitary system so that an excess of gonadotrophins circulates and is excreted in the urine. Purification produces human menopausal gonadotrophin (HMG) which shows primarily follicle-stimulating (but also some luteinising) hormone activity: prescribed as FSH (Fig. 15.1).

For the treatment of infertility:
1 In hypothalamo-pituitary failure give both FSH and HCG or gonadorelin (gonadotrophin-releasing hormone, LHRH) to procure
• in the male, spermatogenesis and androgen release
• in the female (usually given sequentially—as in a normal cycle), oestrogen and progestogen release but, more important, ovulation; excessive ovulation with subsequent multiple births did occur before stringent monitoring procedures to detect the number of stimulated follicles were introduced.

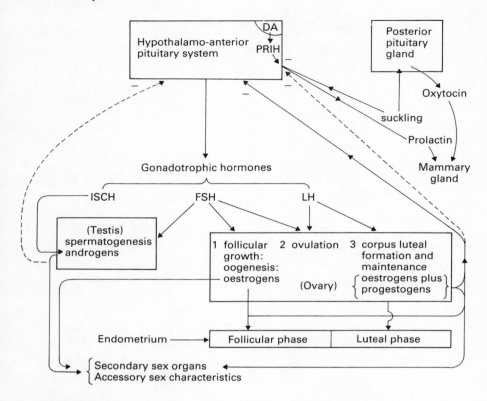

Fig. 15.1 Hormonal control of important reproductive activities (simplified). FSH, follicle-stimulating hormone; LH, luteinising hormone (female) *is equivalent to* ICSH, interstitial cell-stimulating hormone (male); PRIH, prolactin release-inhibiting hormone is activated by dopamine (DA) released from the median eminence (p. 161). Continuous lines indicate activation, except −, inhibition; interrupted lines show probable (rather than proved) pathways. 1–3, successive phases of ovarian function during a normal menstrual cycle with the corresponding endometrial changes shown below.

2   If there is some pituitary function intact, an alternative in the female is clomiphene which blocks the negative feed-back of oestrogens on the hypothalamo-pituitary system. It can produce nausea and vomiting, blurring of vision and hot flushes.

Prolactin
The essential role of this hormone in lactation is clearly demonstrated in Table 15.1. During later pregnancy (together with placental lactogen) and especially postnatally, when oestrogen and progestogen feed-back is minimal and suckling exerts reflex release (Fig. 15.1), prolactin activity results in mammary maturity with synthesis and secretion of milk constituents. Prolactin has marginal effects on the gonads of both sexes but these are unimportant pharmacologically.

Table 15.1 Major factors affecting mammary development and function

Female (or child) stage	Hormone(s) involved*	Origin of hormone(s)	Effects on the mammary gland
Menstrual cycle			
follicular phase	Oestrogen	Ovary (theca interna)	Growth of ducts
luteal phase	Oestrogen plus progestogen	Ovary (corpus luteum)	Growth of ducts and alveoli
Pregnancy			
all stages	Oestrogen plus progestogen	Corpus luteum (early); placenta (later)	More growth of ducts and alveoli
later	Lactogen	Placenta	Further development
	Prolactin	Anterior pituitary gland	Further development: milk production and secretion*
Suckling	Prolactin	Anterior pituitary gland	As above
	Oxytocin	Posterior pituitary gland	Ejection of milk by contraction of myo-epithelial cells of mammary ducts
Weaning	Oestrogen	Contraceptive tablet	Antagonism of prolactin release and/or function (Fig. 15.1)

* Other hormones necessary for complete mammary function are somatotrophin (growth); corticotrophin (salt and water constituents) and parathyroid hormone (calcium content) of milk.

Prolactin is closely related to somatotrophin (14.5) in chemical structure and is similarly produced by acidophil, anterior pituitary cells. However, it differs in that the main control is *inhibitory* and dopamine-mediated (Fig. 15.1). Some therapeutic consequences have already been stated in 14.1. Bromocriptine (a dopamine receptor agonist, *see* Table 6.4) is used to curtail lactation
• immediately post-delivery. Bromocriptine is preferable to an oestrogen (which opposes prolactin release and action on the breast, Fig. 15.1, but also causes endometrial growth and encourages thromboembolism)
• at weaning. Here decreased fluid intake plus the contraceptive tablet are preferred (Table 15.1).

15.2 Gonadal hormones and related compounds

As shown in Fig. 15.1, these encourage the development of secondary sexual organs (including the mammary gland, Table 15.1) and accessory sex characteristics. Their actions are most readily appreciated by studying their uses and side-effects as shown in Table 15.2.

Table 15.2 Uses and side-effects of gonadal hormones and related compounds

Type of drug	Oestrogen	Progestogen	Androgen	Anabolic steroid
Example	Ethinyloestradiol	Norethisterone* (US: norethindrone)*	Testosterone	Nandrolone (19-nortestosterone)†
Route of administration	Oral	Oral	Sublingual, s.c. (implant), i.m.	i.m.
Uses	Ovarian hypofunction‡ Menopausal symptoms‡ Vulvovaginitis (juvenile/senile) Contraception Cancer prostatic mammary (postmenopausal) Osteoporosis (in the elderly female)‡	Ovarian hypofunction‡ Menopausal symptoms‡ Contraception Mammary (premenopausal) Osteoporosis (in the elderly female)‡	Testicular hypofunction	Osteoporosis (in the elderly male)
Side-effects	Nausea (vomiting, diarrhoea) Feminisation (gynaecomastia) } (in the male) Thromboembolism Salt and water retention Decreased glucose tolerance Carcinogenesis (*see* text) Porphyria (20.6)		Epiphysial closure (children) Amenorrhoea Masculinisation (acne, hirsutism, deeper voice) } (in the female) Salt and water retention (only high doses continuously) (Illegal use also . . . decreased male sperm production)	

* Has some androgenic activity and is partly metabolised to an oestrogenic compound: side-effects uncommon.
† Less androgenic activity than testosterone.
‡ Cyclical therapy to simulate natural release (hormone replacement therapy, HRT).

Oestrogens

Their possible indications may be subdivided into the following:

1 Replacement therapy both (in the younger patient) for ovarian hypofunction or juvenile vulvovaginitis and (in the older patient) for menopausal symptoms, senile vulvovaginitis or osteoporosis (*see* later).

2 Negative feed-back on the hypothalamo-pituitary axis (*see* suppression of lactation, under prolactin, 15.1, and oral contraceptives 15.4).

3 Creation of a hostile environment (19.10)

- male prostatic neoplasms
- certain inoperable mammary cancers.

Finally, oestrogens have some anabolic effect (accounting for their use in osteoporosis)—less than that of androgens but additive with the latter in this respect (*see* end of this section; growth production in cattle).

The type substance, *ethinyloestradiol*, is only slowly inactivated in the liver, so that it is effective orally. It has a half-life of about 1 day.

The possible side-effects are listed in Table 15.2: nausea is the commonest; others are discussed under oral contraceptives (15.4).

A note on carcinogenesis. Postmenopausal women given prolonged oestrogen therapy (without concomitant cyclical progestogen treatment—*see* footnote to Table 15.2) show an increased incidence of endometrial cancers. *Regarding the combined 'pill'* (15.4) there have been conflicting reports but the general consensus suggests slight but definite trends as follows

- a slightly increased liability to cervical and/or mammary cancers: the latter particularly in younger nulliparae taking higher dose (50 μg) oestrogens for longer periods (4 years or more). Therefore, regular cervical smears and breast scans are a wise precaution—preferably in all users
- conversely, use of the 'pill' may afford marginal protection against ovarian or endometrial neoplasms.

Tamoxifen is an antagonist at the (intracellular, p. 91) oestrogen receptors: it is an important drug in the treatment of mammary cancers (p. 425).

Progestogens

These act physiologically only on tissues which have been oestrogen-primed (Fig. 15.1) and are particularly important with respect to pregnancy. Adequate production from the corpus luteum (in the second half of the menstrual cycle and during early pregnancy) and from the placenta (in later pregnancy) ensures

- *decreased uterine contractility* (15.3) with correspondingly less chance of abortion or premature labour.
- *prevention of ovulation* by negative hypothalamo-pituitary feed-back (so that superfetation is avoided). This is the basis of their main use—

along with an oestrogen—in the contraceptive tablet. Additionally, they can also render the cervical mucus inimical to spermatozoa (as progestogens do naturally at the end of the cycle) by increasing viscosity and making it more acid (*see* Fig. 15.2)

• *mammary development* (*see* Table 15.1).

Pharmacologically, progestogens are particularly used in contraception, ovarian hypofunction and senile oesteoporosis. They are also employed in gynaecological and early pregnant situations for a variety of purposes.

Androgens

Androgens (e.g. testosterone) are mainly prescribed as replacement therapy but do not cure hypothalamo-pituitary male sterility which requires both FSH and HCG (or gonadorelin, p. 353) to achieve satisfactory spermatogenesis and testicular androgen production.

Anabolic steroids (e.g. nandrolone) possess the protein anabolic effect of testosterone with reduced androgenic activity. They are chiefly used medicinally to increase the protein content of bone (i.e. the treatment of oesteoporosis in the elderly male with insufficient androgen secretion).

Derivatives of testosterone which are *alkyl*-substituted in the 17-position (e.g. 17-methyltestosterone) can produce a dose-related cholestatic jaundice (13.9). The compounds shown in Table 15.2 lack the deleterious substituent and are, accordingly, free of this particular side-effect.

Cyproterone is a partial agonist on androgen receptors which it blocks in the presence of the natural agonist (testosterone). *See* its use in prostatic cancers (Fig. 19.13).

Non-medical usage of gonadal hormones and similar compounds

Anabolic steroids have been taken (illegally) to enhance muscular development and performance in athletes (particularly weight-lifters and field eventers) and given to racehorses ('to improve condition'). A recent (mad) development is the use of pituitary preparations. Much more controversial is the routine employment of this type of drug to improve weight gain in livestock, particularly cattle, for human consumption: an androgen plus an oestrogen is the most effective. The main concern is residual sex hormone concentrations in the finished product, e.g. meat, which—if high—could have serious repercussions (*see* oestrogens, earlier). The administration of hormone growth promoters to animals is now prohibited but there is an exemption for specified hormones for 'therapeutic treatment or for certain other matters concerning fertility and reproduction'. *See also* veterinary use of bovine somatotrophin (BST, p. 352).

15.3   Uterine motility and its modification by drugs

A synopsis is given in Table 15.3.

The uterine (body) smooth muscle often shows spontaneous activity, generating action potentials which can initiate rhythmic mechanical contractions. The autonomic innervation is normally of negligible significance compared to hormonal control which is fundamentally exerted by the balance of female sex hormones (Table 15.4). Assume that the action potential threshold for the *rat* uterus is -40 mV. In the oestrogen-primed uterus only a small change (e.g. $+5$ mV) in membrane potential, which can readily occur spontaneously or easily be induced by drug action, is sufficient to generate an action potential with

Table 15.3   Factors affecting uterine (body) smooth muscle activity

Factor	Excitation	Inhibition	Reference
Nervous (autonomic)			
Innervation	Parasympathetic	Sympathetic	
Receptors			
cholinergic	Muscarinic		Table 2.3
adrenergic*	α	β_2	Table 2.3
Hormonal			
Adrenaline*	α	β_2	
Female sex		Progestogens	
Posterior pituitary	Oxytocin		
Autacoids			
Histamine	H_1	H_2 (rat/mouse)	Table 5.2
5-Hydroxytryptamine	$+$		Table 5.2
Bradykinin	$+$		Table 5.7
Prostaglandins			
non-pregnant human	$F_{2\alpha}$	E_2	Table 5.11
pregnant human	E_2, $F_{2\alpha}$		
Drugs			
Ergometrine	$+$		Table 15.5
β_2-adrenoceptor agonists		$+$	Table 2.3

$+$, present.
* Varies with species, stage of oestrus or menstrual cycle, pregnant or non-pregnant (*see* qualitative variation in receptors, p. 106).

Table 15.4   Rat uterus: effects of different female sex hormone pretreatments

Pretreatment (for several days)	Resting potential (average, in mV)	Spontaneous activity (electrical and mechanical)	Responses to oxytocic agents
Oestrogen	-45	Present	Good
Progestogen	-55	Absent	Poor

resultant muscular contraction. The case is quite different in the progesterone-dominated uterus (but *see* later in women at term).

The uterine body muscle only needs to be active within the female reproductive period of life

- at menstruation (primates only): to expel discarded endometrial layers
- during labour: to deliver the child(ren) and the afterbirth. (Conversely, it has to remain quiescent during pregnancy in spite of a massive increase in its size and stretching by the developing fetus and its associated structures)
- in the puerperium: to eject lochia.

In these three situations circulating progestogen content is low in many animals (in women, however, the fall only occurs immediately *after* labour). So a rationalisation would be that, during pregnancy, the high progestogen level hyperpolarises the uterine cell membrane and decreases the responses to oxytocic drugs (though exogenous prostaglandins are effective in producing therapeutic abortion, *see* later). At low progestogen levels, natural oxytocics (oxytocin, endogenous prostaglandins) act strongly.

Oxytocic agents

The term oxytocic (Gk: *oxys*, keen, sharp; *tokos*, childbirth) is used for substances which contract uterine muscle.

Oxytocin

This is synthesised in the paraventricular and supraoptic nuclei of the hypothalamus. During the last months of pregnancy, the myometrium becomes more sensitive to oxytocin (which indicates that the explanation suggested by the data in Table 15.4 is an oversimplification, for women, as the plasma progestogen level is still high). But the *major* outpouring of oxytocin occurs during labour (by stretch of the cervix and the vagina) and during suckling (by pressure on the nipple area). These stimuli activate reflexes which probably act via autonomic receptors (nicotinic, cholinergic excitatory, 6.2) on the appropriate hypothalamic nuclei and their tracts to the posterior pituitary gland to release oxytocin. The hormone then produces uterine contractions and milk ejection (Table 15.1).

Oxytocinase activity in the blood (probably from the placenta) increases greatly towards term, so reducing the half-life of the hormone to a few minutes. To induce labour, therefore, the oxytocin is infused intravenously in stepwise increments until 'natural' contractions followed by relaxations are obtained (the latter periods allow maintenance of an adequate placental–fetal circulation); excess can produce a sustained contraction of the uterus, which is dangerous. Subsequently suckling produces sufficient endogenous oxytocin to expel lochia and thus aid normal involution of the uterus.

Prostaglandins

There is evidence that

- oxytocin could exert its characteristic actions via prostaglandin release
- prostaglandins are the initial triggering agents for the onset of normal labour.

In any case, prostaglandins $F_{2\alpha}$ (dinoprost) or E_2 (dinoprostone), or their 15-methyl derivatives, which are not catabolised by prostaglandin dehydrogenase, are useful oxytocics, used in the following:

1 *Therapeutic abortion.* Abortion is legally defined as loss of the fetus occurring before the 29th week of pregnancy. For the first 12 weeks, surgical removal of the conceptus—by dilation of the cervix and curettage (D & C)—is preferred. Prostaglandins are useful from the 12th week onwards.

2 *Induction of labour.* From 29 weeks up to term, prostaglandins may still be indicated but oxytocin is increasingly preferred the nearer 40 weeks is approached (or exceeded). This is because of the increasing sensitivity to oxytocin (mentioned earlier) and its lower incidence of side-effects. Given systemically, prostaglandins produce far too much nausea, vomiting, colic and diarrhoea; they are preferably injected into or around the amniotic sac (14 weeks onward) or, at term, applied as a vaginal gel or tablets.

Ergot derivatives

These will be discussed in detail in 15.6, but the preferred oxytocic compound is ergometrine (US: ergonovine) principally because it has fewer side-effects than other ergot compounds. The characteristic response to this drug consists of a tonic spasm—which would be lethal to a fetus if given before its birth—but which is of inestimable value thereafter. Thus this drug is very useful in the treatment of post-partum haemorrhage (incipient or established). It can be given by any route (depending on the exigency of the situation) in the following order of increasing urgency: orally, i.m.; i.m. with hyaluronidase (Fig. 1.4, e); i.v. For auxiliary staff who are not permitted to give i.v. injections, the best alternative in an emergency is i.m. Syntometrine®; this contains oxytocin which acts in about 2 minutes but only for a short time, and ergometrine which has a delayed onset (5–10 minutes) but a prolonged action. The major side-effects of ergometrine are nausea and vomiting but it should be used with care in patients with (pre-)eclamptic toxaemia due to the tendency of ergot derivatives to cause vasocontriction (*see* Table 15.5).

Uterine relaxants

Under certain obstetrical conditions it is necessary to delay the onset of labour. The preferred drugs nowadays are the β_2-adrenoceptor agonists (Table 15.3) such as salbutamol.

15.4   Contraceptive methods

Coitus interruptus and the rhythm method belong to folklore.

Apart from physical barriers, e.g. (male) condom/(female) Dutch cap or sponge plus spermicide or a vaginal ring which releases a progestogen, which are reasonably efficient if used correctly and are still indicated for older women (*see* later), all currently used medical methods are oriented towards females. This is not wholly acceptable in our present society where responsibility for precautions is expected to be equally shared, and much research is being devoted to chemical contraception in the male (as an alternative to vasectomy). The 'AIDS scare' has given the condom a 'second life'.

Oral contraceptives

A great advance in freedom from the possibility (and worry) of an unwanted pregnancy has been the development of oral contraceptives which are taken in the form of a tablet but are universally known as 'the pill'. Possible sites of action are illustrated in Fig. 15.2 and are as follows.

1 *Prevention of ovulation.* A combined negative feed-back of an oestrogen and a progestogen on the hypothalamo-pituitary system is very successful in inhibiting the release of gonadotrophic hormones, so that the surges of follicle-stimulating and luteinising hormones which induce ovulation are eliminated.

2 *Hostility of cervical mucus.* If a progestogen is given during the first half of the menstrual cycle (unlike the normal situation when it is only released in the second half) or continuously, it thickens the cervical mucus and makes it more acid—both of which changes delay or prevent the passage of spermatozoa into the uterine cavity.

3 *Implantation defects.* The deficiencies of gonadotrophins (mentioned under **1**) also result in very thin and immature endometria so that implantation of a fertilised ovum is unlikely to be fruitful. Intra-uterine devices also prevent successful attachment of the blastocyst.

4 *Increased Fallopian tube activity*, e.g. by high doses of oestrogens, prostaglandin $F_{2\alpha}$ (Table 5.11). These substances encourage rapid expulsion of the fertilised egg which passes the implantation site before the latter is sufficiently prepared to receive the conceptus.

Types of oral contraceptive

The oral contraceptives currently available (*see* British National Formulary) are:

Combined oestrogen and progestogen. This is the most widely used form. The oestrogen is usually ethinyloestradiol at a daily dose of 20–50 μg (30–50 mg combines effectiveness with minimal risk of thrombo-embolic complications. The progestogen is commonly norethisterone

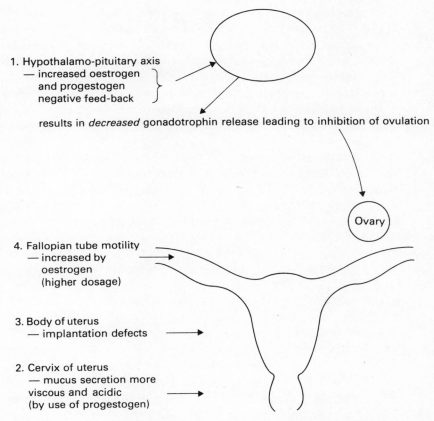

1. Hypothalamo-pituitary axis
   — increased oestrogen
   and progestogen
   negative feed-back

results in *decreased* gonadotrophin release leading to inhibition of ovulation

Ovary

4. Fallopian tube motility
   — increased by
   oestrogen
   (higher dosage)

3. Body of uterus
   — implantation defects

2. Cervix of uterus
   — mucus secretion more
   viscous and acidic
   (by use of progestogen)

Fig. 15.2 Sites of action of oral contraceptives in the female. Numbers refer to mention in text.

(*see* Table 15.2, footnote*). The regime consists of one tablet a day for 3 weeks, then 1 week drug-free (during which a tenuous 'period' occurs): repeat as required. Phased formulations in which tablets 8–21 contain twice the progestogen content of tablets 1–7 provides 'closer' control of the cycle. Protection is unreliable until the second or third drug cycle and, during this time, nausea, breast tenderness and 'breakthrough' bleeding in mid-cycle (all usually slight) are more evident than later.

Other possible side-effects can be seen in Table 15.2 (*re* carcinogenicity, *see* under oestrogens, 15.2). Weight gain may be due to salt and water retention, an anabolic effect or merely relief from worry. Lessened glucose tolerance (14.4) necessitates care in the diabetic. A multiplicity of minor reported effects cannot with certainty be attributed to usage of 'the pill'.

Cardiovascular dangers must be appreciated. There is an increased incidence of venous and arterial *thromboembolism* (related to the oestrogen content: prime factors involved are decreased antithrombin III, an increase in some clotting factors (particularly factor VII) and enhanced platelet aggregation). There can also be a gradual, but definite, sustained *rise in blood pressure* (which usually returns slowly to its original level following drug discontinuance). All the above circulatory sequelae are more common if the woman is over 34 years old, hypertensive, overweight, diabetic or a smoker; in such cases alternative methods (physical barrier techniques or progestogen-only preparations, *see* below) should be recommended.

Decreased liver function (and sometimes a—reversible—jaundice) can be produced by oral contraceptives which interdicts their use in hepatic disease. Conversely, some microsomal enzyme inducers (e.g. rifampicin, phenytoin—p. 439) can increase the destruction and, thereby, lessen the efficacy of the contraceptive: *see also* diarrhoea, p. 438.

On stopping 'the pill', ovulation should return in 2–3 months.

In conclusion, the combined oestrogen and progestogen contraceptive tablet provides a simple and reliable means of preventing pregnancy usually with 'fringe' benefits such as fewer premenstrual symptoms and less pain and blood loss at the menses. Regular gynaecological examinations and checks of, for example, blood pressure, weight, should be made and alternative methods considered as age increases.

Progestogen-only preparations. These mainly act on the cervical mucus. They are either taken orally in low dosage (lay term, the 'minipill') continuously or as a depot preparation ('the shot') i.m. every 1–3 months. They are slightly less reliable than 'the pill' (but useful during lactation) and largely avoid oestrogen side-effects but may produce irregular bleeding. The depot preparation can be given long-term in women 'for whom other contraceptives are unsuitable'.

Other possibilities

Intra-uterine devices (e.g. copper wire coiled round a plastic carrier) act mainly on implantation (*see* earlier). They release copper ions (which probably act locally to be inimical to the embryo or receptive endometrium). They are less effective than 'the pill' and rarely, if pregnancy occurs, it may be ectopic.

Post-coital contraceptives ('morning-after pill'). Very short courses of higher dose oestrogen (usually in the form of one of the combined tablets) desynchronise the ovum reaching its uterine receptive site at the necessary stage of development of the latter, possibly by increasing fallopian tube movements. They produce much nausea and vomiting, and should only be used under *direct* medical supervision.

15.5   Side- and toxic effects in relation to reproductive activity
These may be classified as follows (add further examples as you meet them).

Those associated with child-bearing
Pregnancy. The chief danger is passage of drugs across the placenta in sufficient amount to cause embryopathic effects (1.11). Important considerations regarding teratogenicity, together with drug examples, are detailed in 20.7. Abortion (or premature labour) may follow fetal damage or direct uterine stimulation (e.g. with ergot derivatives, 15.6). *See also* smoking (Table 2.5).

Labour. The main deleterious effects—exerted on mother and/or fetus/child—are those associated with general anaesthesia (for caesarean section), local analgesia (caudal, or infiltration, e.g. prior to episiotomy), central analgesia (e.g. pethidine, 7.12 and Table 7.15), rapid lowering of the blood pressure (Table 10.3, e.g. in pre-eclamptic toxaemia), or anticonvulsant treatment (Table 7.1, e.g. in eclampsia).

Puerperium. Most problems arise either because of immaturity of the infant (Table 1.9) or passage of drugs in the breast milk. The latter is a relatively uncommon source of difficulty. Charts are available and indicate care with the following drugs: indomethacin (*see* 7.9), anthraquinone purgatives (colic, diarrhoea: 13.6), carbimazole (goitre: 14.3), ergotamine (vasoconstriction: 15.6), chloramphenicol (grey baby syndrome, p. 30), and 'antimitotic agents' (for possible effects, *see* Table 19.2).

Effects on specific sexual organs, characteristics or function

Feminisation or masculinisation (*see* Table 15.2).

Gonads. Sterility due to antimitotic drugs (Table 19.2).

Uterus. Contraction (e.g. ergotamine, 15.6), producing abortion. Relaxation (e.g. the vasodilator diazoxide given in severe pre-eclamptic toxaemia to lower the blood pressure can relax the uterus and stop labour; restart with Syntometrine®, 15.3). Carcinogenesis (*see* under oestrogens, 15.2).

Penis. Erection (*see* Table 2.3) is produced by muscarinic cholinergic innervation via the 'nervi erigentes' (pelvic splanchnic nerves). In the treatment of hypertension, loss of erection was usual when ganglion-blocking agents (e.g. hexamethonium, *see* Table 10.2) were used: nowadays, it can occur with saluretic thiazides.

Ejaculation (*see* Table 2.3) partly depends on sympathetic innervation via α-adrenoceptors. So, loss of emission is a possible side-effect of α-blockers, 3.4.

Mammary gland. Gynaecomastia in the male may be caused by oestrogens used in prostatic cancer (Table 15.2) or spironolactone (p. 308). Galactorrhoea may be caused by chlorpromazine by inhibition of the dopamine receptor controlling the prolactin release-inhibiting hormone (Fig. 15.1).

15.6   Ergot and related substances
The fungus *Claviceps purpurea* infects cereal plants (especially rye) to produce a purple-black, banana-shaped sclerotium (*c.* 2 cm long) on the grain. This is ergot and it contains many common pharmacological compounds, such as histamine, tyramine and acetylcholine, but also more specific constituents. Effects of these latter have long been known because of the characteristic manifestations ('ergotism') sporadically produced by accidental ingestion of infected rye products (bread)
• central nervous system symptoms: nausea and vomiting (dopamine receptor agonism, 13.4 and *see* Fig. 13.1)
• vascular insufficiency: angina pectoris, gangrene of the extremities (due to intense vasoconstriction which is aggravated by intimal damage resulting in thromboembolism)
• uterine contractions: abortion or premature labour in pregnant females.
These actions are mainly due to the principal naturally occurring constituents, ergotamine and ergometrine. Their effects and those of their derivatives, bromocriptine and methysergide are compared in Table 15.5. Many responses (but not all of them) can be seen to be dependent upon interactions with either dopamine, 5-HT or α-adreno-receptors. A brief discussion of each agent follows.

Ergometrine is used in post-partum haemorrhage because its uterine contraction (mainly direct but also partly via 5-HT and α-adrenoceptors) is much greater than any of its other actions so that it has few side-effects (*see* 15.3). It is a relatively weak inhibitor of dopamine-mediated vasodilation (p. 89).

Ergotamine has a complex series of effects. Its vasoconstrictor action appears to be mainly direct but there is an element of 5-HT plus α-adrenoceptor partial agonism. When used in the treatment of migraine (10.6) it is not markedly hypertensive, although its vasconstrictor action is a contraindication to chronic therapy or its employment in patients with vascular insufficiency.

Table 15.5   A comparison of four lysergic acid derivatives

	Ergometrine (US: ergonovine)	Methysergide	Ergotamine	Bromocriptine
Chemical structure				
Lysergic acid *plus*	Amine	Amine	Dipeptide	Dipeptide
Dopamine receptors				
CNS: CTZ (D_2) stimulation giving vomiting (Fig. 13.1)	+ +	0	+ + +	+ +
Peripheral: vaso-dilation (p. 89)	−	0	0	0
5-HT receptors				
vasoconstriction (Table 5.3)	P.ag.	− −	P.ag	0
α-Adrenoceptors				
vasoconstriction	P.ag.	±	P.ag.	0
Overall vasoconstriction	±	0	+ + +	0
Uterine contraction (Table 15.3)	+ + +	0	+ + +	0
Use(s)	Post-partum haemorrhage	Migraine (but *see* p. 260)	Migraine (acute attack)	Suppression of lactation (15.1) Parkinsonism (7.2) Acromegaly (14.5)

CTZ, chemoreceptor trigger zone. P.ag, partial agonist. *Only main actions specified.*
Agonist actions: + + +, strong; + +, moderate; +, present; ±, weak; 0, negligible.
Antagonist actions: − −, moderate; −, present.

Methysergide is more closely related chemically to ergometrine, yet its use in migraine is more like that of ergotamine. Its major properties are shown in Table 5.3.

Bromocriptine is related chemically to ergotamine. Pharmacologically it shows negligible 'ergot effects' except dopamine receptor agonism (for uses, *see* parkinsonism, 7.2; acromegaly, 14.5; suppression of lactation, 15.1).

Finally, *lysergic acid diethylamide* (LSD) is an amine derivative of lysergic acid and is chiefly remarkable for its psychotomimetic effects, which are described in 7.6 and are considered to be mainly due to decreased 5-HT transmission at relevant CNS sites.

16 Vitamins

Table 16.1 summarises, for the major vitamins, their prime functions and results of deficiencies.

16.1 Hypo- and hypervitaminoses
Except in Third World countries, normal diets contain adequate supplies of all these essential substances and vitamin deficiencies therefore occur mostly when there is
- *increased requirement*: during pregnancy and lactation, a relative vitamin D deficiency will result in inadequate calcium intake
- *decreased intake*: in those who are impoverished, down-and-out, or alcoholic (multiple deficiencies); in the elderly, especially if living alone (insufficient fresh fruit and vegetables—C lack); or in vegans (B_{12} deficiency)
- *poor absorption*: in cases of alcoholic gastritis (B_{12} and other B components); in malabsorption syndromes (water-and/or fat-soluble vitamins may be affected); where there is lack of bile salts, e.g. obstructive jaundice; e.g. cholestyramine, 13.8 (fat-soluble deficiencies); or in prolonged liquid paraffin usage, 13.6 (fat-soluble lack).

While frank cases of the vitamin deficiencies shown in Table 16.1 are easily recognisable, it is often difficult to diagnose 'subclinical' (often multiple) inadequacies presenting with poorly defined signs and symptoms.

There is a tendency for the laity to dose themselves with 'multiple vitamin' preparations in an attempt to 'stay young' or to avoid 'vitamin deficiency'. Usually this is harmless, as excessive amounts of water soluble vitamins are excreted in the urine, but large doses of fat-soluble vitamins given repeatedly can produce
- vitamin A toxicity with bone overgrowth (in experimental animals this has been severe enough to compress nerves and blood vessels passing through skull foramina)
- vitamin D toxicity with resultant hypercalcaemia and metastatic calcification (most dangerous in the kidney).

16.2 Fat-soluble vitamins
Vitamin A. Retinol (*see* Fig. 9.2), a primary alcohol, is the main active form either taken in the food or produced from dietary β-carotene. It is

Table 16.1 Vitamins: physiological actions and consequences of lack

	Vitamin	Necessary for	Deficiency results in
Fat-soluble (stored especially in the liver)	A	Scotopic vision Epithelial integrity	Night blindness Xerophthalmia } Total blindness (in Keratomalacia } extreme deficiency) Hyperkeratosis
	D	Bone growth control Maintenance of plasma calcium content	Rickets Osteomalacia
	K	Blood clotting	Bleeding
Water-soluble (not significantly stored: excess excreted in the urine)	B_1 (thiamine) B_2 (riboflavine, US: riboflavin) B_6 (pyridoxine) Nicotinic acid* (US: niacin) B_{12} (cyanocobalamin)	Intracellular enzymic activity (all are essential components of co-enzymes)	Beriberi Angular stomatitis, glossitis, dermatitis, anaemia, neuropathy Neuropathy, anaemia, dermatitis Pellagra Megaloblastic (pernicious) anaemia (17.1)
	Folic acid		Megaloblastic (folate-deficiency) anaemia (17.1)
	C (ascorbic acid)	Intracellular redox reactions	Poor wound healing, scurvy

* Activated in the body to nicotinamide (US: niacinamide) which is preferred therapeutically as it lacks side-effects (e.g. vasodilation, *see* nicotinic acid, p. 328).

an essential drug for primary health care (prevention of blindness) in developing countries.

Vitamin K (*see* p. 382 and Fig. 17.4)

Vitamin D. This is intimately involved with the homeostasis of calcium in the body. As shown in the table at the foot of Fig. 16.1, two major Vitamin D compounds—closely related chemically—occur naturally: D_2 in the diet and D_3, either produced by solar irradiation of the skin or taken in the diet. These are activated by successive hydroxylations on the 25 and 1 positions by the liver and kidney, respectively. Thus, activated 'vitamin' D is (strictly) a hormone. 1,25-dihydroxycholecalci-ferol (calcitriol), an active form, cannot be synthesised in renal rickets—where the chronic kidney failure results in poor 1(alpha)-hydroxylase function: this problem is now overcome by the administra-tion of 1(alpha)-hydroxycholecalciferol (alfacalcidol), which only requires hepatic activation. Further hydroxylation, principally on the 24 position, lessens activity.

The actions of vitamin D derivatives are most clearly defined in the small intestine where they increase the synthesis of a calcium-binding protein (and probably enzymes necessary for calcium transport) in the mucosal cells. Two corollaries are
- the effects appear relatively slowly
- about 10% of sarcoidosis patients develop hypercalcaemia (? due to the formation of a vitamin D-like substance) and can be treated with prednisolone (*see* Table 14.4) which opposes the small intestinal action of vitamin D. This also accounts for the osteomalacia induced by adrenal corticoids (*see* Table 14.1).

Decreased effectiveness of 1,25-DHCC may be the cause of osteo-malacia occurring during prolonged anti-epileptic therapy (p. 170).

16.3   Calcium homeostasis: hormonal control

Major factors which control calcium plasma concentration are shown in Fig. 16.1. The specific hormone mechanisms involved are indicated in Table 16.2, and will now be specified for each agent.

Activated vitamin D derivatives produce hypercalcaemia by increased calcium
- absorption from the small intestine (as described in 16.2)
- reabsorption from the renal tubular fluid
- mobilisation from bone, by potentiation of parathyroid hormone action.

Parathyroid hormone (PTH, parathormone) produces hypercalcaemia by increased calcium

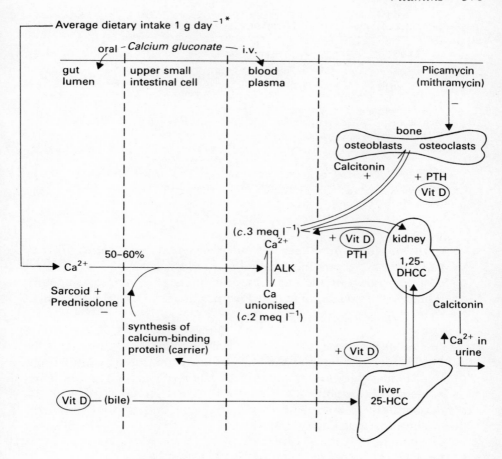

Vitamin D: sources and activation (D_1 was a mixture of compounds; D_4 is a reduced derivative of D_2)

Vitamin	Usual name	Produced by irradiation of	Mammalian source	Converted in Liver to	Kidney to
D_3	Cholecalciferol	7-Dehydro-cholesterol	Diet Sunlight on the skin	25-Hydroxy cholecalciferol (calcidiol, US: calcifediol)	1,25-Dihydroxy cholecalciferol (calcitriol)
D_2	Ergocalciferol (calciferol)	Ergosterol (in plants)	Diet	Similar compounds	

Fig. 16.1 Pharmacokinetics of calcium with main modifying hormones, drugs and pathological condition: +, increased; −, decreased. *More required during pregnancy or lactation. PTH, parathyroid hormone; Vit D, vitamin D; ALK, alkalosis.

Table 16.2   Hormonal control of plasma calcium content

Function affected	Hypercalcaemic factors		Hypocalaemic factor: calcitonin
	Activated vitamin D	Parathyroid hormone	
Absorption from gut	+ +	(+)	0
Mobilisation	(+)	+ +	− −
Reabsorption from kidney tubular fluid	+	+	−

Effect: + +, major increase; +, marked increase; (+), minor increase; − −, major decrease; −, marked decrease; 0, negligible decrease.

- mobilisation from bone (via increased cAMP, *see* Table 4.5)
- reabsorption from the renal tubular fluid
- absorption from the small intestine. Indirectly, by increasing renal 1(alpha)-hydroxylase function which results in enhanced activation of vitamin D.

Calcitonin (originally extracted from the parafollicular 'C' cells of the thyroid but also now known to be additionally produced by similar cells in the human parathyroid and thymus glands) produces hypocalcaemia by increased calcium
- deposition in bone
- excretion in the urine.

16.4   Treatment of abnormalities in calcium distribution

Tetany

Tetany (generated by low *ionised* calcium in the plasma, *see* Fig. 8.6) is of two types which require radically different treatments.

1   *Hypocalcaemic* (low total calcium resulting in low ionised Ca^{2+} content), e.g. due to hypoparathyroidism. In the short-term, administer calcium gluconate either i.v. *slowly* (otherwise cardiac dysrhythmias may occur—*but must monitor plasma calcium concentrations*) or orally (if less urgent). In the long-term, calcium gluconate plus a vitamin D preparation should be given orally.

2   *Eucalcaemic* (alkalotic tetany). From Fig. 16.1 it can be seen that alkalosis, such as that caused by overbreathing in hysteria (or in the early stages of salicylate overdosage, 7.9), diminishes the ionised in relation to the unionised calcium plasma concentration, so that tetany is precipitated. In these cases there is no deficit in total plasma calcium, and reversal of the alkalosis by simply increasing blood CO_2 (rebreathing into a bag) plus sedation is effective in the hysterical situation.

Hypercalcaemia

As indicated in Table 16.3, chelation or renal elimination of the ion is generally effective in reducing plasma Ca^{2+} levels to normal (*monitor with repeated estimations*); other more specific methods are shown: combine all with appropriate treatment of the cause.

Idiopathic hypercalciuria responds to
- dietary restriction of calcium
- sodium cellulose phosphate (a divalent cation-exchange resin which binds calcium in the gut, and, thereby, prevents its absorption)
- thiazide diuretics (*see* Table 12.4) which diminish renal calcium excretion.

Table 16.3   Treatment of hypercalcaemia

Agent	Mechanism	Cause of the condition			
		Hyperpara-thyroidism	Sarcoidosis	Vitamin D overdose	Bone malignancy
Trisodium edetate	Chelation	+	+	+	+
Prednisolone	Decreased gut absorption		+	+	
Calcitonin* Plicamycin† Disodium etidronate*‡	Decreased bone mobilisation	+		+	+ + +
Frusemide§ (Table 12.4)	Decreased reabsorption from renal tubular fluid	+	+	+	+

* Also used in Paget's disease of bone.
† An alkylating agent (Fig. 19.8).
‡ This (and related diphosphonates) decreases the turnover of calcium hydroxyapatite which is increased in Paget's disease.
§ Plus fluid supplements—as dehydration (due to vomiting and polyuria) is usually present in acute hypercalcaemia.

16.5   Water-soluble vitamins

B complex

Vitamin B_{12} and folic acid (*see* 17.1)

Vitamin B_6 (pyridoxine) is indicated
- for deficiency prophylaxis, e.g. to prevent peripheral neuropathy during treatment with isoniazid (19.2) or penicillamine (pp. 148, 172)

- to activate enzymes for which its derivative pyridoxal phosphate is a co-factor, e.g. in homocystinuria to increase the formation of cysteine (normally lacking in this condition).

Vitamin C. This is useful clinically in scurvy and to acidify the urine (12.10). As a powerful reducing agent it is commonly added in low concentration to solutions of oxidisable substances such as catecholamines to prevent their inactivation during laboratory testing.

17 Blood

17.1 Red blood cell formation

Iron

The economy of the body with respect to this essential element is shown in Fig. 17.1. The normal dietary requirement is about 10 mg day^{-1} which, assuming 10% absorption, produces the 1 mg day^{-1} adequate to replace the amount lost via the bile, epithelial cells of gut and skin on desquamation, and in the urine. Menstruating females (loss 5–80 mg per period) or others suffering from a chronic *loss* of blood (e.g. patients with haemorrhoids) require iron supplements. The latter may also be needed when there is an increased *requirement* (e.g. pregnancy, dietary lack, marrow hypofunction or increased red cell destruction).

Absorption occurs almost entirely in the ferrous form, mainly in the upper small intestine, by the intermediation of the carrier molecule apoferritin which combines with iron to form ferritin. In the plasma, iron
- is attached to a protein (transferrin) which is normally only about one-third saturated (this becomes saturated in iron poisoning, *see* later)
- is present in a negligible amount compared with that in circulating erythrocyte haemoglobin.

The total body iron is *c.* 50 mg kg^{-1} (male); *c.* 35 mg kg^{-1} (female). Thus, a 70 kg man has 3.5 g of the element, divisible (approximately) into

6% (0.2 g).	*Fixed*, e.g. in essential enzymes (such as cytochromes and catalase), e.g. in myoglobin: not available for haemoglobin synthesis.
24% (0.8 g).	*Storage*: as ferritin in the reticulo-endothelial system.
70% (2.5 g).	*Erythrocytic*: as haemoglobin in red blood cells both circulating and along with their precursors in the red bone marrow.

Therefore in iron-deficiency anaemia, to increase the haemoglobin by 1% per day—which is the usual aim, except in emergencies—25 mg of elemental iron is required. As the 200 mg ferrous sulphate tablet contains 60 mg of iron, about a quarter of which is absorbed (Fig. 17.1, footnote), 15 mg per tablet is available within the body so that 2–3 tablets every day are adequate. Side-effects are mainly gastrointestinal

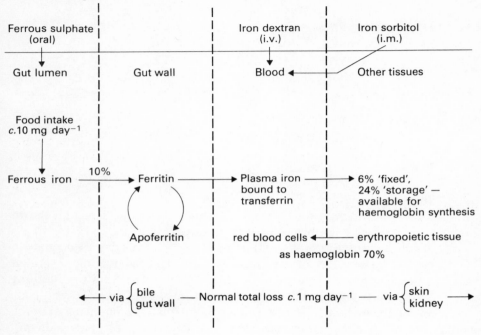

Fig. 17.1 (*Top*) iron preparations. (*Below*) pharmacokinetics of iron.
Note: Different intake requirements, e.g. menstruating (*see* text). Different absorptions from gut of *dietary* iron—normal person, 5–10%; iron deficiency anaemic patient, 10–20%: of *medicinal* iron, 20–30%.

(nausea and vomiting; constipation is more common than diarrhoea—unlike poisoning, *see* below) and may be induced by suggestion (e.g. talking to other prospective mothers at the antenatal clinic), but if genuine, they may often be alleviated by the prescription of an alternative preparation such as ferrous gluconate.

Poisoning
Iron sulphate tablets are pale green in colour and shaped like similarly coloured Smarties®—though in fact less than half the size. Nevertheless, the resemblance means that they are sometimes eaten by younger children in sufficient amounts to produce poisoning. The brunt of the damage falls on the gastrointestinal tract (vomiting, colic, diarrhoea); accompanying blood losses orally, rectally or intraperitoneally (by perforation) lead to haemorrhagic shock (hypotension, pallor, tachycardia). The passage of large amounts of iron into the blood overloads the transferrin capacity so that the metal is precipitated out in several organs, particularly the liver which is on the direct portal route. Acidosis (with hyperventilation) and coma can result. Death may occur

at any point, though there is commonly a stage of apparent recovery between the initial and terminal stages.

Treatment must be prompt and consists of
• first-aid. Raw egg or milk to precipitate the iron as the albuminate or the caseinate
• chelation with desferrioxamine (US: deferoxamine). This is best given i.v. but there is a maximum dose, as it can liberate histamine (20.9) and thus, dangerously, intensify the hypotension: i.m. injection is a safer but less immediate route
• stomach washout. Care must be taken because of the perforation risk. Use sodium bicarbonate solution (to precipitate iron carbonate) and follow by the retention administration of desferrioxamine.

Parenteral iron
Sometimes, in iron-deficiency anaemia, oral iron preparations are unsatisfactory or contraindicated. For example there may be proven malabsorption of the element, patient disobedience, or iron preparations may be too irritant. Under such conditions parenteral iron therapy is indicated. This will replenish the body stores rapidly but not significantly increase the rate of haemoglobin synthesis. *A test dose should preferably be given first.* Suitable preparations are
• i.m. iron sorbitol. This contains iron which is well absorbed with a low occurrence both of local irritant effects and general toxic actions (e.g. allergy, *see* below). Iron dextran is an alternative but about 10% may remain for some time at the injection site and—although it is perfectly safe in humans—repeated i.m. usage in rats has produced sarcomata
• i.v. iron dextran is satisfactory. Given either as single injections or as a total dose infusion (this does not procure more rapid erythropoiesis but ensures adequate medication in disobedient patients); it has a low incidence of allergic responses (rash, fever, bronchospasm).

Folic acid, vitamin B$_{12}$
These substances are essential for DNA/RNA formation and lack particularly manifests itself on erythrocytes resulting in megaloblastic anaemias.

Folic acid
This is an essential precursor for the folinic acid co-enzyme necessary to achieve the one-carbon transfers requisite for purine and nucleotide production (Figs 19.4–19.6). As its name implies, this vitamin is present in 'leaves' (green vegetables) as well as most other foods, and diets are adequate except in

- malnutrition or malabsorption syndromes
- chronic haemolytic anaemias (where there is a rapid red cell turn-over).

In these situations, oral replacement therapy is entirely satisfactory.

Complications arise in the following circumstances

- when red (or white) cell toxicity occurs with an agent which inhibits dihydrofolate reductase (e.g. methotrexate, trimethoprim; *see* Fig. 19.5). Here, fol*in*ic acid (5-formyltetrahydrofolic acid; US: leucovorin) is preferable to folic acid for avoidance of the blood disorder without nullification of the chemotherapeutic action
- with antiepileptic agents (e.g. phenytoin) which are inactivated by hydroxylation (requiring a folic acid co-factor), folate-deficiency anaemias can occur (*see* p. 170) but administration of the vitamin can result in greater drug breakdown
- in pernicious anaemia (*see* immediately below).

Vitamin B₁₂ (cyanocobalamin)

This is the 'extrinsic factor', present in the diet, which cannot be absorbed from the small intestine unless the mucoprotein ('intrinsic factor') is elaborated by the appropriate cells in the gastric mucosa (these are non-functional in pernicious anaemia). The vitamin only occurs in animal (including microorganismal) tissues and is therefore absent from the diets of vegans, who abstain from all animal products. Functionally, cyanocobalamin forms a co-enzyme essential for erythro-poiesis, its actions interdigitating with those of folinic acid in a complex, but collaborative, fashion. In pernicious anaemia, the diffi-culty of absorption of the vitamin can readily be overcome by the parenteral administration of cyanocobalamin or preferably, as the treatment is for life, injections of the longer-lasting (because more heavily plasma protein bound, p. 9) hydroxocobalamin.

However, particular caution must be exercised if subacute combined degeneration of the spiral cord is present. Hydroxocobalamin is the correct therapy but must *not* be accompanied by concomitant folic acid administration, as Fig. 17.2 makes clear. While folic acid and vitamin B₁₂ act together to achieve erythropoiesis, they are antagonistic with regard to the formation of myelin (the factor lacking in the neurological complication). Normally, the latter is produced via a triple methylation of ethanolamine to choline by a B₁₂-dependent pathway which is opposed if folic acid is also given. Therefore, in pernicious anaemia accompanied by subacute combined degeneration, folic acid must *not* be given routinely as, although it will alleviate the anaemia, it will worsen the neurological disorder.

To summarise, the indications for parenteral hydroxocobalamin are

- pernicious anaemia
- malabsorption syndromes

Red blood cell formation

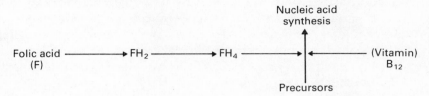

Transmethylation reactions in nervous tissue

Fig. 17.2 Treatment of pernicious anaemia. Vitamin B_{12} and folic acid (F) help each other in the correction of the blood disorder but are antagonistic in the formation of myelin. So, *don't* give folic acid in the presence of subacute combined degeneration of the spinal cord.

- cyanide poisoning (including tobacco amblyopia, 18.4). The aim is to chelate the toxic ion (Table 20.5).

The Schilling test is useful in the assessment of the efficiency of orally administered vitamin B_{12} absorption. Oral radiolabelled compound is followed by immediate, parenteral non-radioactive vitamin (to encourage excretion): lack of radioactivity in the urine indicates defective alimentary absorption.

17.2 Thrombosis

Platelet aggregation

There are two main types of thrombus
- platelet-dominated clot (a primary aggregation of thrombocytes)
- fibrin-dominated clot (a primary precipitation of fibrin strands).

In all thrombi both kinds of aggregatory activity are present, but in conditions of rapid blood flow the platelet interaction predominates whereas in stagnant vascular (usually venous) situations fibrin is the major constituent. However, both types mutually activate each other.

A simplified scheme for platelet aggregation is illustrated in Fig. 17.3. Adhesion of thrombocytes to an injured or pathologically affected blood vessel wall or interaction with collagen or thrombin results in:

1 Activation of *phospholipase C* which produces (from phosphatidyl inositol diphosphate, Fig. 4.7)

a *inositol triphosphate* which increases the free Ca^{2+} ion concentration resulting in

• change in platelet shape from discoid to spheroid with pseudopodia which encourages more aggregation and enables fibrinogen or one of its products to entangle more platelets

• the release of ADP and 5-HT which cause other platelets to become cohesive ('sticky'), autorelease ADP/5-HT and aggregate

b *diacylglycerol* which (*via* protein kinase C) can induce secretion of ADP/5-HT independently of an increase in free internal Ca^{2+} ions. It

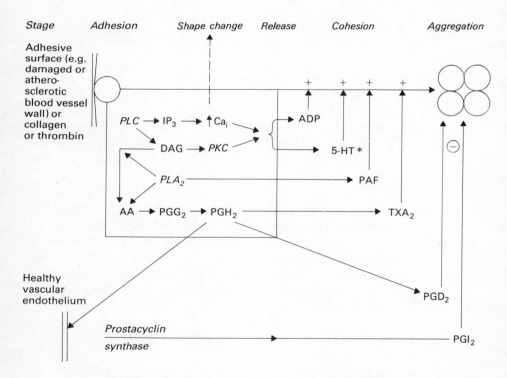

Fig. 17.3 Platelet aggregation. For explanation *see* text. All actions excitatory unless designated (⊖). Interrupted line indicates probable mechanism. AA, arachidonic acid; DAG, diacylglycerol; IP₃, inositol triphosphate; PAF, platelet activating factor; PG, prostaglandin; PKC, protein kinase C; PL, phospholipase (A₂ or C); TX, thromboxane. * 5HT₂ action, *see* Table 5.3.

will also produce some arachidonic acid when hydrolysed by phospholipase A_2 (*see* next).

2 Activation of *phospholipase A_2* which produces

a *platelet activating factor* (Fig. 4.7b). This, in turn, causes further activation of both phospholipases C and A_2

b *arachidonic acid either* from membrane phospholipids (*see* Fig. 5.6) *or* by hydrolysis of diacylglycerol (*see* Fig. 4.7a). Consequent production of eicosanoids mainly involves thromboxane A_2 (TXA$_2$) although prostaglandin D_2 is also formed (and PGI$_2$, *see* next).

TXA$_2$ is a potent inducer of irreversible platelet aggregation *but some collagen-induced aggregation can occur in its absence*: it also constricts vascular smooth muscle. There is a safety mechanism, however, inasmuch as healthy vascular endothelia (but not platelets) contain prostacyclin synthase which forms the potent anti-aggregatory agent and vasodilator, prostacyclin (PGI$_2$). Some races (e.g. Eskimo, *strictly* Inuit) whose diet contains fats with an extra double bond (thus producing, instead of arachidonic acid—*see* Fig. 5.6—an eicosa*penta*enoic acid) preferentially form TXA$_3$, which is only weakly aggregatory and PGI$_3$, which is a good inhibitor of aggregation: this might account for their lower incidence of myocardial infarction. PGI$_2$ also has *fibrinolytic* and *'cytoprotective'* (e.g. protects myocardial cells against hypoxia) effects: these are not dependent on cAMP. The anti-aggregatory action is dependent on cAMP and, therefore, can be duplicated (weakly) by β_2-adrenoceptor agonists and phosphodiesterase III inhibitors. Other endothelium-derived products which decrease platelet aggregation are endothelium-derived relaxing factor (which produces its effects via GMP, Fig. 10.5) and 13-HODE (13-*h*ydroxy-9, 11-*o*ctadeca*di*enoic acid, formed from dietary linoleic acid).

Possible drugs to diminish platelet aggregation in the treatment of thromboembolic conditions

• prostacyclin (epoprostenol) has a very short $t_{1/2}$ (few minutes) and produces too much general vasodilation, causing fainting. Attempts are being made to develop derivatives without these disadvantages

• a specific inhibitor of thromboxane synthetase (dazoxiben) is being tested clinically but remember that some collagen-induced aggregation is TXA$_2$-independent

• aspirin (*in low dosage*) is used as an antithrombotic. Its major effect is to inhibit cyclo-oxygenase function irreversibly, and it is stated to achieve a beneficial response by preventing platelet microsomal enzyme activity for the life of the cell (several days) but vascular intimal enzyme action for a much shorter period (several hours for new enzyme synthesis to occur); thus, TXA$_2$ is depressed more than PGI$_2$ (this differential effect appears to be enhanced at lower drug dosage). Aspirin may also act by other mechanisms, e.g. decreased liberation of ADP (and ? 5-HT, p. 260) from platelets, e.g. depression of TXA_2-independent pathways.

Some other drugs affecting platelet function are shown in Table 17.2.

Fibrin formation (Fig. 17.4)

Vitamin K
This is an essential co-factor for the conversion of glutamic acid to γ-carboxyglutamic acid which is essential for the production of factors II (prothrombin), VII, IX and X in the liver. There are two main natural forms, differing only in their side-chain substituents, namely
• *vitamin K_1* (phytomenadione; US: phytonadione). As its name suggests, this is derived from plant sources (e.g. green vegetables). It is the main dietary source of this vitamin and is absorbed in the small intestine with the help of bile salts.
• *vitamin K_2*. Is formed by microorganisms in the gut and also requires bile salts for its absorption.
    Deficiency presents, and so indications are, in *hypoprothrombinaemias* (the other three factors are also depressed, *see* under oral anticoagulants, later in this section) e.g. due to malabsorption, liver disease or drugs (warfarin; aspirin toxicity, 7.9). Most vitamin K preparations take several hours to act so, in an emergency, fresh blood or freeze-dried plasma is given (antidote to warfarin, Table 17.1).

Anticoagulants
These are used for the prevention or treatment of blood clotting. As shown in Table 17.1, they are divisible into the following:
1 *Parenteral anticoagulants*: type substance, heparin, which
a acts *directly* upon clotting factors (Fig. 17.4) and thus is effective
• immediately: use for initial therapy *in vivo*
• also *in vitro*: use in extracorporeal circuits, e.g. heart–lung preparations. Platelets are activated by *artificial* surfaces which cannot produce prostacyclin; therefore add PGI_2 (epoprostenol) as well as heparin
b is relatively short-lasting.
2 *Oral anticoagulants*: type substance, warfarin, which
a acts *indirectly* to inhibit synthesis of vitamin K-dependent clotting factors and thus is effective only
• when circulating clotting factors have been sufficiently depleted
• *in vivo*
b is longer-lasting: use for continuation therapy.
Haemorrhage is the chief side-effect of both groups.

Heparin. The anticoagulant effect of heparin is mainly achieved by inducing a conformational change in (inactive) plasma antithrombin III

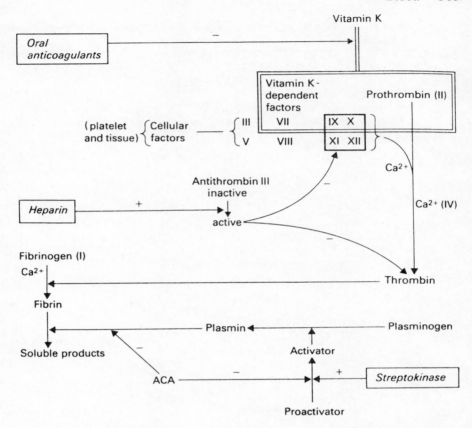

Fig. 17.4 Drugs acting on the formation and breakdown of fibrin. Roman numerals indicate clotting factors which are *activated* in cascade fashion to products designated by an additional 'a', e.g. factor XIIa. ACA, aminocaproic acid; +, excitation; −, inhibition.

to generate the active form which, in turn, now attaches to the proteases thrombin and *activated* factors IX, X, XI and XII to neutralise their actions. *Note*: oestrogens reduce plasma levels of antithrombin III.

Heparin is present with histamine in mast cells (5.1) and is prepared from animal sources: yet allergic responses seldom occur. Chemically, it is a mucopolysaccharide containing many acidic (negatively charged) sulphonyl groups. An effective antidote is the strongly positively charged protein, protamine, although it is rarely required due to the relatively short half-life of heparin. (*c.* 90 minutes after the usual i.v. dose). Protamine is given i.v. *slowly* (to avoid cardiovascular collapse) and in equal dose to that of the heparin (as in excess it is itself an anticoagulant).

Oral anticoagulants. These drugs are structural analogues of the naphthoquinone end of the vitamin K molecule and they antagonise its

Table 17.1 Anticoagulants: comparison of the pharmacological properties of heparin with those of warfarin

	Heparin	Warfarin
Pharmacokinetics		
Route of administration	i.v. (injection or infusion), s.c.	Oral
Distribution: cross placenta	No. Can use drug during pregnancy	Yes—can cause fetal haemorrhages. Avoid during pregnancy
Plasma protein binding	High	High (95–99%)
Hepatic metabolism	Mainly	Mainly
Renal excretion (unchanged)	Slight	Slight
Pharmacodynamics		
Effect		
anticoagulant	*In vitro* and *in vitro*	*In vivo* only
onset	Immediate (given i.v.)	1–3 days
offset	3–5 h (after i.v. injection)	3–5 days
mechanism	Antithrombin Anti-*activated* factors IX, X, XI and XII	Interference with production of factors II, VII, IX and X
control test(s)	Activated partial thromboplastin time	Prothrombin time or percentage*
Side- and toxic effects:		
bleeding	Can occur	Can occur
antidote	Protamine (excess can cause bleeding)	Fresh blood; freeze-dried plasma (prothrombin-preserved); vitamin K preparations (slower)
allergy	Rare	Uncommon

* This test is invalid during a heparin infusion.

actions reversibly. The type substance, warfarin, is a coumarin and shows significantly less allergic reactions (including renal involvement, type III, Table 20.1) than the structurally similar indandione, phenindione, which is now obsolete.

Warfarin depresses the formation of factors II, VII, IX and X and, as prothrombin (II) has the longest half-life among these, its reduction to and maintenance at a requisite plasma level is the most sensitive indicator of the continuation dose to be given (Table 17.1).

As the amount of free warfarin in the plasma has to be so closely controlled, interactions with other drugs become very critical and the difficulties are intensified because this anticoagulant is

• mainly metabolised (in the liver)

• given as the racemate which consists of two isomers (R- and S-warfarin) with different potencies—S greater than R—and different mechanisms of hepatic breakdown. Phenylbutazone decreases the breakdown of S-warfarin (as do metronidazole and co-trimoxazole) but increases the plasma clearance of the less active R-isomer with a resultant overall potentiation of warfarin action.

Further possibilities of interactions with commonly administered drugs are legion but in Table 17.2 an attempt has been made to classify some of the more illustrative examples. Most drugs exert consistent effects (even if via more than one factor): e.g. aspirin, clofibrate— potentiation; e.g. oestrogens—antagonism. Some do not; for example rifampicin is usually antagonistic due to increased breakdown of warfarin but this may be opposed by displacement from plasma proteins (only temporary) or an allergic thrombocytopenia (p. 436).

Ethanol is usually interdicted during warfarin therapy. Undoubtedly, in the chronic alcoholic, liver function is depressed and compliance

Table 17.2 Possible drug interactions with warfarin

	Drugs which tend to cause the anticoagulant effect of warfarin to be	
Site and mechanism of interaction	Increased	Decreased
Gut		
Absorption of vitamin K: decreased	Liquid paraffin	
Absorption of warfarin: decreased		Cholestyramine
Liver		
Metabolism of warfarin		
Microsomal enzyme activity:		
increased		Rifampicin
		Phenytoin
Microsomal enzyme activity:		
decreased	Allopurinol	
Competition for microsomal		
enzymes	Tolbutamide	
Breakdown of S-warfarin: decreased	Phenylbutazone*	
	Metronidazole	
	Co-trimoxazole	
Blood		
Clearance of R-warfarin: increased	Phenylbutazone*	
Plasma protein binding of warfarin:		
decreased†	Clofibrate	
	Rifampicin	
Alteration in clotting factors		
platelet aggregation		
decreased	Aspirin	
	Clofibrate	
increased		Oestrogens
antithrombin III: decreased		Oestrogens
Thrombocytopenia (type II allergy)	Rifampicin	

* *See* text.
† Only slight temporary effect because of increased distribution and renal excretion (p. 15).

is poor, but relatively few patients fall into this category and only a minor amount of ethanol metabolism occurs within the hepatic microsomal system (1.9) which is, however, initially stimulated but later depressed by indulgence in alcohol. Moderate ethanol intake might be allowable.

Warfarin is a rat poison and resistant strains have appeared; some humans show a similar proclivity (*see* Table 20.4,4).

Fibrinolytics and their antagonists
The basic situation is portrayed in Fig. 17.4. The fibrin clot is broken up (solubilised) by plasmin which is activated from its precursor, plasminogen. Fibrinolytic agents generate the activating enzyme. An example is streptokinase which is injected near a massive pulmonary embolus for 3 days and may produce recanalisation (monitored by angiograms) within a week. This drug is very expensive and, because it is obtained from a streptococcus, may produce allergic reactions to the bacterial protein. An alternative preparation, stated to be non-allergenic, is urokinase (now obtained synthetically but still very expensive). In either case, therapy results in systemic plasminogen depletion so that, on cessation of treatment, heparin cover is indicated for about a week until the fibrinolytic system has been restored to normal. If serious bleeding should take place during (or after) fibrinolytic therapy, the antidotes are aminocaproic acid (Fig. 17.4) or an analogue, tranexamic acid.

Attempts to avoid systemic defibrination (and therefore bleeding) by the use of preparations with a relatively greater ability to activate *fibrin-bound* plasminogen such as anistreplase (APSAC, *a*nisoylated *p*lasminogen-*s*treptokinase *a*ctivator *c*omplex) or alteplase (*t-PA*, recombinant human *t*issue-type *p*lasminogen *a*ctivator) have not proved wholly successful. But APSAC has a significantly longer functional half-life than streptokinase while t-PA is less antigenic. Each of the three can improve survival when infused in acute myocardial infarction and clinical trials are in progress to compare t-PA, APSAC and streptokinase as 'life-savers'.

17.3   Side- and toxic effects upon formed elements of the blood
Representative drug examples follow: add others as you meet them.

All red marrow-produced cells, i.e. erythrocytes, granulocytic leucocytes and platelets, are depressed (pancytopenia) by, for example, 'antimitotic' agents (*see* Table 19.2); or, rarely, with gold salts or penicillamine (*see* Table 5.13). This response can be allergic in origin, e.g. with chloramphenicol, 19.6.
Red blood cells. These may show
- abnormalities of haemoglobin synthesis: porphyrias (20.6).
- changes in the haemoglobin molecule: formation of carboxyhaemo-

globin (e.g. carbon monoxide poisoning) or methaemoglobin (e.g. 'nitrites', primaquine). Methaemoglobinaemia is due to the conversion of ferrous to ferric iron in the haemoglobin molecule which renders it incapable of oxygen carriage. Most cases are slight but, if treatment is necessary, the most satisfactory reducing agent is methylene blue: this is not suitable in patients with glucose-6-phosphate dehydrogenase deficiency (20.6).

• reduced blood erythrocyte content due to *either* decreased marrow production (aplastic anaemia) e.g. due to chloramphenicol (19.6), *or* haemolysis e.g. α-methyldopa (Type II allergy, *see* Table 20.1), e.g. primaquine (glucose-6-phosphate dehydrogenase lack, *see* Table 20.4, 7).

White blood cells. Granulocytopenia (leucopenia) may be dose-related or an allergic response. It can occur, for example, with phenytoin or ethosuximide (*see* Table 7.1), chlorpromazine (*see* Table 7.6), captopril (10.5), carbamizole (14.3), chlorpropamide or tolbutamide (*see* Table 14.9) and chloramphenicol (19.6). Patients taking such drugs should be told to report immediately if they get a sore throat, mouth ulcers or a raised temperature: stop the drug and institute anti-infective therapy.

Platelets. Thrombocytopenia from a type II allergic reaction (e.g. caused by rifampicin) or a pancytopenia results in purpura. Some drugs affecting platelet aggregation are shown in Table 17.2.

18 Eye and Skin

18.1 Physiological backgound (Fig. 18.1; Table 18.1)
The pupil is
- constricted via parasympathetic fibres arising in the oculomotor (IIIrd cranial) nerve nucleus in the brainstem, the postganglionic fibres of which activate the constrictor (sphincter) pupillae muscle of the iris through muscarinic, cholinergic receptors

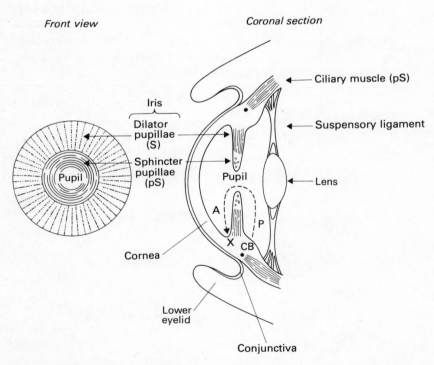

Front view   *Coronal section*

Ciliary muscle (pS)

Iris

Dilator
pupillae
(S)

Suspensory ligament

Sphincter
pupillae
(pS)

Pupil

Pupil

Lens

A

P

X CB

Cornea

Lower
eyelid

Conjunctiva

Fig. 18.1 Anatomy of the eye (anterior parts: diagrammatic). A, anterior chamber; P, posterior chamber—both containing aqueous humour; interrupted line indicates circulation of the latter fluid from ciliary body (CB) to filtration angle (X). Innervation: pS, parasympathetic; S, sympathetic.

- dilated via sympathetic fibres traversing the superior cervical ganglion to cause *contraction* of the iridal dilator (radial) pupillae muscle by activation of postganglionic α-adrenoceptors.

The pupil size is modified reflexly by several mechanisms; the most important pharmacologically are

- *light reflexes*. Light shone into one eye elicits pupillary constriction in the same (direct reflex) or the opposite (consensual reflex) eye. The pathways involved are: afferents—optic nerves; superior colliculi; efferents—oculomotor nerves (parasympathetic)
- *accommodation reflex*. When a near object is focused, the pupil is automatically constricted to aid definition. Similar pathways to the above but greater central involvement is necessary, via the lateral geniculate bodies and occipital (visual) cortices.

Accommodation for near vision to ensure clear focusing is achieved by activation of efferent parasympathetic (IIIrd nerve) fibres producing contraction of the right and left ciliary muscles. Each of the latter has the shape of a truncated cone with the origin of the muscle at the end of smaller radius (Fig. 18.1): contraction of the muscle, therefore, results in it adopting a smaller overall circumference with consequent slackening of the suspensory ligaments so that the lens (under less external tension) is allowed to adopt its more globular (natural) configuration.

Table 18.1 Autonomic control of visual activity

	Parasympathetic	Sympathetic
Smooth muscle receptors involved	Muscarinic, cholinoceptor	α-adrenoceptor
Iris		
sphincter pupillae	Contraction	
dilator pupillae		Contraction
resultant effect upon pupil	Constriction (miosis)	Dilation (mydriasis)
Ciliary muscle	Contraction	
near point of vision*	Nearer	Slightly further†
Intraocular blood vessels	Dilation	Constriction
Intraocular pressure (*if raised*)‡	Decreased	Decreased§
Levator palpebrae superioris		Contraction
Nictitating membrane		Contraction

* Simplest measure of maximum degree of accommodation to a near object which can be achieved.
† Due to pupillary dilation (*see* text).
‡ Effects of drugs rather than nerve stimulation.
§ Probably due to vasoconstriction decreasing both the intraocular and vascular volume and the rate of formation of aqueous humour.

From the pharmacological viewpoint, the important consideration is that, while parasympathomimetic drugs or their antagonists affect accommodation significantly, sympathomimetic agents or their antagonists only do so marginally (e.g. as the pupil becomes dilated, the near point of vision—*see* footnote[†] to Table 18.1—moves slightly further away).

Intraocular pressure. This is measured by external instrumentation of the conjunctiva and represents the balance between formation, capacity and absorption in the aqueous humour system.

Formation, which occurs primarily at the ciliary bodies, is similar in many respects to cerebrospinal fluid production, i.e. mainly passive but with some active (Na^+ ions) or facilitated (D-glucose) processes. Lipid solubility is the major prerequisite for drugs to cross the blood–aqueous (analogous to the blood–brain) barrier. *Capacity* of the system is increased by intraocular vasoconstriction and lessened by vasodilation. *Absorption* of the bulk of aqueous humour occurs at the iridocorneal (filtration) angle into the spaces of Fontana, canal of Schlemm and the long ciliary veins.

Glaucoma (Gk: *glaukos*, bluish-green; the colour of the chronically affected eye) is due to raised intraocular pressure and is dangerous because of pressure on the optic nerve which, if maintained, can cause blindness. Acute glaucoma requires surgical relief: the more common chronic glaucoma can be controlled by decreased formation or increased absorption of aqueous humour. The fall in production is usually initially brought about by β-blockers, e.g. timolol, given as eye-drops: mechanism of action unclear. Other drugs which decrease aqueous humour formation are adrenaline (p. 392) and acetazolamide. The latter—given orally—is a carbonic anhydrase inhibitor which is considered to act by prevention of sodium bicarbonate, and hence water, passage into the aqueous humour (similarly to its action on the renal tubular cells, p. 305). Miotics (18.2) lower intraocular pressure mainly by stretching the iris centrally thus allowing freer access of aqueous humour to the filtration angle (especially in narrow-angle glaucoma): conversely, mydriatics (e.g. atropine) can precipitate glaucoma in some patients.

Eyelids. The eye is opened mainly by withdrawal of the upper eyelid using the levator palpebrae superioris which is innervated both somatically (therefore, eyelid closure with D-tubocurarine) and autonomically (sympathetic: α-adrenoceptors mediating contraction). In many mammals (e.g. cat) there is a 'third eyelid' called the nictitating membrane (L: *nictitare*, to wink). This has its origin near the inner canthus of the eye and in the relaxed state covers approximately the *medial* third of the conjunctiva. Stimulation of its sympathetic innervation results in its retraction nasally. (*Aide-mémoire*: in the 'fight or flight' situation, the eye should be fully 'open'.) The nictitating membrane can easily be attached to a recording system and used as a marker of either superior cervical ganglion or α-adrenoceptor activity (Fig. 2.8).

18.2 Effects of drugs modifying ocular autonomic mechanisms

A knowledge of these is not only essential for correct therapeutic usage but is also valuable for revision of autonomic pharmacology which can, in many cases, be reinforced in the experimental laboratory using human subjects. A simple scheme based on pupil changes is shown in Table 18.2 and will now be discussed further.

Miotic drugs are indicated to reverse mydriatic actions and in the treatment of glaucoma. They are given as eye-drops (which are suitably buffered to avoid local irritation) into the lower conjunctival sac, from which ocular absorption is satisfactory: subsequent absorption from the eye or nasolachrymal duct occasionally happens at high concentrations with resultant systemic effects. The latter is most likely to occur with the long-acting ecothiopate, less so with the shorter-acting parasympath-omimetic miotics, e.g. eserine (p. 48), pilocarpine (p. 53). Additionally, long-term treatment with ecothiopate commonly results in cataract (18.4).

Table 18.2 Comparison of miotic and mydriatic mechanisms

Mechanism	Miotic example(s)	Mydriatic example(s) With cycloplegia*	Without cycloplegia	Reference
Parasympathetic				
Central (stimulation of IIIrd nerve nucleus)	Morphine			Table 7.15
Muscarinic agonist	Pilocarpine			Table 2.4
Muscarinic antagonists		Atropine Homatropine Tropicamide		Table 2.8
Anticholinesterases	Eserine (physostigmine) Ecothiopate			2.6
Sympathetic				
Adrenergic neurone block	Guanethidine†			p. 83
α-Adrenoceptor agonism			Phenylephrine	Table 3.2
Uptake₁ block			Cocaine	Table 8.2

* Cycloplegia means paralysis of ciliary muscle function and, thus, inability to accommodate for near vision.
† Usually an initial *mydriasis* occurs (*see* p. 392).

Mydriatic and cycloplegic drugs. These are muscarinic antagonists (Table 2.8). Atropine is indicated in acute iridocyclitis. For general use, homatropine is preferable but is being replaced for routine retinoscopy by tropicamide—which has a much shorter action (a few hours).

Mydriatic drugs. Sympathomimetic substances (e.g. phenylephrine, an α-adrenoceptor agonist, 3.3) can be used as mydriatics. Strangely, adrenaline instilled into the conjunctival sac is a weak mydriatic because constriction of the conjunctival vessels (readily seen in the human eye—'white eye'; compare with 'red eye' due to atropine vasodilation, 18.4) limits absorption to the iris. However, adrenaline can lower a *raised* intraocular pressure. (Table 18.1, footnote§). Guanethidine has a similar action but initial accompanying mydriasis *reverts to miosis* later (this drug is also used to alleviate lid retraction in exophthalmic goitre, p. 337). Cocaine is unique among local anaesthetics in that it also blocks uptake$_1$ and, therefore, has additional sympathomimetic actions. These effects can easily be shown in the human subject and may be used in eye surgery to produce pupil dilation and vasoconstriction (less bleeding) *with local analgesia.*

18.3   Miscellaneous drug actions on the eye

Infections of the conjunctiva, cornea (keratitis) or eyelids (blepharitis) are usually treated with anti-infective drugs by local application which avoids systemic effects. Antibacterial agents are neomycin (19.6), chloramphenicol (19.6) and sulphacetamide. This latter compound in solution can be brought to neutrality without precipitation (unlike most other sulphonamides) and thereby made non-irritant to the eye. The antiviral agent acyclovir is used in herpes simplex keratitis (19.9).

Allergic conjunctivitis may be treated with a preparation of sodium cromoglycate. The use of locally applied adrenal glucocorticoids as anti-inflammatory agents requires care as they can increase the spread of infection and also may produce glaucoma by an increase in the intraocular pressure, due to interference with aqueous outflow.

Retinal sensitivity is increased by strychnine. Given experimentally to human subjects at dosage well below that which produces any effects upon spinal reflexes (9.7), it results in an expanded visual field with greater colour discrimination, especially in the blue/yellow range.

18.4   Ocular toxicity and side-effects

It is important to realise the possibilities here as monitoring is simple in most cases.

Allergy. The commonest offenders are locally applied antimicrobial agents and atropine. For example, the latter often produces a 'red eye' due to local vasodilation which subsides in about 10 minutes (20.3) and is thus readily separable from the persistent vasodilation of atropine poisoning (Table 2.7).

Glaucoma. Adrenal glucocorticoids and atropine both interfere with removal of aqueous humour.

Cataract means loss of transparency of the lens or its capsule. It can occur with prolonged use of ecothiopate (2.6), chlorpromazine (Table 7.6), or adrenal glucocorticoids (Table 14.1).

Retina. Digoxin overdosage (p. 271) commonly produces visual disturbances (particularly changes in colour perception, haloes round objects, scotomata or decreased acuity), which are considered to be primarily mediated at the photoreceptor level.

Chloroquine (19.8) causes corneal opacities and retinal pigmentation: the latter is a good early sign of toxicity.

Retina/optic nerve. The lesions arise either in bipolar or ganglion cells of the retina or the IInd cranial nerve itself. They commonly present as scotomata and may lead to optic atrophy.

Ethambutol (p. 418) is a drug of first choice in the treatment of pulmonary tuberculosis but the dose must be kept fairly low (which it can be with triple therapy) to minimise the above side-effects: repeated monitoring of visual acuity, especially in the red/green, is necessary.

Chronic methanol poisoning leads to optic atrophy (*see* p. 233).

Tobacco amblyopia (*see* Table 2.5) appears to be related to cyanide intake from tobacco smoke and can be treated with hydroxocobalamin (*see* Table 20.5).

Fibrosis of eye structures may occur in combination with some of the above conditions; further specific examples are as follows.
* *retrolental fibroplasia* occurs when 40% oxygen is given to premature babies for prolonged periods (11.6)
* *oculomucocutaneous syndrome* associated with the chronic use of practolol (p. 87) is manifested in the eye by fibrosis of the conjunctiva and cornea (with opacities) and diminished tear secretion. It probably has an immunological basis.

Jaundice due to hepatotoxic drugs (13.9) tinges the conjunctivae yellow.

Corneal microdeposits develop during amiodarone therapy (p. 283).

SKIN

18.5 Physiological background
Much of this has already been detailed elsewhere, *see* sensory function (local anaesthetics, 8.1), vitamin D production (16.2), temperature control (7.8) and skin colour (p. 245).

Extravascular darkening of the skin results from melanocytes passing melanin-containing granules into their epidermal cytoplasmic extensions. Melanins (polymers of indole quinone, synthesised from tyrosine in the melanocytes) are dark pigments (Gk: *melas*, black). Melanocyte-stimulating hormones (MSH) from the intermediate lobe of the pituitary gland increase melanin formation in human skin. Alpha-MSH (Table 6.8) consists of the first 13 amino acids of corticotrophin—which itself has weak MSH activity: this, however, may be sufficient to account for the characteristic 'bronzing' (at pressure points) seen in chronic adrenal insufficiency (Addison's disease), when lack of adrenal glucocorticoid 'negative feed-back' on the hypothalamo-pituitary system raises circulating corticotrophin levels. In *frog* skin the melanin granules are contained in special cells, called melanophores. Under dark conditions, MSH spreads the granules with resultant darkening of the skin and camouflage; in light conditions, melatonin (produced from 5-hydroxytryptamine in the pineal gland) aggregates the granules and lightens the skin coloration. **NB** In mammals, where melatonin probably has a different function, light *decreases* its formation (p. 162) and it does not antagonise MSH action on the melanocytes.

18.6   Pharmacokinetics and the skin

Route of administration
For a local effect, topical (skin) application is usually satisfactory—not least to the patient's psyche. A notable exception is that anti-(H_1) histamines are often given orally, e.g. in urticaria. But, beware of photosensitisation (with anti-(H_1)histamines, antimicrobials), spread of infection (glucocorticoids) or systemic absorption from large areas of abraded skin (antimicrobials, glucocorticoids).

For a systemic effect, the skin is an unusual route. Relatively few drugs penetrate the intact epidermis (the stratum corneum is the significant barrier). However, the percutaneous route avoids hepatic first-pass metabolism and may be used to produce a modest but sustained action, e.g. glyceryl trinitrate (patch or ointment) for anginal prophylaxis, particularly overnight, p. 268.

Cutaneous metabolism. Important in the production of vitamin D_3 (Fig. 16.1, lower).

Excretion. Secretion in the sweat is an unimportant route generally (1.10).

18.7   Drug actions in dermatology (*see* Itch, p. 148)
Emollients (e.g. calamine lotion) soothe by leaving a protective powder after evaporation of the water vehicle, which has a cooling effect.

Anti-(H₁) histamines are specifically indicated in type I allergic skin reactions, particularly urticaria and angioneurotic oedema (as histamine is the predominant autacoid released in these conditions).

Eczema is of two main types
• a type IV hypersensitivity reaction (*see* Table 20.1) leading to inflammation, irritation and itching of the skin
• atopic. This is a familial type I hypersensitivity reaction and the sufferers often develop bronchial asthma later in life. Treatment consists of removal of possible causes, emollients (milder cases) or topical anti-inflammatory glucocorticoids (more severe cases) and antimicrobial therapy if there is superimposed infection.

Treatment of skin infections (sensitivities should first be determined if possible)
• *antibacterial.* Neomycin, an aminoglycoside (19.6) which is too toxic for systemic use, can be applied topically
• *antifungal.* Dermatophytoses (e.g. athlete's foot) are treated locally by pedal hygiene with the application of an imidazole, e.g. clotrimazole or miconazole (p. 406). To treat nail infestations, griseofulvin can be given *orally.* This drug enters the keratin of new nail growth which it clears of fungi but prolonged therapy is required. Unlike most antifungal agents, which mainly act on the cell membrane of the invader (19.4), griseofulvin probably interferes with fungal mitosis (p. 413). The commonest side-effect is headache; it potentiates ethanol and is porphyrogenic (20.6). Prolonged treatment of pregnant rats with much higher dosage of griseofulvin than is given to humans has produced fetotoxicity and teratogenicity; therefore, do not use during pregnancy.

Skin disinfectants
• for a minor procedure, e.g. blood sampling, ethanol, 70% is optimal; higher concentrations precipitate proteins in the microbial cell wall and hinder penetration
• for a major procedure, e.g. surgical operation. Ethanolic solution of iodine (tincture of iodine) or chlorhexidine are used
• surgeon's hands should be cleaned with soap and a chlorhexidine scrub followed by 70% alcohol rinse.

Psoriasis. The major defect is an increase in epidermal mitotic activity which can be depressed by adrenal glucocorticoids, coal tar preparations, dithranol, psoralens (*see* below) or (*under specialist advice*) topical glucococorticoids or oral etretinate. The latter is teratogenic so contraception must be effective. (*See also* psoralens, below.)

*Psoralens.*The skin, on exposure to sunlight, is particularly affected by ultraviolet (UV) radiation as follows

- UVA (320–400 nm wavelength) immediate darkening of melanin; superficial browning
- UVB (290–320 nm), sun*burn*, i.e. redness and blistering on initial exposure with longer-term melanin production.

Both types cause ageing of the skin. UVA is now considered to be more carcinogenic.

Psoralens, such as 8-methoxypsoralen, increase the dermatological responses to UV light. Thus the aim in 'tanning' should be to use a screening agent, which eliminates UVA and UVB; ? along with a psoralen. In psoriasis, UVA plus a psoralen (which cross-links DNA) decreases mitoses. The psoralen may be used alone in vitiligo—a patchy whiteness of the skin, usually on the limbs, where there is a deficiency of melanocyte function.

18.8   Side- and toxic effects of drugs on the skin

Allergic responses
Almost any drug can produce allergic phenomena in the skin whether given topically or systemically. Reactions (*see* Table 20.1) may be
- type II. Uncommon, e.g. purpura with rifampicin
- type I. More common, e.g. with penicillins or aspirin
- type IV. Most common, can occur with gold salts (*see* Table 5.11); phenobarbitone, phenytoin (*see* Table 7.1); chlorpromazine (*see* Table 7.6); phenolphthalein (p.323); carbimazole, iodide (14.3); penicillins (19.3); or sulphonamides (p.408). These effects usually follow systemic administration of the drug and result in allergic eczema, which in severe cases can progress to exfoliative dermatitis. Contact dermatitis (ie. a type IV allergic response to a locally applied agent) can occur with anti-(H_1) histamines (5.7), which are preferably given orally; or with local anaesthetics (*see* Table 8.2).

Photosensitivity
Table 18.3 is descriptive.

Other eruptions
The cutaneous toxicity with practolol (3.5) appears to be like psoriasis—with increased mitoses in the epidermis. Vesicular lesions are present along with redness in erythema multiforme and its more severe manifestation, Stevens–Johnson syndrome, which can occur with, for example, sulphonamides (p.408), especially in elderly patients.

Miscellaneous
1   Acne is a side-effect of treatment with androgens (*see* Table 15.2), androgenic adrenocorticoids (*see* Table 14.1) or corticotrophin (Table 14.3).

Table 18.3 Different types of skin photosensitivity and their properties

	Photoallergy	Phototoxicity
Sunlight acting on	Drug or a metabolite	Drug or a metabolite
Produces	Antigen	Activated compounds
Resulting in	Allergic eczema	Severe sunburn-like reactions
Onset	Delayed—or only on subsequent dose of drug or further exposure to sunight	Rapid—within a few hours
Offset	Slow	Rapid—within a few hours
Other points	Increased sensitivity may persist for a long period	Dark-skinned less affected than fair-skinned; suntan is protective
Therefore	Never give again	Can give again if protect skin from ultraviolet light
Common causes externally applied	Coal tar derivatives; anti-(H_1)histamines (5.7).	
systemically given	Chlorpromazine (Table 7.6)	Chlorpromazine, sulphonamides, tetracyclines, amiodarone Drugs precipitating cutaneous porphyria (20.6)

2 Hirsutism (in the female) can result from treatment with the same drugs or minoxidil (*see* Table 10.3). The latter has been used in baldness.

3 Alopecia is an almost inevitable accompaniment of 'antimitotic' therapy (Table 19.2).

4 Jaundice is an obvious manifestation of drug hepatoxicity (p.329).

19 Chemotherapy

Most therapy nowadays employs drugs whose chemical identity is known and is, therefore, *chemo*therapy; but by convention this term is usually restricted to those medicaments used in the treatment of infective and neoplastic diseases, and as immunosuppressive drugs. Similarly the distinction between chemotherapeutic agents produced by microorganisms (antibiotics) and those produced by the organic chemist (antibacterial substances, e.g. sulphonamides) has been rendered ludicrous by terms such as 'semi-synthetic' penicillins, indicating mould products which have been modified by the chemist.

19.1 Advantages and disadvantages of chemotherapy

Advantages are
- a decrease both in mortality and in morbidity attributable to infectious or neoplastic conditions
- preventive exhibition. Examples: malaria prophylaxis, prior to gastrointestinal surgery (p. 325), to prevent recurrence of rheumatic fever or as an immunosuppressant.

These far outweigh the *disadvantages* which, however, do indicate the areas where caution is necessary in the use of these drugs, namely
- development of resistance by the 'invader' cells
- side-, allergic and toxic effects of the chemotherapeutic agent (including opportunistic infections, *see* under tetracyclines, 19.6)
- production of chronic conditions, e.g. carrier states, 'cold' abscesses
- masking of infection, e.g. PUO (*pyrexia of uncertain origin*); syphilis not diagnosed because of treatment for gonorrhoea
- removal of an antigenic stimulus which produces natural immunity: for example, do not give antimalarial therapy prophylactically to indigenes of countries in which this disease is endemic (except groups at special risk, e.g. under 5-year-olds in present trials in The Gambia).

19.2 Fundamental actions of chemotherapeutic agents

These are shown in Fig. 19.1, and will now be amplified. Major side/toxic effects are described under representative individual drugs in this chapter: for hypersensitivity reactions, *see* 20.2.

Death of the invading organism or cell is obviously the primary concern and may be achieved by a

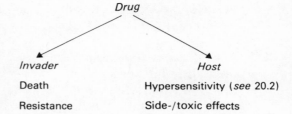

Fig. 19.1 Chemotherapeutic drug action in relation to the invading process and the host (patient).

- 'cidal' effect: the drug directly kills the microorganism or cancer cell
- 'static' effect: the chemotherapeutic substance stops cell multiplication and the injurious agent is then destroyed by natural body defence mechanisms.

Using *in vitro* microbiological tests it can be shown that
- a given agent is lethal to some organisms or cancer cells but only prevents growth in others; or that the effect varies with the concentration used, i.e. the above terms may only be comparative
- a bacteriostatic drug (e.g. chloramphenicol) prevents the action of penicillin which only acts on *multiplying* organisms. Thus, theoretically, combinations of bacteriostatic and bactericidal agents should not be given together.

Such observations and generalisations are valuable but not invariably applicable in practice due to other factors (e.g. defence mechanisms, drug distribution) which complicate such simple relationships. Therapeutically, the drug of first choice is given *immediately after* taking specimens for culture and *in vitro* drug sensitivity tests performed using the patient's own organisms from a swab of the infected area, suitable secretion (e.g. sputum) or tissue extract (cancer cells). If the initial treatment is unsuccessful, alternatives of proven efficacy are thus available. The range of antimicrobial effects is indicated by the terms '*broad-spectrum*' (if a wide variety of organisms is affected) and '*narrow spectrum*' (if only relatively few genera are attacked).

'*Selective toxicity is the basis of chemotherapy*'
This is the fundamental tenet and, obviously, is the more difficult to achieve the closer the relationship between the invader and the host. Thus antibacterial agents, which can exploit major differences in structure and function between the prokaryotic (not having a discrete nucleus, i.e. bacterial) and the eukaryotic (nucleated, i.e. mammalian) cell, have so far been more successful than antiviral (19.9) and anticancer (19.10) chemotherapy.

Sites of action of chemotherapeutic agents may be classified as effects on
1   The cell wall.
2   The cell (plasma) membrane.

3 Nucleic acid synthesis and/or cell division.

4 Messenger RNA (m-RNA) formation and subsequent protein synthesis.

5 Miscellaneous. Two examples follow

- the anthelmintic drugs, Table 19.6

- isoniazid (isonicotinic acid hydrazide) which might form a 'false' NAD (nicotine adenine dinucleotide) and thereby disrupt carbohydrate and fat metabolism, particularly in *Mycobacterium tuberculosis*. Another possibility is that this drug hinders the formation of mycolic acid in the cell wall of the same organism. As this drug is structurally similar to pyridoxine it interferes with the function of and encourages excretion of the latter resulting in peripheral neuritis, which can be prevented by prophylactic administration of the vitamin (B_6). Acetylation is an important process in the inactivation of isoniazid and normal (as opposed to 'slow', 2, *see* Table 20.4) acetylators may be at a disadvantage if the drug is given intermittently, e.g. bi-weekly or less often.

19.3 Cell wall actions

This is a fruitful source of selective toxicity as all bacterial walls contain peptidoglycans which are not present in eukaryotic cells. A typical peptidoglycan synthesis is shown in Fig. 19.2: it forms most of the wall in Gram-positive organisms, usually much less in Gram-negatives.

Penicillins and related substances

The major drug acting to disrupt the peptidoglycan formation in the cell walls of most cocci, some Gram-positive bacilli (e.g. *Clostridium tetani, Bacillus anthracis, Actinomyces israelii*) and spirochaetes is benzylpenicillin (penicillin G). The final stage in the wall synthesis (occurring on its outer side) consists in a cross-linking of a NAG-NAM-pentapeptide (produced internally) by a bridge—pentaglycyl in *Staphylococcus aureus*—to a terminal D-alanyl-D-alanine molecule of the existing wall, with the elimination of one D-alanine residue (Fig. 19.2). The spine of the penicillin molecule is similar to that of D-alanyl-D-alanine (Fig. 19.3, upper) and the drug combines with and inhibits one or more of the enzymes (certainly a transpeptidase and possibly a carboxypeptidase) necessary for the cross-linkage, thus preventing cell wall formation. This function is particularly required when the cell is dividing and therefore, penicillin is most effective against *multiplying* organisms (but *see penems*, p. 405). Under these conditions, the cell wall deficiencies result in osmotic lysis when the cell membrane is unsupported by the wall and the drug is bactericidal. The plasma membrane of *mammalian* cells does not require the additional protection of a cell wall to maintain its integrity: thus, a high degree of selective toxicity is achieved.

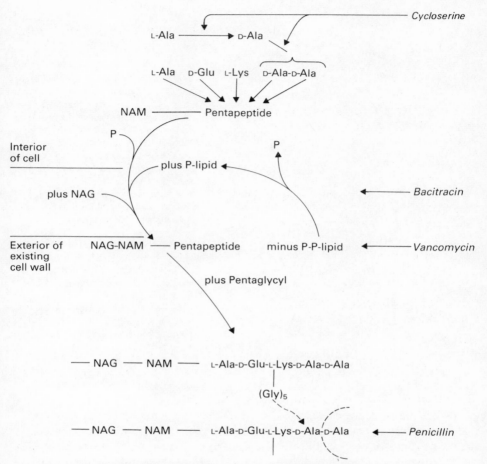

Fig. 19.2 Bacterial cell wall peptidoglycan synthesis (*Staphylococcus aureus*): sites of *inhibition* by drugs. NAM, *N*-acetylmuramic acid; NAG, *N*-acetylglucosamine; Ala, alanine; Glu, glutamic acid; Lys, lysine; Gly, glycine; P, phosphate. P-P-lipid is necessary to pass the NAG-NAM-pentapeptide to the outside of the existing cell wall to which it then attaches via an acquired pentaglycyl side-chain which affixes to the penultimate D-Ala of the pentapeptide (*transpeptidase* action) with loss of the terminal D-Ala (*carboxypeptidase* action).

Molecular structure

The fundamental penicillin molecule consists of fused thiazolidine and β-lactam rings (Fig. 19.3, lower) and important structure–activity relationships are as follows.

If *the sulphur atom* in the 1-position is replaced by–CH_2–(desthiopenicillin) activity is lost. The sulphur atom can be in a 6-membered dihydrothiazine (in place of the thiazolidine) ring (*see* cephalosporins, below) or attached to the N of a β-lactam ring (monobactams).

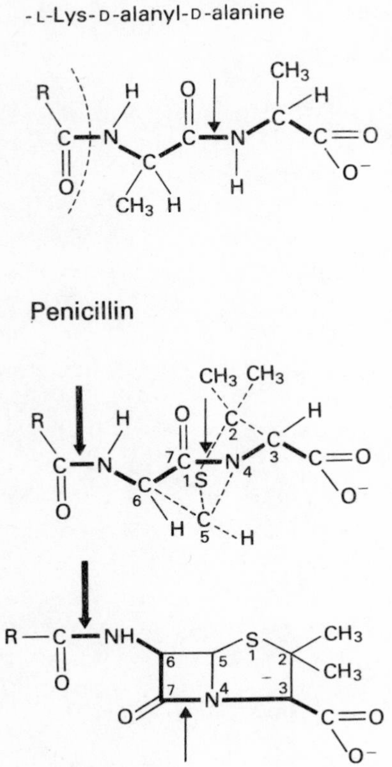

- L-Lys- D-alanyl- D-alanine

Penicillin

Fig. 19.3 A chemical basis for the bactericidal effects of a penicillin. (*Upper*) Similarity of D-alanyl-D-alanine and penicillin molecules. The *thin* arrows represent the sites of cleavage of the peptide bond in the final stage of normal peptidoglycan formation and the analogous inactivation of the penicillin by *penicillin β-lactamases (penicillinases)*. The *thick* arrows indicate the site of hydrolysis on the 6-position side-chain by penicillin amidase, use of which allows the original mould product to be modified by the addition of the requisite groups by the organic chemist.
(*Lower*) Penicillin skeleton shown diagrammatically to illustrate the essential backbone (thicker line) and to allow structure–activity relationships to be considered (*see* text). Type substance, benzyl-penicillin, has $R = C_6H_5.CH_2-$.

The carboxylic acid on the 3-carbon atom must be unsubstituted (as it corresponds to the terminal carboxyl group of the D-Ala-D-Ala dipeptide). This fact has the important corollary that, as this organic acid group accounts for the rapid excretion of the drug by the mechanism in the proximal renal tubule shown in Fig. 1.5, c, it is impossible by chemical manipulation of the structure to overcome this defect. Conversely, the 3.COOH group *can* be esterified to allow better absorption from the gut, e.g. pivaloyl derivatives (Table 19.1) which are hydrolysed to active agents in the body.

The 4–7 β-lactam connection is vital. This corresponds to the peptide link between the two D-alanine molecules and, as it is the bond broken by the penicillin β-lactamase isoenzymes (penicillinases), these enzymes destroy the drug's chemotherapeutic action.

The 6-position side-chain has only a weak action if it merely consists of an unsubstituted amine group (6-aminopenicillanic acid) but becomes therapeutically effective by conversion either to an amide (corresponding to the peptide linkage between the penultimate D-alanine and L-lysine), to an imide (e.g. mecillinam) or to an aminoacy-lureide (e.g. azlocillin)—see Table 19.1.

Penicillins

Benzylpenicillin is a very important drug which is still used therapeutically when a very potent action is necessary (e.g. subacute bacterial endocarditis, p. 14) and in the slow-release preparation, procaine penicillin (p. 10). However, it has some disadvantages which can be overcome, to varying degrees, by chemical manipulation of the molecule (as shown by illustrative examples in Table 19.1).

It is not very active orally, partly because it is broken down by acid in the stomach and partly due to poor absorption from the gastrointestinal tract. Orally active derivatives are acid-stable and well absorbed from the gut.

It is destroyed by penicillin β-lactamases. This deficiency can be remedied by the attachment of a large substituent in the R-position (Fig. 19.3), e.g. a bulky, substituted isoxazolyl group in flucloxacillin (Table 19.1) which most probably prevents approximation and combination of the enzyme to the drug by steric hindrance. An alternative strategy is to add *clavulanic acid*, a β-lactamase inhibitor (unfortunately not effective against all β-lactamase isoenzymes)—in combination with, for example, amoxycillin.

It is relatively restricted in its antibacterial spectrum. This can be broadened to include Gram-negative bacilli (e.g. carbenicillin against *Proteus* and *Pseudomonas* species, e.g. ampicillin/amoxycillin have

Table 19.1   Penicillin β-lactam variants which overcome some of the defects of benzylpenicillin

Name	Orally active	Staphylococcal penicillinase resistant	Broader spectrum
Flucloxacillin (US: floxacillin)	+	+	
Carbenicillin	O+ (carfecillin)*		+
Ampicillin	+ (pivampicillin)*		+
Amoxycillin (US: amoxicillin)	+		+
Mecillinam (US: amdinocillin)	O+ (pivmecillinam)*		+
Azlocillin			+
Cefuroxime		+†	+
Cefotaxime		+†	+

+, effective
O, parent substance not orally active.
* Hydrolysed to parent drug after absorption from gut; carfecillin is phenyl ester, others are pivaloyl compounds.
† Shows slight sensitivity to staphylococcal penicillinase.

been used in typhoid carriers as they are excreted in the bile). Structurally, it is difficult to see how these drugs gain their advantage. The mere substitution of a carboxyl (carbenicillin) or an amino (ampicillin) group should not modify their mechanism of chemotherapeutic action and (by introducing an ionisable group) should decrease passive absorption. However, the β-lactam antibiotics are known to combine in bacterial cell walls with several specific binding proteins (PBPs 1–7: the major transpeptidase and carboxypeptidase are PBP1B and PBP4, respectively) and increased affinity for one or more of these probably accounts for the wider spectra. Many Gram-negative bacilli have a predominance of teichoic acid (rather than peptidoglycans) in their cell walls and are only affected by the broadest spectrum penicillins.

It is excreted very rapidly by the renal proximal tubular mechanism described in Chapter 1, so that the plasma half-life is about 30 minutes. To maintain an adequate therapeutic concentration with normal spacing (4–6 hourly) of i.m. injections, large doses are given. This is possible because penicillin is generally non-toxic. In fact when the drug was initially administered experimentally to assess the LD_{50} (the dose which would kill 50% of the animals), the toxicity was found to be that of the sodium or potassium ion, depending on which salt was given. Direct intracerebral injection of high concentrations of benzylpenicillin (in animals) or intrathecal injection in man can cause fits (? due to GABA antagonism or NMDA agonism, p. 165). This situation could also arise therapeutically if large systemic doses of penicillin were administered to a patient with severe renal insufficiency but, even then, the chances are slight since the drug (being highly charged) would only cross a blood–brain barrier which had been rendered unusually permeable (e.g. by meningitis). An alternative to avoid the high sodium or potassium content of very large doses of penicillin is to administer the drug with probenecid (*see* Fig. 1.5, c). Remember that it is not possible to modify the molecule so that active renal tubular excretion is prevented (as explained earlier).

It is able to act as (or to form) an allergen (*see* p. 391). A preparation of benzylpenicillin is available from which a highly allergenic fraction of mould protein has been removed; this is useful in patients who are allergic to this particular constituent. However, most cases are due to hypersensitivity either to the pencillin molecule itself or to one of its derivatives present as a contaminant or produced by metabolism within the body.

Variations on the penicillin/β-lactam theme (Table 19.1)
• *substitution on a 6-imide (amidino) group.* The representative drug is mecillinam which shows a broader spectrum (against Gram-negative organisms) and, as its pivaloyl derivative, is effective orally

- *substitution of a 6-aminoacylureido group.* These 'ureido' penicillins e.g. azlocillin will attack a wider range of Gram-negative organisms than, for example, amoxycillin
- *cephalosporins.* These contain a 6-membered dihydrothiazine ring fused to the β-lactam moiety but act in a similar manner to the penicillins. In general they have a broader spectrum of Gram-negative activity, are not destroyed by penicillinase, (although resistant organisms may develop cephalosporinase which also attacks the β-lactam bond) and, uncommonly, produce hypersensitivity reactions in penicillin-sensitive patients. The original 'first generation' cephalosporins are rarely used. Cefuroxime is an example of the 'second generation' (less susceptible to β-lactamases) and cefotaxime 'third generation' (even less susceptible to β-lactamases and broader spectrum especially against Gram-negative bacteria): both must be injected
- *monobactams* (*mono*cyclic *bac*terially produced β-lac*tams*) are unusual in having only a single ring structure. They particularly affect penicillin binding protein 3 (a transpeptidase which controls synthesis of the cell septum) and therefore produce filamentous forms of, for example, coliforms. Aztreonam is an example: active *parenterally* against Gram-negative aerobes
- *penems*, e.g. carbapenem, are unusual β-lactams in that they can clearly kill *non-growing* bacteria. This property appears to be associated with attachment to penicillin binding protein 2 (necessary for the maintenance of the rod shape) in *Escherichia coli*.

Other drugs which act on peptidoglycan synthesis (Fig. 19.2)
- cycloserine (rarely used in the treatment of tuberculosis). It is a structural analogue of alanine, which interferes with the earlier stages of cell wall peptidoglycan synthesis by preventing the formation of D-(from L-)alanine and its combination to D-alanyl-D-alanine
- bacitracin prevents pyrophospholipid breakdown to the monophosphate lipid which acts as the carrier for peptidoglycan elements to cross the cell wall. It is too toxic to use in practice
- vancomycin prevents removal of the lipid once externalisation of the NAM-NAG-pentapeptide has been achieved. It is indicated (orally) in pseudomembranous colitis (19.6).

19.4 Cell membrane actions: antifungal drugs
The plasma membrane, which consists in most cases of a phospholipid bilayer (possibly with some carbohydrate attachments, as in Fig. 1.2), is common to most cells so that selective toxicity is difficult to achieve. The drugs used clinically are mainly active against fungi and they disorganise the pathogen's membrane so that it loses small, vital molecules (ions, sugars, amino acids) with lethal results. These agents are divisible into

• polypeptides with fatty acid side-chains which act essentially like detergents (e.g. polymyxin—US: polymyxin B—disrupts the lipoprotein organisation of *Pseudomonas* species)

• polyenes. Nystatin (applied locally) and amphotericin (also used systemically, often with the addition of 5-fluorocytosine, *see* later) attack *ergosterol*-based *fungal* cell membranes to produce pores. However, following systemic use, amphotericin can produce serious toxic effects upon the cholesterol-based mammalian plasma membranes particularly of the kidney. Perhaps the sterol to phospholipid ratio is the necessary factor in the (weakly) selective toxicity of the polyenes.

• imidazoles, e.g. miconazole, clotrimazole, cause leakage through the fungal cell membrane but, additionally, block ergosterol synthesis by inhibition of the cytochrome P_{450}-mediated sterol demethylase. They also inhibit mitochondrial cytochrome oxidase and ATPase.

Summary of antifungal agents (antimycotic drugs)
• *nystatin*: particularly used locally in candidal infections
• *amphotericin*: systemic use against a range of fungi
• *clotrimazole, miconazole*: commonly used locally against dermatophyte infections, e.g. athlete's foot, p. 395
• *flucytosine* is a systemic antimycotic which inhibits the formation of fungal DNA selectively (Table 19.3) but occasionally it can depress human bone marrow: check by blood counts
• *griseofulvin* in the treatment of chronic athlete's foot has been described on p. 395. Its mechanism is interference with microtubular function, i.e. it is a spindle poison, p. 413.

19.5   Drugs affecting nucleic acid production and cell division
Possible sites of action are illustrated in Fig. 19.4. Agents may conveniently be subdivided into those *primarily* affecting
a   purine and/or pyrimidine nucleotide formation
b   nucleic acid synthesis
c   DNA replication
d   cell division (spindle poisons).
Some drugs have effects in more than one category.

Interference with purine and/or pyrimidine nucleotide formation

Folate pathways
These are very important (Fig. 19.5, *see* footnote [†] and Fig. 19.6). Drugs indicated *above* the reaction series in Fig. 19.5 show selectivity. Susceptible bacteria cannot absorb folic acid and therefore must synthesise it from paraaminobenzoic acid. Sulphonamides are structurally very similar to this precursor and so interfere with the folic acid production. Dapsone acts similarly and is used in the treatment of leprosy (p. 418). Humans are not affected by this mechanism because

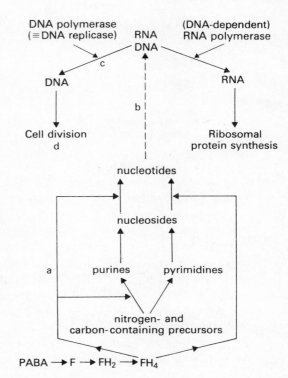

Fig. 19.4 Available effector sites for chemotherapeutic agents which interfere with nuclei acid (NA) production, cell division or protein synthesis. D (deoxyribo-) NA and R(ribo-) NA are shown at the top centre. On the bottom left, folic-folinic acid production is via PABA (paraaminobenzoic acid), F (folic acid), FH_2 (dihydrofolic acid) and FH_4 (tetrahydrofolic acid), respectively (*see* Fig. 19.5). **a**, **b**, **c** and **d** as in text.

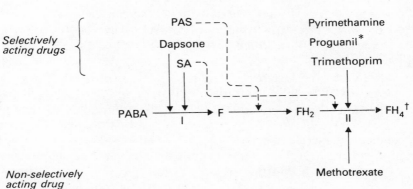

Fig. 19.5 How drugs may interrupt folic–folinic acid synthesis. Vertical lines indicate inhibition of an enzyme (directly by the drug—full lines; or after conversion to a false substrate—interrupted lines): PAS, paraaminosalicylic acid; SA, a sulphonamide. Reaction I is a two-stage process from PABA, adding successively pteridine (to form dihydropteroic acid) and then glutamic acid to produce folic acid (F); the drugs SA and dapsone act mainly at the first stage, i.e. on the enzyme dihydropteroic acid synthase. Reaction II involves a complicated series of enzymes which are most conveniently described by the portmanteau title 'dihydrofolate reductase'.

*Proguanil (US: chloroguanide) has to be activated in the body before it can act at this site.

†Tetrahydrofolic acid (FH_4) via its formyl derivatives (the 5-formyl compound is *folinic* acid) acts as a one-carbon transfer agent in the synthesis of purines and some nucleotides, including inosine monophosphate (*see* Figs. 19.4 and 19.6)

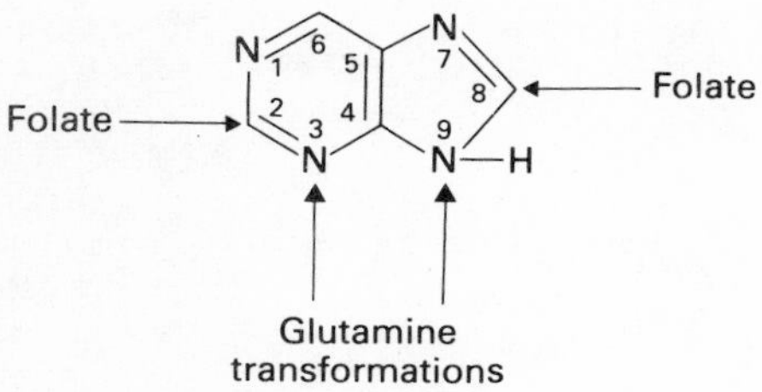

Fig. 19.6 Factors necessary in the genesis of the purine molecule.

they absorb preformed folic acid from the gut. A small amount of any sulphonamide may additionally act by synthesis to a 'false dihydrofolic acid' which will inhibit dihydrofolate reductase. This latter type of mechanism is more clearly manifested by paraaminosalicyclic acid (a former antituberculous agent) as shown in Fig. 19.5.

Sulphonamides are relatively narrow-spectrum, bacteriostatic, antibacterial agents. Most are inactivated by acetylation (and thus are susceptible to pharmacogenetic differences, 2, Table 20.3 and *see* 7): also, the acetyl derivatives, like the parent compounds, can precipitate in the urinary tract—this is minimised by adequate fluid intake and alkalinisation of the urine. Some sulphonamides are converted to glycuronides and avoid the difficulties just mentioned. The length of action of sulphonamides varies from several hours to a week. In general, the longer-acting compounds are more plasma protein bound. Side-effects are chiefly gastrointestinal (nausea, vomiting) or allergic rashes but if a relatively uncommon though serious reaction occurred (e.g. blood dyscrasia, e.g. Stevens–Johnson syndrome—severe erythema multiforme, 18.8), it would not be easy to remove a long-acting sulphonamide (*see* 20.8).

Selective inhibitors of dihydrofolate reductase include the antimalarial drugs, pyrimethamine and proguanil (19.8); and trimethoprim. This latter compound binds much more strongly (about 50 000 times) to many bacterial, compared with the human, isoenzymes. Its use in combination with a sulphonamide (sulphamethoxazole plus trimethoprim results in co-trimoxazole) is synergistic. Further advantages of the combination over a sulphonamide alone are stated to be
• bactericidal, rather than bacteriostatic, action
• wider antibacterial range (as the two individual spectra do not exactly overlap)
• less chance of resistance developing. Two steps to be bypassed instead of one (for possible mechanisms, *see* Table 19.5). Resistance to trimethoprim *alone* is not very common and this drug is often used as *sole* therapy, as it has fewer side-effects than sulphonamides.

However, it can be seen from Fig. 19.5 that interference by trimethoprim, however slight, is with a pathway common to humans and so side-effects (e.g. folate-deficiency anaemia) are possible. Therefore, blood counts are necessary during long-term therapy.

Table 19.2 Side-effects of 'antimitotic'* drugs

Tissue or organ	Effect of depression
Red bone marrow	Aplastic anaemia, granulocytopenia, thrombocytopenia
Lymphoid tissue	Lymphocytopenia, lack of immune response(s)
Digestive tract	Oral ulceration, nausea and vomiting, haemorrhagic enteritis
Hair follicle	Loss of hair (alopecia)
Skin	Delay in healing of wounds
Gonadal germinal epithelium	Mutation of sex cells, sterility
Embryonic mesenchyme	Fetal abnormalities

* 'Antimitotic' indicates that the drug interferes with cell division. The term is far too imprecise except for general use, as here.

Methotrexate (Fig. 19.5) is the classical example of a folic acid antagonist which does *not* show selective toxicity. It is used therapeutically in the treatment of neoplasms but will inevitably produce side-effects upon rapidly dividing tissues in the host (Table 19.2). Use fol*in*ic acid against the haemopoietic effects (p. 378).

Glutamine transformations

These are essential to introduce the nitrogen atoms at positions 3 and 9 in the purine molecule (Fig. 19.6). This transfer can be prevented by either DON (*d*iazo-*o*xo-*n*orleucine) or azaserine (diazoacetylserine), but these agents are insufficiently selective to have any clinical use.

Inhibitors of nucleic acid synthesis

Analogues of purines and/or pyrimidines must be sufficiently similar to the natural substances if they are to enter the relevant chemical pathways. They may then (Table 19.3)
• inhibit enzymes either directly or after transformation to a further 'false' compound and/or
• form a 'false' RNA or DNA which is unable (or slower) to replicate due to the presence of extra binding groups which interfere with uncoiling of the spiral molecule or its correct use as a template.

The type substance here is 6-mercaptopurine which, by the presence of a thiol (SH) group in place of a hydrogen substituent on the 6-position of the purine ring, is converted to *thio*inosine monophosphate which then prevents the formation of both AMP and GMP (Fig. 19.7). 6-thioguanine acts similarly. These agents (Table 19.3)—except flucytosine and acyclovir—do not generally show much selective toxicity and, therefore, if given systemically, produce the side-effects shown in Table 19.2.

Table 19.3 Major mechanisms of action of some representative drugs affecting nucleic acid synthesis

Drug	Conversion to	Action		Forms 'false'
		Inhibits	Prevents formation of	
6-Mercaptopurine	Thioinosine monophosphate	Several enzymes	DNA/RNA (Fig. 19.7)	
6-Thioguanine	Thioguanosine monophosphate	Several enzymes	DNA/RNA	
8-Azaguanine				RNA
5-Fluorouracil	5-Fluorouridine monophosphate			RNA
	5-Fluorodeoxyuridine monophosphate	Thymidylate synthetase	DNA	
Flucytosine (5-fluorocytosine)	5-Fluorouracil in many fungi (which possess cytosine deaminase)		(*see* above)	
Idoxuridine (5-iodo-2-deoxyuridine)	Mono-, di- and triphosphate*		DNA	DNA
Acyclovir (Acycloguanosine)†	Mono-, di- and triphosphate*		DNA	DNA
Cytarabine (Cytosine arabinoside)†		Cytidine monophosphate reductase	DNA	
Bleomycin		Thymidine incorporation into DNA	DNA‡	

* The initial phosphorylation is carried out by thymidine kinase. This enzyme in the herpes group of viruses shows a selective affinity (compared with the mammalian enzyme) for *acyclovir* but not for idoxuridine. Resistance to acyclovir can occur by the development of thymine kinase-deficient mutants.
† Also prevents DNA replication by inhibition of DNA polymerase.
‡ Also causes fragmentation of DNA molecules (*see* p. 413).

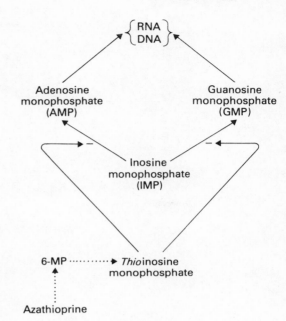

Fig. 19.7 How 6-mercaptopurine (6-MP; given for immunosuppression as the pro-drug azathioprine, *see* Table 19.9) interrupts nucleic acid production by inhibition (−) of (a number of) essential enzymes. Dotted lines indicate biotransformations of the administered agent.

Prevention of DNA replication
There are several mechanisms by which this may occur.

Formation of a 'false' DNA (idoxuridine, acyclovir—*see* Table 19.3).

Alkylating agents (Fig. 19.8, left). The two alkyl groups form an irreversible (*covalently bonded*) bridge, most commonly between the nitrogen atoms (e.g. in the 7-positions, Fig. 19.6) of two guanine residues on the same or on adjacent DNA strands, thus preventing replication or causing miscoding. The type substance is mustine (a nitrogen mustard, US: mechlorethamine) but this is extremely irritant (p. 14) and has mainly been replaced by a phosphorylated derivative, *cyclophosphamide*. The original concept here was to target the drug on to rapidly metabolising cells of tumours. These have a high energy requirement, mainly supplied through phosphates, and accordingly contain more phosphatases than other cells; thus, preferential release of the active nitrogen mustard by dephosphorylation should occur in their vicinity. In fact, cyclophosphamide is mainly activated in the liver to a mustard derivative which is an effective alkylating agent especially for lymphoblastic neoplasms. Its side-effects are those shown in Table 19.2 plus cystitis, due to bladder irritation caused by another metabolite, acrolein (increase fluid intake to dilute and inactivate with mesna, 2-*m*ercapto-*e*thane *s*ulphonate sodium, *Na*). Other nitrogen mustard

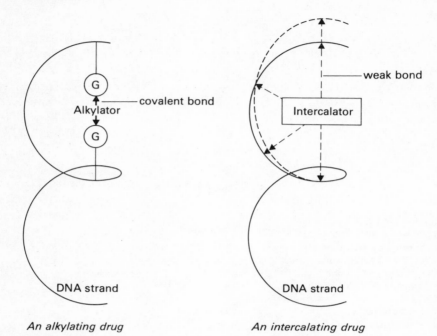

An alkylating drug   *An intercalating drug*

Fig. 19.8 How drugs may interfere with the template function of DNA. G, guanine residue. Interrupted lines indicate modifications produced by an intercalating agent (*see* text).

derivatives are *chlorambucil* (used in chronic lymphatic leukaemia) and *melphalan* (for multiple myeloma).

Chronic myeloid leukaemia is usually treated by a chemically unrelated alkylating drug, *busulphan*; its trade-name, Myleran®, indicates its use. *Nitrosoureas*, e.g. carmustine (*bi*schloroethyl*ni*trosou*rea, BCNU) act mainly by alkylation. Not only are they strongly myelo-suppressive but have also been implicated in the production of secondary cancers (leukaemias, *see* p. 444 and Fig. 20.3). Finally *cisplatin* links two guanine molecules by a diamine platinum bridge. There are the usual side-effects, particularly nausea and vomiting (p. 317); additionally, otic, renal and neural manifestations can occur.

Intercalating agents (Fig. 19.8, right). As their name implies these are flat molecules which interpose themselves between the coils of the DNA strands and, by forming *weak bonds*, cause partial unwinding (which can be used quantitatively as a measure of the number of molecules interposed) and hinder the correct uncoiling and exposure of the DNA and/or RNA (19.6) templates. Thereby, they may be cytostatic or cytocidal. Some show selective toxicity, such as *chloroquine* against the malarial parasite; others do not, e.g. the anticancer drug *doxorubicin*. The latter, in addition to the side-effects shown in Table 19.2, is cardiotoxic. This is because it produces oxygen free radicals which are normally inactivated by catalase and glutathione peroxidase (Fig. 1.10): the former is in low concentration in heart tissue and the latter enzyme is inhibited by doxorubicin. Therefore, monitor cardiac function.

Metronidazole (a nitroimidazole) shows selectivity for *anaerobic* protozoa (e.g. *Trichomonas vaginalis, Entamoeba histolytica*) and *anaerobic* gut bacteria because, after entry into the microorganism, it is reduced to active metabolites which disrupt DNA structure and function. Patients taking this drug may show ethanol sensitivity (9.2).

Bleomycin (*see* also Table 19.3) mainly acts by producing fragmentation of DNA molecules. It causes relatively little bone marrow suppression but marked cutaneous reactions and a dose-related pulmonary fibrosis. *Clofazimine* (antileprotic drug, p. 418) also disrupts DNA function.

Inhibitors of DNA gyrase. 4-Quinolones prevent resealing of *bacterial* DNA strands after supercoiling which results in loss of stability and unwinding of the supercoils with ultimate cell death. Human DNA gyrase is not affected by these drugs. *Nalidixic acid* was an early example of this group and it is still used in urinary tract infections. *Ciprofloxacin*, a more potent derivative, is an important orally-active antipseudomonal drug but is not used in children (because of arthropathies in *young* experimental animals).

Inhibitors of DNA polymerase. Acyclovir (via its mono-, di- and triphosphate derivatives) inactivates the viral (particularly herpes simplex) enzyme (19.9). Cytarabine (Table 19.3) can also act here.

Spindle poisons

An essential preliminary to cell division is the formation of the proteins, α- and β-tubulins, necessary for the spindle structure (p. 121). This process is prevented by substances extracted from a periwinkle (Vinca) plant, e.g. vincristine, vinblastine. In their presence, the chromosomes cannot orientate themselves coherently at the metaphase stage and mitosis is arrested. Strangely, the expected side-effects (Table 19.2) are not all present: the erythrocytes, platelets and gut epithelium are relatively spared and the brunt of the damage falls on the granulocytes and the hair follicles *plus* a peripheral neuropathy (due to interference with microtubular function in nerves, p. 121).

In the treatment of chronic athlete's foot, griseofulvin (p. 395) acts by disruption of microtubular function.

19.6   Drugs preventing protein synthesis (Fig. 19.4)

Possible sites of action and mechanisms follow.

(DNA-dependent) RNA polymerase, which is essential for the production of messenger RNA (transcription) may be inhibited
- by *intercalation*, e.g. with actinomycin D (US: dactinomycin). Not selective and used in certain tumours, e.g. Wilms' kidney neoplasm
- *selectively*. Rifampicin depresses this bacterial enzyme, particularly in *Mycobacterium tuberculosis* or *leprae*, without significant effect upon the mammalian isoenzyme. Its most common side-effects are allergic (including a type II destruction of platelets, Table 20.1). There is often some induced deterioration in liver function, normally reversible on stopping the drug but a definite contraindication to its use in the presence of hepatic insufficiency (e.g. alcoholics). However it can induce liver microsomal enzymes and thereby decrease the effectiveness of warfarin (Table 17.2), or the contraceptive 'pill' (15.4). The latter interaction is important because rifampicin is contra-indicated during pregnancy due to a risk of neonatal bleeding. Rifampicin can cause an orange-red coloration of secretions: warn the patient. Also, this can be used as a test of compliance, which may become wayward in long-term antituberculous or antileprotic therapy (p. 418).

Ribosomal function. Protein synthesis at the bacterial ribosome (70S, with fragments separable as 50S and 30S) is shown in Fig. 19.9. Selective toxicity (Table 19.4) usually depends upon the circumstance that most mammalian ribosomes (except those in mitochondria) are 80S (separable into 60S and 40S subunits). Note that puromycin (a valuable biochemical tool to determine the precise site of action of other ribosomal blockers) is insufficiently selective for clinical use. Some important untoward effects of individual agents follow.

Aminoglycosides (e.g. streptomycin) can cause eighth nerve damage,

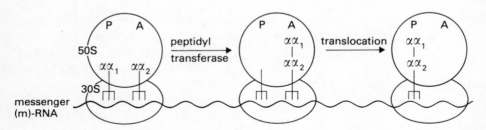

$\alpha\alpha_1$-t-RNA (⊓) combines at P site; then $\alpha\alpha_2$-t-RNA combines at A site: need elongation factor (EF)-T and GTPase

$\alpha\alpha_1$ transfers to A site and forms a peptide link with $\alpha\alpha_2$

peptidyl-t-RNA transfers from A site to P site: need EF-G and GTPase

Fig. 19.9 Protein synthesis at the bacterial ribosome (schematic). $\alpha\alpha_1$ and $\alpha\alpha_2$ are amino acids. t-, transfer (RNA); A, aminoacyl (acceptor) site; P, peptidyl (donor) site.

Table 19.4 Drugs acting on ribosomal functions

Drug	Binding site(s)	Selective toxicity	Major action(s)	Primary effect
Streptomycin*, gentamicin*	30S subunit	70S > 80S	Prevents binding of aa-t-RNA or causes miscoding (distortion of the codon triplets resulting in misreading)	Bactericidal
Tetracycline†	30S subunit	Increased concentration in prokaryotic cell	Prevents binding of aa-t-RNA	Bacteriostatic
Chloramphenicol	50S subunit	70S > 80S	Prevents peptide bond formation	Bacteriostatic
Clindamycin	50S subunit	70S > 80S	Inhibits peptidyl transferase	Bacteriostatic
Puromycin	50S subunit	Negligible	Complexes with peptidyl-t-RNA so that incomplete proteins are released	Not applicable (*see* text)
Fusidic acid‡	50S subunit	70S > 80S	Prevents translocation by sequestering elongation factor-G	Bacteriostatic
Erythromycin§	50S subunit	70S > 80S	Prevents translocation	Bactericidal/bacteriostatic (dose-dependent)

* An aminoglycoside.
† The simplest representative of the 'tetracycline' group.
‡ Still a valuable agent usually in combination with flucloxacillin for serious staphylococcal infections, e.g. septicaemia.
§ A possible alternative in patients who are allergic to penicillin. Major side effects: gastrointestinal upsets.

especially upon the vestibular division, and nephrotoxicity. In high dosage they can potentiate competitive neuromuscular blocking actions by preventing mobilisation of acetylcholine-containing vesicles at the junction (p. 64). The development of resistance is a major problem with streptomycin: it is far less of a difficulty with the currently preferred gentamicin. Neomycin can be applied locally, e.g. to eye, skin or gut (pre-operatively): it is too toxic for systemic use.

Tetracyclines. These are broad-spectrum drugs which, by destroying the normal microorganismal balance (e.g. in the gut or upper respiratory tract) can result in opportunistic infections ('superinfections'), such as candidosis, staphylococcal enteritis, pseudomembranous colitis (due to *Clostridium difficile*), which are often difficult to treat: also in gut, irritation causing vomiting or diarrhoea. The tetracyclines can act as chelating agents (*see* Table 20.5), especially for calcium and iron which, by precipitation, prevents absorption of both antibiotic and mineral ions from the gut following oral administration (20.5). A further corollary of calcium ion chelation is that if given during pregnancy the drug can pass the placental barrier and produce skeletal abnormalities; also, if administered during the first 12 years of life, yellow-coloured metabolites of tetracyclines (which turn brown on exposure to light) are deposited in the teeth: therefore, avoid in these situations.

Chloramphenicol has a sinister reputation. It is safe if applied to surfaces (e.g. eye-drops) but, if used systemically, it may produce
• a dose-related decrease in red cell production (aplastic anaemia) which is reversible on cessation of the drug. This appears to be due to depression of *70S* ribosomal function in mammalian mitochondria particularly of the bone marrow erythroid cell series.
• total bone marrow depression (pancytopenia) by an allergic reaction: often fatal but fortunately rare. Most likely caused by the *para*-nitro (p-NO_2) group of the drug forming intermediate compounds (*see* Fig. 20.3) which produce the response (? idiosyncratically) in susceptible patients.

Thus, its systemic indications are limited to those infections for which it is the best available agent, such as *Haemophilus influenzae* meningitis or typhoid fever. In the newborn this drug must not be used because inadequate metabolism (by glucuronyl transferase) and inefficient renal excretion can produce toxic actions upon several organs. This dangerous situation is called the 'grey baby' syndrome (1.9) because of the pallor associated with the characteristic cardiovascular collapse. Also remember that this drug is secreted in breast milk (15.5).

Clindamycin can produce pseudomembranous colitis (*see* under tetracyclines).

19.7   Resistance

This term describes the condition in which invading cells are invulnerable to the chemotherapeutic agent. It may be:

1 *Natural*. That is, the drug is not interfering with some process essential for a particular pathogen. This accounts for limitations of antibacterial spectra. Even within sensitive species, e.g. Gram-positive cocci, there can exist (at least *in vitro*) individuals which do not lyse under conditions of cell wall deficiency produced by the action of penicillin: these 'persisters' are naturally unaffected by this antibacterial agent but are apparently insignificant in practice.

2 *Acquired. In the presence of the drug*, the invading cell alters its genetic structure to produce a resistant phenotype either
• by natural selection of particular mutants or
• by transfer of genetic material (DNA which codes for a particular phenotype) by release to and uptake from the environment (transformation), by the intermediation of a bacteriophage (transduction) or by a resistance transfer factor (RTF, conjugation).

In each case the drug resistance may be multiple, i.e. directed against more than one chemotherapeutic agent.

The genotype having modified, the mechanistic change (phenotype) can be divided into three broad categories (shown, with examples, in Table 19.5), namely
• destruction or prevention of activation of the chemotherapeutic agent

Table 19.5 Phenotypic mechanisms of resistance to chemotherapeutic agents

Decrease the concentration of the active agent	Prevent the drug getting to its site of action	Oppose the chemotherapeutic action directly
Inactivate, e.g. penicillin, by β-lactamases or amidases (Fig. 19.3); streptomycin, acetylation or adenylation; chloramphenicol, acetylation	Render the cell wall impermeable to the drug so that it cannot enter to exert its effects, e.g. isoniazid or streptomycin with the tubercle bacillus; sulphonamides, penicillin, or tetracyclines with other organisms	Increase the amount of enzyme (by less derepression), e.g. DHF reductase against methotrexate
Prevent the formation of the active nucleotide, e.g. 6-mercaptopurine conversion to thioinosine monophosphate (Fig. 19.7)		Produce an enzyme with lower affinity for the drug (compared with the natural substrate), e.g. dihydropteroic acid synthetase for sulphonamides; dihydrofolate reductase for trimethoprim or methotrexate
		Lower the drug's affinity for its ribosomal binding site by loss or other alteration of the S_{12} protein of the 30S subunit, e.g. streptomycin; L_6 protein of the 50S subunit, e.g. chloramphenicol

Note: one particular chemotherapeutic agent may induce *different* phenotypic mechanisms.

- interference with the drug reaching its site of action
- antagonism of the agent at its effective site.

Resistance development is encouraged by inappropriate treatment and can be minimised by correct drug usage (*see* Table 21.2). To particularise, *antimicrobial agents should be given in adequate dosage for sufficient time against diseases for which they are specifically indicated.* Their exhibition in insignificant situations, e.g. against possible bacterial sequelae of the common cold, or in veterinary practice to lessen the number of handlers and (theoretically) increase the meat yield in cattle, is not recommended.

The emergence of resistance to *antituberculous* agents is slowed by the simultaneous administration of three drugs (triple therapy)—usually isoniazid, rifampicin and ethambutol. The mode of action of *ethambutol* is at present unknown but it can produce a decrease in visual acuity and red/green blindness: these are reversible, so perform regular optical tests during the course of treatment (18.4). Similarly, *antileprotic* triple therapy consists of dapsone (p. 406), rifampicin and clofazimine. The latter interferes with the template function of DNA in the bacterium. Like rifampicin (p. 414), it can produce red urine—also, red skin and a bluish-black discoloration of leprotic lesions.

19.8   Antiprotozoal and anthelmintic drugs

The major protozoal and some worm (helminth) diseases are endemic in certain tropical countries but increased communications have resulted in an appreciable number of sporadic cases in temperate countries. Illustrative examples follow.

Malaria (*Plasmodium* species)
The life cycle (simplified) is shown in Fig. 19.10.

Therapy may conveniently be divided into the following:

Suppressant (prophylactic). Pyrimethamine (weekly) or proguanil (daily) should be taken immediately before, during and for a month after being in an endemic malarial area. These drugs are selectively toxic against plasmodium dihydrofolate reductase (bind about 2000 times more strongly than to human isoenzymes, Fig. 19.5) and act as schizonticides in the liver and red blood cells. Chloroquine (*see* below) is now extensively used as a prophylactic agent (weekly). Suppressants are curative in *Plasmodium falciparum* infestation—in which there is not a recurrent hepatic cycle.

Acute attack. Chloroquine—an intercalator (p. 412)—is less toxic than the classical agent, quinine, and kills erythrocytic schizonts more rapidly than the other suppressants just mentioned. However, care must be exercised due to:

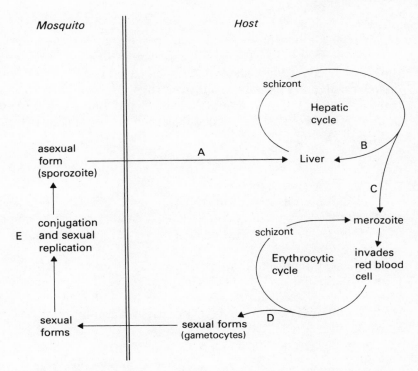

Fig. 19.10 Malarial life cycle. A, sporozoites (from an infected mosquito bite) invade host hepatic parenchymal cells and replicate asexually forming schizonts. B, persistent infection may be maintained by repeated cycles of replication in the liver: not present in *Plasmodium falciparum* infection. C, merozoites (released by rupture of hepatic schizonts) invade erythrocytes and undergo repeated cycles of erythrocytic schizont formation. Acute attacks are associated with red cell destruction and merozoite release. D, sexual forms also develop in erythrocytes and are ingested by biting mosquitoes. E, sexual replication in the mosquito stomach leads to the development of asexual sporozoites, which pass to the salivary glands to repeat the cycle.

1   Its visual dangers, only significant on prolonged therapy, namely
•   corneal opacities: reversible on stopping the drug
•   retinal pigmentation: may be permanent.
2   A gradual spread of *P. falciparum* resistance to this antimalarial world-wide. If so, treat the acute attack with quinine.

Radical cure. Chloroquine (with the caveats just stated) *plus* primaquine. The latter depresses the recurrent hepatic cycle (stage B): note its production of red cell haemolysis and methaemoglobinaemia in patients with low glucose-6-phosphate dehydrogenase (*see* Table 20.4, 7).

Amoebic dysentery
Metronidazole (p. 413) is the main agent used.

Worms

Those which are commonly encountered in medical or veterinary practice (with their usual therapy) are shown in Table 19.6. All the drugs shown are selective for the helminth indicated with minimal side-effects on mammals. A subsequent purgative may be necessary to ensure expulsion of the worm (examine the faeces) and to avoid cysticercosis, by absorption of ova set free on disintegration of the parasite, in the case of *Taenia solium*.

19.9   Antiviral chemotherapy

Alternative safeguards include:

• natural immunity, e.g. against the common cold. It is certainly not worth administering a drug (with however small a degree of potential toxicity) to the whole population as a preventive measure against this infection

• artificial immunisation. *Active*, e.g. by the ingestion of an attenuated form of the poliomyelitis virus. This is effective if only a few strains exist, which can be contained in the vaccine, and if the immunity is relatively long-lasting (several years). Also, *passive* immunisation, e.g. with antisera.

Chemotherapy is indicated if none of the above preconditions exist. It is much more successful prophylactically than therapeutically since, by the time the signs and symptoms present themselves, the virion has passed its replication peak and 'beaten the system'. Possible sites of antiviral action are shown in Fig. 19.11. It must be realised, however, that most of the drugs indicated are insufficiently selective for clinical use, the basic difficulty being that the invader nucleic acids 'take over' the mammalian cell control of protein synthesis and force the host cell ribosomes to produce compounds essential for *viral* reproduction and structure, including the ability to invade (infect) other cells.

The above points are illustrated by the following agents.

Amantadine is effective against all strains of influenza virus *type A* and is valuable preferably prophylactically, but also therapeutically, in patients with a significant risk of mortality or serious complications, or in essential hospital personnel. (For use in parkinsonism, *see* p. 173)

Idoxuridine (a thymidine analogue) is converted to the triphosphate which is incorporated into both viral and mammalian DNA. Therefore, it is too toxic for systemic use but may be applied locally to treat herpes simplex keratitis: however, recurrences are common. These are less likely with *acyclovir* (Table 19.3) which is also used for systemic or genital herpes simplex and varicella-zoster infections. *Acyclovir* is more selective against the herpes group of viruses both at the initial

Table 19.6 Important anthelmintic drugs

Type of helminth	Example	First-line drug	Mechanism of action	Significant absorption from gut	Main side-effects
Threadworm	*Enterobius vermicularis*	Mebendazole	Decreased helminth microtubular function	No	Gastrointestinal
Threadworm/ roundworm		Piperazine	Flaccid paralysis of worm (membrane hyperpolarisation: GABAergic agonist)	Yes*	Gastrointestinal (rare) neurological
		Pyrantel	Spastic paralysis of worm (membrane depolarisation: cholinergic agonist)	No	Gastrointestinal
Roundworm	*Ascaris lumbricoides*	Levamisole	Nicotine-like stimulation followed by depolarising block	Yes†	Gastrointestinal
Tapeworm	*Taenia saginata* (beef) *Taenia solium* (pork)	Niclosamide	Uncouples formation of adenosine triphosphate in anaerobes	No	Gastrointestinal
Fluke	*Schistosoma mansoni*	Oxamniquine	Unknown	Yes†	Gastrointestinal (rare) neurological

* Mainly excreted in the urine; therefore, care in renal disease.
† Main inactivation in the liver; therefore, care in hepatic insufficiency.

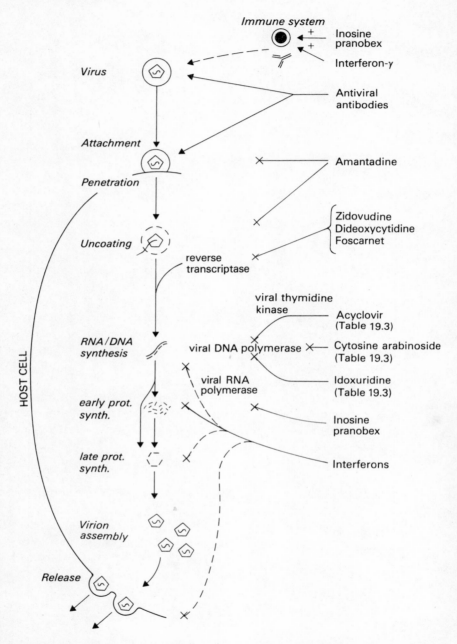

Fig. 19.11 Sites of action of potential antiviral agents. All are inhibitory except inosine pranobex and interferon-γ which enhance (+) immune processes. Lower interrupted lines indicate additional possible sites of actions. Prot., protein.

Table 19.7 Major groups of interferons.

Interferon type	Inducing mechanism	Site of production
I (α): IFN-α	Viral invasion of cell	Leucocytes
I (β): IFN-β	Viral invasion of cell	Fibroblasts
II (γ): IFN-γ	Immune response	Lymphoblasts

phosphorylation stage (*see* footnote to Table 19.3) and also because the phosphorylated derivative *selectively* inhibits the *viral* DNA polymerase. *Inosine pranobex*, which acts as an immunostimulant by the production of T-killer lymphocytes and is also stated to have a subsidiary action against viral RNA polymerase (Fig. 19.11), has also been used in herpes simplex treatment.

Interferons are glycoproteins produced by virus-infected cells (Table 19.7). They are not virus-specific but are relatively *species*-specific. One overall picture of α-interferon action is shown in Fig. 19.12. The glycoprotein produced by the first cell binds to specific receptors on the surface of the second cell which results in the formation of 'translation-inhibiting proteins', which are enzymes interfering with ribosomal protein production of the *virus* but not of the host cell. Original preparations (e.g. from *human* fibroblasts) were weak. Nowadays 'pure' human interferons are widely available—produced by recombinant DNA technology. Clinical trials are in progress against viral infections, e.g. hepatitis B, and the interferons are used in hairy cell leukaemia. In the latter case, interferons are thought to be both immunostimulant and to exert direct inhibitory effects on tumour cell growth. The interferons are potent substances and can produce a severe influenza-like syndrome (some 'flu' symptoms ordinarily are probably due to interferon release, *see* Fig. 7.4), haematological and CNS side-effects.

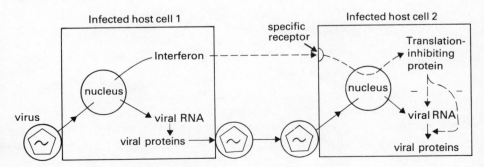

Fig. 19.12 Broad mechanism of interferon action. −, inhibition.

AIDS treatment

AIDS is an immunodeficiency condition produced by infection of a specific sub-population of T-lymphocytes by human immunodeficiency viruses. These have a single-stranded RNA which, after entry into the host cell, has to be converted by *reverse transcriptase* to proviral DNA which is then inserted into the DNA of the infected cell. Present therapy only delays (prevents) the development of the disease and the most useful drugs available at the moment are inhibitors of reverse transcriptase. Zidovudine (3′ *az*ido-3′-deoxy*t*hymidine, AZT) is the best but is only used in severe cases because it produces serious depression of red and white blood cell counts. Other inhibitors of reverse transcriptase are 2′, 3′-dideoxycytidine (the most promising of the dideoxynucleosides) which is presently undergoing clinical trials; and foscarnet (phosphonoformate) still used for the treatment of cytomegalovirus infections (*see* later). Other approaches to prevent AIDS spread and development include various different vaccines and antisense oligonucleotide inhibitors. The latter are tailored to bind with specific target sites of the viral genome and thus interfere with different stages of viral replication. Secondly, drugs are required to treat the opportunistic infections which occur in AIDS patients. The commonest of these is *Pneumocystis carinii* pneumonia for which co-trimoxazole (p. 408) is indicated; for cytomegalovirus infections, foscarnet or ganciclovir (a guanine derivative acting similarly to acyclovir, *see* above) are used.

19.10 Treatment of neoplasms

The main methods available (with their general indications) are
- *Surgery* for a readily removable growth, e.g. most mammary tumours
- *Radiotherapy* for neoplasms or secondary deposits which are radio-sensitive
- *Chemotherapy*. For chemosensitive tumours or for widespread conditions, e.g. leukaemia.

These techniques are often used advantageously in combination.

For chemotherapy, the overriding aim is to achieve a *selective* kill of neoplastic cells.

Specific agents
These can act by:

1 *Changes in endocrine control,* e.g. in hormone-dependent cancers (for side-effects of sex hormones used, refer to Table 15.2).
- prostatic. Figure 19.13 shows the hormonal control of the primary tumour and its metastases, namely androgens from the testis and adrenal cortex plus precursors from the adrenal cortex which are converted to androgens in prostatic tissue. Only 75% of prostatic

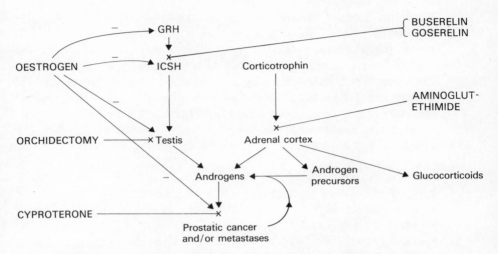

Fig. 19.13 Therapy (names in capital letters) used in prostatic cancer treatment. For explanation *see* text. GRH, gonadotrophin-releasing hormone; ICSH, interstitial cell-stimulating hormone. X or −, inhibition.

cancers are hormone-dependent. For these, possible first-line treatment is either orchidectomy or an oestrogen. The latter exerts a negative feedback on the hypothalamo-pituitary axis, decreases testicular secretion of androgens and antagonises the androgenic drive to prostatic tissue. An alternative strategy is to administer an analogue of gonadotrophin releasing hormone (luteinising hormone releasing hormone), e.g. buserelin or goserelin, both of which down-regulate pituitary receptors to decrease release of interstitial cell-stimulating hormone. However, either treatment usually initially stimulates the relevant system which will require the addition of cyproterone (p. 358) to the regime at first. In resistant cases adrenal cortical production of androgens may be reduced with aminoglutethimide but, as this also prevents glucocorticoid synthesis (*see* p. 333), concomitant replacement therapy (prednisolone) for the latter is necessary

• mammary (oestrogen-dependent). *Tamoxifen* is the most useful drug. It acts by blocking oestrogen receptors (which in hormone-dependent cancers stimulate growth) but can have some cytotoxic effect even in the absence of oestrogens. If premenopausal, second/third line therapy is oophorectomy or a progestogen; if postmenopausal, it is an oestrogen (which paradoxically can result in regression of the breast tumour) or aminoglutethimide plus glucocorticoid (see under prostatic cancer treatment, above). In postmenopausal women oestrogens result from conversion of androgens in peripheral tissues by the enzyme oestrogen synthase: aminoglutethimide blocks this enzyme.

2 *Concentrating the lethal agent* in the vicinity of the new growth

• by preferential uptake into specific tissues, e.g. ^{131}I into thyroid carcinoma cells (p. 338)

• by perfusion of a non-specific agent (*see* below) through the 'isolated' circulation of the tumour area ('regional perfusion'). In this case, 'scavenger' molecules may be used either to 'mop up' any of the drug reaching the general circulation or to oppose its deleterious effects, ('rescue' therapy, e.g. fol*in*ic acid 12–24 hours after methotrexate)

• by using monoclonal antibodies against specific tumours which could also act as targeting carriers for drugs (experimental).

Non-specific agents
It is necessary to appreciate that neoplastic cells
• lack contact inhibition
• often show cellular aneuploidy
• have growth rates which range from fast to slow (compared with unaffected host cells).

Cells showing excessive chromosome development and/or rapid division have increased nucleic acid requirements and are, accordingly, susceptible to drugs inhibiting nucleic acid synthesis and replication (19.5, usually with the inevitable side-effects shown in Table 19.2). Some of these drugs are only effective during certain phases of the cell cycle (Fig. 19.14 and Table 19.8), while others (e.g. actinomycin D,: also, alkylating agents, doxorubicin) are cell-cycle independent as they act during most phases, i.e. G_1, S and G_2. Such information has been used to help in devising suitable drug combination schedules, e.g. use several drugs which act during different phases.

Conversely, if the tumour cells grow slowly, it is possible to exploit the difference in rate of growth by the use of pulse therapy. As shown in Fig. 19.15, this involves the administration of antineoplastic agents at

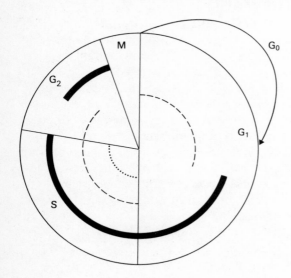

Fig. 19.14 Phases of the cell cycle (diagrammatic: read in combination with Table 19.8). Products of synthesis are shown as follows: dotted line, DNA; dashed lines, RNA; thick lines, protein. G_0 indicates a dormant phase during which the cell is not growing and, therefore, all non-specific chemotherapy is ineffective.

Table 19.8 Anticancer drugs acting on various phases of the cell cycle

Phase		Major cell product(s)	Inhibitory drug(s) as example(s)	Reference
G₁	Growth of cell (Presynthetic)	RNA/protein	Actinomycin D	p. 414
S	Synthesis (of DNA)	DNA	Cytarabine	Table 19.3
		DNA/RNA	Methotrexate	p. 409
		DNA/RNA	6-Mercaptopurine	p. 409
		RNA/protein	Actinomycin D	p. 414
G₂	Growth of cell (Postsynthetic, premitotic)	as G₁	as G₁	
M	Mitosis prophase metaphase anaphase telophase	Microtubules (*see* 4.13)	Vincristine*	p. 413

* Mainly inhibits cell division at metaphase.

intervals which favour recovery of rapidly dividing normal host tissues (Table 19.2) at the expense of less recovery (relative destruction) of the tumour cells.

Further aspects of cancer chemotherapy
With some tumours complete cell kill is necessary, i.e. one cell remaining can re-establish the neoplastic process. However, for many

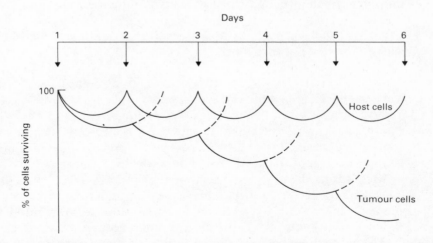

Fig. 19.15 The strategy of pulse therapy. If rapidly dividing host cells recover in 24 hours but tumour cells only in 36 hours, repeated selective kills may be achieved by administration of the chemotherapeutic agent every day. Interrupted lines indicate potential recovery processes (in absence of drug).

new growths the major aim is to kill at least 90% of the invading neoplastic cells in the hope that macrophages and cytotoxic T-cells will exterminate the remainder. As already mentioned (p. 423), any antineoplastic activity of interferon is probably mediated by a combination of direct cytotoxicity and immunostimulation.

Combinations of drugs are often used initially (e.g. in the treatment of leukaemias or lymphomas) to obtain a remission. Advantages are
• multiple modes and phases of action which may increase tumour cell kill and, possibly, slow the development of resistance
• lower doses of individual agents can be given thus minimising side-effects which also may show less overlap with different drugs.

Subsequent maintenance therapy then involves minimal chemotherapeutic drug usage to prevent recrudescence of the neoplastic process. This is attempted curative treatment: in cases where the patient is unable to stand the rigours of such heroic chemotherapy, palliative treatment may be the most that is possible.

As may be appreciated, cancer chemotherapy is often empirical but, overall, it has achieved mainly modest—though important—successes, particularly when specifically acting drugs can be used.

19.11 Immunosuppressive agents

These are used
• to prevent rejection of organ transplants
• to treat auto-immune diseases.

The immune process of graft rejection principally involves the recruitment and proliferation of cytotoxic T-lymphocytes in response to major histocompatibility (MHC) antigens suddenly introduced by the transplant or endogenously exposed in auto-immune conditions.

Graft-versus-host reaction. Lymphocytes from the graft attack host cells and are the cause of early rejection.

Host-versus-graft reaction. MHC antigens from transplanted tissue reach the host lymph nodes, where they induce the formation of a large number of cytotoxic T-lymphocytes. These latter, by entry into the graft and reaction with (resulting in destruction of) cells bearing the appropriate specific MHC antigen, probably represent the most important mechanism of transplant rejection in the longer term.

Methods used to prevent rejection are shown in Table 19.9. Most transplant centres use a 'triple therapy' of azathioprine, prednisolone and cyclosporin, each given at a relatively low dose to avoid individual toxicity but to contribute to an additive immunosuppressive effect.

The development of monoclonal antibodies against cytotoxic T-cells is a recent, more specific approach.

Table 19.9 Immunosuppressive therapy

Drug	Mechanism of action	Possible side-effects
Azathioprine*	Destruction of lymphocytes (Fig. 19.7)	Side-effects on other rapidly dividing cells (Table 19.2)
Prednisolone	Decreased production of cytotoxic	Many side-effects (Table 14.1)
Cyclosporin	T lymphocytes (by interference with Interleukin-2)	Mildly nephrotoxic, therefore not suitable alone if renal function is impaired

* *Im*uran®. This is a pro-drug forming the active agent 6-mercaptopurine.

Part 4
Therapeutic Considerations

20 Toxicology

Toxicological ('poisonous') or adverse effects may conveniently be divided into those attributable to

- side-effects
- overdose
- idiosyncrasy
- hypersensitivity (allergy, 20.2)
- teratogenicity (20.7)
- carcinogenicity (20.7).

20.1 Distinction between side-effects, overdose and idiosyncrasy

This is illustrated in Fig. 20.1. The usual therapeutic dose range shows a normal distribution of effective responses. A discontinuity in the graph indicates a *genetic* factor resulting in *idiosyncrasy* so that the patient is unusually sensitive (c_1) or abnormally resistant (c_2) to the drug action: examples will be detailed in 20.6.

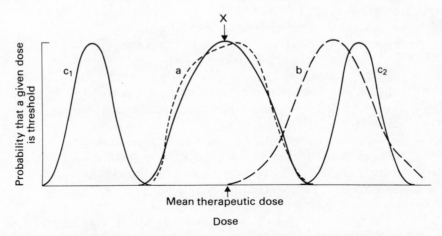

Fig. 20.1 Some types of toxic effect in relation to the effective therapeutic dosage of a drug (full line, centre — average value, X) in diagrammatic form. Side-effects (a) usually occur over a similiar dose range to the required action, while absolute overdose effects (b) are indicative of higher doses in the normal individual. A discontinuity in the graph signifies monofactorial idiosyncrasy more sensitive (c_1) or less sensitive (c_2).

Side-effects may be defined as 'those responses not required clinically, which occur at doses of the drug within the therapeutic range.' Thus, whether an action is a side-effect or not depends upon the particular use of the agent (20.3). However, if the drug requires an extended period to exert its beneficial response, e.g. an antidepressant such as imipramine (p. 182), the antimuscarinic side-effects (e.g. blurred vision, dry mouth) usually appear first and may discourage the patient from continuing with the therapy unless the situation is explained beforehand. Side-effects are manifest expressions of concomitant actions upon other organs or tissues due to lack of specificity. For example, cytotoxic agents used in the treatment of neoplasia inevitably affect host cells (*see* Table 19.2). Similarly, broad-spectrum antibiotics (such as tetracyclines) lead to superinfections and gut disturbances due to their production of microorganismal imbalances (19.6).

Overdose can be
1   Absolute (b, Fig. 20.1), i.e. too large a dose of the drug has been administered by accident, suicide or homicide
2   Relative, i.e. the given dose has been a correct one but its effects have been unduly accentuated by:
a   *pharmacokinetic* interactions resulting in an increase in free drug concentration due to
•   excessive absorption or activation *or*
•   decreased plasma protein binding, inactivation, redistribution or excretion, either in the particular individual (idiosyncrasy) or due to the presence of the same drug (pharmacokinetic tolerance, p. 188) or of other drugs (20.5).
b   *pharmacodynamic* considerations due to
•   recent use of the same agent. For example, digoxin (p. 271) has a half-life of *c.* 1.5 days: if given too frequently it collects in the body—termed *cumulation*. Therefore do not give a *'loading'* dose (*see* Fig. 1.9) of this drug until that previously given has been effectively removed from the body i.e. within five half-lives (p. 25)—about a week for digoxin
•   concomitant effects of another drug, e.g. frusemide, by increasing potassium ion excretion will precipitate digoxin ventricular extrasystoles (p. 283) if potassium supplements are not given.
   Overdose manifestations vary from acute to chronic and may produce toxicity by:
1   A quantitatively enhanced action which can be an extension of
•   the therapeutic action, e.g. neostigmine in excess in the treatment of myasthenia gravis resulting in a depolarising block; ergotamine giving limb vessel constriction, p. 260
•   of a side-effect, e.g. morphine producing respiratory depression, 7.11.

2 A qualitatively different action, e.g. streptomycin affecting vestibular function and causing dizziness, 19.6.

3 A poisonous effect *ab initio*, e.g. strychnine inducing spinal fits (9.7), e.g. cyanide producing histotoxic hypoxia (11.6) by inhibition of cytochrome oxidase.

The estimation of plasma drug levels is valuable in a number of potentially toxic situations such as lithium carbonate therapy (7.5) or paracetamol poisoning (1.9).

Side-effects, overdose responses and idiosyncratic reactions are characteristic for any given drug. This is in contrast to the next category.

20.2 Hypersensitivity reactions

Many of these are due to allergies. The remainder are unusual responses which are not idiosyncratic, e.g. asthmatic reactions to aspirin, p. 192.

The final manifestations of allergy are usually limited to one of the four reactions originally described by Gell and Coombs. Fundamentally, the drug or one of its metabolites acts as a hapten (Gk: *haptein*, to fasten) which combines with a body protein to produce an antigen which, in turn, produces antibodies and/or antigen-reactive (sensitised) T cells. These latter then react with any antigen remaining or subsequently formed (by further administration of the same or a related compound) to elicit one (or more) of the characteristic responses shown in Table 20.1. Here, it can be seen that allergy to penicillin, for example, may produce different responses in individual cases.

Natural allergies are usually investigated by skin testing with relevant possible antigens (e.g. in hay-fever; bronchial asthma, 11.5). This procedure is also usually satisfactory for drugs but may fail if, for example, the metabolite essential to the development of allergy is not formed in the skin but is produced, for example, by hepatic transformation, when the agent is subsequently given systemically.

Desensitisation, i.e. the deliberate administration of small amounts of the antigen gradually to induce a state of non-reactivity (by producing circulating IgG blocking antibodies), can be valuable in hay-fever (termed specific, preseasonal desensitisation) but is only indicated for a drug if it is the sole treatment for a particular disease. Thus, it is usually unnecessary in modern chemotherapy where satisfactory alternative drugs are almost always available.

Auto-immune diseases arise by similar mechanisms to allergic reactions: the only difference is that, instead of a drug acting as a hapten, components of the host are recognised (abnormally) as antigens.

20.3 Effects of atropine to illustrate the above distinctions

1 The side-effects depend upon the required action, i.e. vary with the use (Table 20.2).

Table 20.1 Characteristics of different allergic responses

Type	Antigen	Antibody	Complement necessary?	Onset	Resultant effect	Commonly used drugs producing this effect
I (anaphylactic)	Free	IgE on mast cells or basophil granulocytes	No	Immediate	Release of vaso- and bronchoactive substances*	Penicillin Aspirin
II (cytotoxic)	On surface of erythrocyte platelet neutrophil	IgG circulating	Yes: for complement-induced lysis but not for cell-mediated killing	Immediate	Direct cell damage haemolytic anaemia thrombocytopenia leucopenia	α-Methyldopa Rifampicin Phenytoin
III (toxic complex formation)	Free	IgG circulating (throughout extracellular fluid)	No: but invariably involved in amplification of the initial reaction	Immediate	Formation of precipitates in and around small blood vessels resulting in lesions of surrounding cells	Penicillin Hydralazine (pp. 256–7)
IV (cell-mediated)	Free or on surface of cell	Antigen-reactive (sensitised) T-lymphocytes	No	Delayed (up to 24 h)	Local cytotoxicity and release of inflammatory mediators from the sensitised lymphocytes	Penicillin

* Usually causing *vasodilation* and *bronchoconstriction*.

Table 20.2   Actions and side-effects of atropine

Use	Eye		Inhibition of cardiac vagal tone	Decreased salivary secretion	Antagonism of CNS effects of acetylcholine
	Dilation of pupil	Loss of accommodation			
Acute iridocyclitis (18.2)	+	+	0	0	0
Pre-operative medication (8.6)	S	S	+	+	0
Parkinsonism (7.2)	S	S	S	+/S*	+

All effects are due to blockade of muscarinic acetylcholine receptors: +, desired action; S, side-effect; 0, not noteworthy (in the case of treatment of acute iridocyclitis, due to *local* application into the conjunctival sac).
* Relieves 'drooling' if present; otherwise is a side-effect.

2   An overdose produces characteristic signs and symptoms (*see* Table 2.7).

3   Idiosyncrasy is shown in about 70% of tame rabbits which, because of a genetic difference, have a plasma esterase capable of catabolising (by hydrolysis) atropine in minutes rather than hours: the latter is the case in about 30% of tame rabbits and most other species, including humans.

4   Allergy can occur when atropine (or homatropine) is dropped into the conjunctival sac (18.4). In under 1% of patients, a 'red eye' develops almost immediately probably due to a type I reaction releasing vasodilator substances which result in conjunctival flushing: this disappears spontaneously within 10 minutes.

20.4   Variations in drug toxicity

Examples of specific toxicity upon particular organs or tissues have already been discussed in previous chapters. As mentioned earlier (1.13) in any individual, toxicological effects can be modified by genetic and environmental factors, age and pathological conditions. The spectrum may now be progressively broadened to include differences in sex (*see*, for example, Table 15.2) and in species (e.g. morphine produces excitement in horses and cats, p. 203). However, of even greater importance are situations where modifications are due to other drugs (or foods) taken concurrently or in succession. Illustrative examples are detailed in the next section.

20.5   Drug interactions

These may be deliberate (e.g. to augment the therapeutic action or to remove poisons from the body) or accidental. The possibilities of accidental interactions are great and can alter either the drug effect or its toxicity. The latter is more common and may vary in severity from lethal to trivial, and in likelihood from common to uncommon—either because of the relative incidence of reactions or because of the relative possibility of the interacting drugs being prescribed together. Excellent wall charts illustrating the possibilities are available.

Important examples, systematised under the pharmacokinetic and pharmacodynamic classifications already established, are shown in Table 20.3. The reader should amplify these with further cases noted personally during clinical study. Responses preceded by numbers 1–8

Table 20.3 Factors affecting the responses to drugs

Resulting in *decreased* effect of drug	Resulting in *increased* effect of drug
ABSORPTION *From the gut*	
Antacids increase the gastric pH and, so, lower the concentration of aspirin in the epithelial cells (Fig. 1.3) resulting in less local toxicity	Metoclopramide increases gastric emptying resulting in more rapid action of antimigraine drugs, p. 260
Diarrhoea, e.g. purgative ($MgSO_4$, 13.6) in removal of poisons, e.g. contraceptive 'pill' less effective	Concomitant constipation, e.g. with morphine increases systemic absorption of digoxin
Tetracyclines (by chelation and precipitation) diminish absorption of calcium and iron ions, and vice versa (19.6 and Table 20.5)	
From s.c. or i.m. sites	
Depot preparations (pp. 9–10), e.g. procaine penicillin gives lower concentration of penicillin in the systemic circulation. Similarly, protamine zinc insulin	Addition of a vasoconstrictor such as adrenaline to a local anaesthetic solution prolongs its local action and decreases systemic toxicity (Table 8.2)
	Conversely, addition of hyaluronidase encourages absorption and increases the systemic action of, for example, ergometrine (p. 361)
PLASMA PROTEIN BINDING	
	Decreased protein available, e.g. liver disease, malnutrition; or displacement by more strongly bound compounds, e.g. clofibrate: all result in enhanced responses to warfarin (*see* Table 17.2).
EXCRETION (*renal*)	
Acidification of urine increases removal of base, e.g. in treatment of gentamicin poisoning	Alkalinisation of urine decreases removal of base e.g. in retention of gentamicin to treat renal parenchymal infection
Alkalinisation of urine facilitates organic acid excretion, e.g. aspirin poisoning, e.g. with uricosuric (12.8)	Probenecid prevents renal secretion of penicillin (p. 404 and Fig. 1.5c)

indicate idiosyncratic reactions, discussed in detail in 20.6; some of these are effects of drugs given *alone*. (Drugs can also interfere with laboratory tests.)

20.6 Idiosyncratic reactions to drugs
As previously stated, genetic differences are involved here and the

Table 20.3 — *Cont'd*

Resulting in *decreased* effect of drug	Resulting in *increased* effect of drug
METABOLISM	
Induction of enzymes, e.g. by phenytoin resulting in increased breakdown of warfarin and contraceptive 'pill' less effective	Depression of enzymes, e.g. by allopurinol resulting in decreased breakdown of warfarin (Table 17.2)
1B High activity plasma cholinesterase: impossible to achieve neuro-muscular relaxation with suxamethonium (extremely uncommon, Table 20.4)	**1A** Low affinity plasma cholinesterase: prolonged apnoea (several hours) following suxamethonium administration
	2 'Slow' acetylators subject to increased therapeutic and toxic effects of, e.g. hydralazine, isoniazid
	3 Patients unable to hydroxylate, and thus inactive, phenytoin normally because of genetically determined lack of epoxide hydrolase (p. 26)
ACTION	
4 Warfarin resistance Antagonism specific, e.g. chelating agents (20.9), e.g. atropine in nerve gas poisoning (2.6) functional, e.g. treatment of acute, severe type I allergic responses (histamine → bronchoconstriction/hypotension) with adrenaline, 5.7	Synergism (4.4) *addition*, e.g. ethanol with either sedative anti-(H_1)histamine or benzodiazepines, producing excessive CNS depression *potentiation*, e.g. (desmethyl)imipramine and (nor)adrenaline (Table 3.3); e.g. neostigmine and acetylcholine (p. 49)
SIDE- AND OTHER TOXIC EFFECTS	
	Potassium-losing diuretics increase incidence of ventricular extrasystoles with digoxin (p. 306)
	5 Porphyria (acute intermittent hepatic) — *see* next page
	6 Abnormal haemoglobins (M types) can enhance occurrence of methaemoglobinaemia
	7 Glucose-6-phosphate dehydrogenase deficiency in erythrocytes
	8 Malignant hyperthermia

characteristic ways in which they are expressed and are transmitted to offspring are shown in Table 20.4. The last four examples (5–8 in Table 20.3) will now be discussed in more detail.

Porphyria

The significant steps in the synthesis of haem (Fig. 20.2) show end-product inhibition of the rate-limiting reaction. In patients liable to develop acute intermittent hepatic porphyria, the feed-back is in a metastable equilibrium (probably due to a deficiency of enzyme(s) in the porphobilinogen →haem reactions) which can be upset by therapeutic doses of substances such as barbiturates, phenytoin, oestrogens (including the contraceptive tablet), sulphonylureas and griseofulvin. *Then* there is increased production of haem precursors but the enzymes in the pathway beyond porphobilinogen rapidly become saturated. This results in high concentrations of δ-aminolaevulinic acid and porphobilinogen in the central nervous system (producing, for example, madness, autonomic symptoms, cardiovascular effects) and in the urine (a diagnostic aid). As potential porphyriacs and porphyrogenic drugs can both be identified, ideally it should be possible to avoid giving the latter to the former.

There are less serious types of porphyria. For example, cutaneous porphyria is most commonly acquired (particularly through alcoholism), is only precipitated by large doses of, e.g, barbiturates, and is manifested as a phototoxicity due to deposition of *haem* products in the skin (see Table 18.3).

Abnormal haemoglobins

Several drugs which are strong oxidising agents (e.g. 'nitrites', p. 269), convert red blood cell ferrous, Fe^{2+}, to ferric, Fe^{3+}, ions (i.e. haemoglobin → methaemoglobin) but, unless doses are excessive, the process is

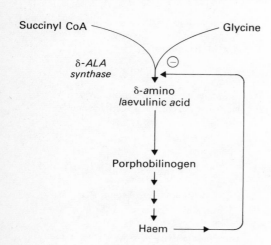

Fig. 20.2 The synthesis of haem. In patients predisposed to acute intermittent hepatic porphyria, the negative feed-back loop is defective and control is lost in the presence of porphyrogenic drugs.

Table 20.4 Drug idiosyncrasies

Key number in text	Phenotype	Clinical response	Inheritance	Occurrence*
1A	Low affinity plasma cholinesterase	Prolonged apnoea with suxamethonium	Autosomal autonomous	2
1B	High activity plasma cholinesterase	Resistance to suxamethonium paralysis of voluntary muscle	Autosomal autonomous	3
2	Deficient hepatic acetyl transferase	Slow acetylation of hydralazine, isoniazid, sulphonamides, phenelzine	Autosomal recessive	0
3	Deficient hepatic epoxide hydrolase	Inability to hydroxylate phenytoin resulting in hepatotoxicity		3
4	?	Resistance to the anticoagulant action of warfarin	Autosoral dominant	2
5	Impaired end-product feedback on formation of δ-aminolaevulinic acid	Acute intermittent hepatic porphyria—CNS, ANS and CVS disturbances with, for example, barbiturates	Autosomal dominant	3
6	Abnormal haemoglobins (M types)	Increased sensitivity to the production of methaemoglobinaemia with, for example, 'nitrites'	Autosomal dominant	2
7	Deficient glucose-6-phosphate dehydrogenase in red blood cells	Haemolytic anaemia and methaemoglobinaemia with, for example, primaquine, sulphonamides	Sex-linked autonomous	1–3†
8	Persistence of calcium ions at their muscle fibril binding sites	Malignant hyperthermia and muscle rigors with, for example, suxamethonium *and* halothane	Autosomal dominant	3

ANS, autonomic nervous system; CVS, cardiovascular system.

* Occurrence: 0, very common (c. 50% of population); 1, common (> 1%); 2, less common (0.1–1%); 3, uncommon (< 0.01%). Ethnic differences occur.

† Incidence proportional to degree of endemicity of falciparum malaria.

normally reversed by intracellular methaemoglobin reductase. This enzyme, however, is ineffectual in patients with abnormal haemoglobins (particularly of M types) so that they show a greatly increased tendency to drug-induced methaemoglobinaemia.

G6PD deficiency

Glucose-6-phosphate dehydrogenase is required in erythrocytes to generate the NADPH necessary to produce sufficient thiol (SH) groups
- to maintain the cellular integrity
- (as reduced glutathione) to keep haem iron in the ferrous form.

Patients with a deficiency of this enzyme are, accordingly, much more sensitive to drugs with a tendency to produce haemolysis and methaemoglobinaemia. The latter cannot be reversed by methylene blue (17.3) because this antidote requires reduced glutathione as an intermediate.

Natural (i.e. not drug-induced) haemolysis due to G6PD deficiency disrupts the erythrocyte cycle of the malarial parasite (see Fig 19.10) and confers some resistance to the disease.

Malignant hyperthermia

This most commonly results from the use of halothane together *with* suxamethonium. It manifests itself as a sudden pyrexia with rigors. The major finding in experimental animals is a tonic spasm of skeletal muscle due to persistence of calcium ions at their binding sites on troponin C (similar to cardiac muscle, 10.7)—whether resultant on increased release or decreased sequestration is uncertain. Give dantrolene (see Table 7.3).

20.7   Teratogenicity and carcinogenicity

Teratogenesis

Teratogenesis (Gk: *teras*, monster) is the production of physical defects in the fetus. The classical example of a teratogenic agent is thalidomide which, given as a hypnotic to pregnant females when ontogenesis of the limb buds was occurring (24–36 days fetal age) produced defects in limb development (e.g. phocomelia—'seal flippers') in *a small number of* human fetuses. This illustrates the factors necessary for a drug to be teratogenic
- itself, or a metabolic product, must cross the placental barrier
- the concentration in the fetus is critical: too little is not embryopathic, too much will result in abortion or still-birth
- the stage of pregnancy will determine the malformation produced
- there is a large individual variation in liability. Further, there are species variations: thalidomide is teratogenic in human and rabbit but not in rat.

After the thalidomide disaster, a number of commonly used drugs were shown to be capable of inducing fetal abnormalities in pregnant animals but many of the findings were invalid as the high doses used often cause maternal deaths.

The lessons to be learnt from this distressing episode are

1 Test all new drugs, acutely and chronically, on a wide variety of fetal tissues at different stages of development.

2 Adopt a very conservative attitude to therapy during human (or veterinary animal) pregnancy, using only drugs which are essential and preferring those of long standing.

3 With all malformed fetuses check the drugs which have been used during pregnancy and report any possible teratogenic connection to the Committee of Safety on Medicines (21.4).

Other possible teratogens include drugs which can (or have been reported to) do the following:

1 Induce chromosomal breakage either in the female (e.g. gold salts) or in the male (e.g. phenylbutazone).

2 Act to reduce fetal development

- generally, e.g. antitumour and other mutagenic agents (*see* later); griseofulvin; etretinate, p. 395
- more specifically, e.g. phenytoin (increased incidence of hare-lip and cleft palate); also sodium valproate in animals: *see* Table 7.1.

It must be stressed that only 2–3% of developmental abnormalities can definitely be ascribed to drug usage during pregnancy but, in the author's opinion, this is far too great a price to pay for the therapeutic benefits gained.

Carcinogenesis
The production of new growths by drugs is, paradoxically, most proven with respect to *agents used in antineoplastic chemotherapy*, indicating their relative lack of selective toxicity (19.10). Particular pharmacological groups involved are radioactive substances, alkylating agents, purine and pyrimidine analogues, non-selective folic acid antagonists (e.g. methotrexate) and some intercalators. They appear to exert their maleficent actions by

1 Mutagenesis, i.e. modifications of the genotype, induced by the drug itself or the formation of toxic compounds (e.g. ethylene imines, epoxides, oxygen free radicals) or by 'scrambling' of the genetic code by transformation, deletion or addition of base pairs.

2 Emergence of oncogenic viruses. This is one possible explanation of the lymphomata which sometimes resulted when antilymphocyte immunoglobulin was used to prevent transplant rejection.

Other carcinogens (actual or potential) include:

1 Oestrogens (15.2).

2 Nitro-compounds (Fig. 20.3). Nitrates or 'nitrites' (p. 269) via intermediate nitrosamines are converted by cytochrome P_{450}-dependent enzymes to carcinogenic diazo compounds which act by alkylation

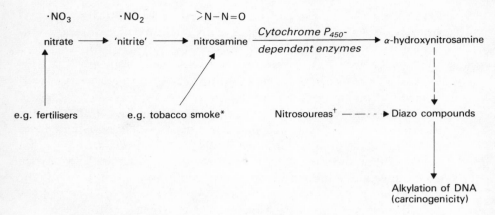

Fig. 20.3 Carcinogenicity of nitro-compounds. Interrupted lines indicate multiple-step processes. * p. 50; † p. 412.

of DNA (Fig. 19.8). Tobacco smoke contains small amounts of nitro-samines. Nitrosoureas (p. 412) form similar diazo derivatives and can produce leukaemia.

3 A number of commonly used drugs, which certainly appear to be safe in humans, but produce tumours in rodents, e.g.

- iron dextran (sarcomata in rats, 8.1)
- metronidazole (various mouse cancers)
- oxazepam (a major metabolite of diazepam—given *for a year* produced some murine hepatomas)
- isoniazid (carcinogenic in mice).

20.8 Treatment of poisoning

If the condition is a *chronic* one, tell the patient to *stop taking the drug* and institute specific and symptomatic measures as necessary.

Acute poisoning

In the acute emergency, regional poisons information services and centres are listed in the *British National Formulary* and are on call at all times.

Recognition of the causative agent is valuable but should not prejudice immediate treatment which consists of:

1 *Life-saving procedures*, especially the maintenance of adequate respiration, circulation and renal function but also including control of fits and maintenance of body temperature.

2 *Administration of specific antidotes*, e.g. atropine and pralidoxime for anticholinesterase poisoning (p. 54), naloxone against opioids (p. 206), chelating agents (20.9), oxygen in carbon monoxide poisoning

(11.6). Or *functional antagonists* such as anticonvulsants in strychnine overdose (9.7).

3 *Attempts to decrease the plasma or tissue concentration of the toxic agent*

• lessen absorption, particularly from the gastrointestinal tract by emesis, gastric lavage, absorption (e.g. activated charcoal), neutralisation (appropriate acid or base), precipitation (raw egg, milk, e.g. iron overdose, p. 377), chelation or purgation (magnesium sulphate). Emesis or gastric lavage is contra-indicated for corrosive substances; in the unconscious patient gastric lavage may be performed if a cuffed endotracheal tube is used to prevent inhalation of vomitus

• increase pulmonary elimination by assisted respiration, especially for overdose of gaseous or volatile anaesthetics

• encourage renal excretion by diuresis (copious draughts of water in mild cases) accompanied by alteration of the urinary pH, if indicated (12.10). *Forced diuresis,* employing frusemide or mannitol, can be dangerous by inducing drastic swings in plasma fluid or ionic concentrations, and should not be undertaken lightly. As the plasma clearance, $CL_p = V_d \times k_{el}$ (see Fig. 1.7), the higher the volume of distribution the slower the elimination by *haemoperfusion* (through a charcoal column) or *dialysis* (from either blood or peritoneal fluid). Dialysis is also slowed by heavy protein binding. These methods are only employed in extremely serious cases of poisoning.

4 *Care of the unconscious patient*

• nurse in semi-prone position

• turn every few hours to prevent hypostatic pneumonia and bed sores

• maintain adequate nutrition by the administration of appropriate fluids intravenously

• monitor urinary output and faecal excretion, and replace vital losses as necessary

• maintain body temperature.

20.9 Chelating agents

Ionised forms of many metals and some other compounds (e.g. epoxides) are poisonous by forming strong (usually covalent) bonds with chemical groups (ligands) which are essential for the normal functioning of body constitutents, particularly enzymes. Chelating agents possess one or, more commonly, two (or more) such ligands with a high affinity for a particular ion (or ions) and, thereby, sequester the toxic substance usually within an organic, heterocyclic ring structure which is biologically inert and will eventually be excreted. The protecting molecule thus neutralises the poison by holding it in a claw-like embrace (Gk: *chele*, claw).

The most commonly encountered chelating agents and their relevant ligands are shown in Table 20.5 alongside ions for which they show

Table 20.5 Chelating agents

Agent	Active ligand(s)		Ion chelated
Dimercaprol	.SH	.SH	Mercury, arsenic, gold
D-penicillamine*	.SH	.NH$_2$	Lead, copper
Trisodium edetate	.COOH	.COOH	Calcium
Sodium calciumedetate	.COOH	.COOH	Lead
Dicobalt edetate	Cobalt		Cyanide (*see* below)
Desferrioxamine (US: deferoxamine)	.CO	N.OH	Iron
Tetracyclines	.CO	.OH	Calcium, iron, magnesium, aluminium
Hydroxocobalamin	Cobalt (already in a ring structure)		Cyanide (including tobacco amblyopia, 18.4)
N-acetylcysteine	.SH	.NH.R†	Epoxide (paracetamol poisoning, 1.9)
Activated compound‡ formed from disulfiram	.SH	.NEt$_2$	Copper

* A chemical misnomer. This *minor* metabolite of penicillin consists of the 1–4 parts of the molecule shown in Fig. 19.3 and is obviously ββ′-dimethylcysteine.
† R = CO.CH$_3$.
‡ Diethyldithiocarbamic acid.

a high affinity. It must be stressed that when used as antidotes

1 Any particular chelating agent has to affect the poison more than it interferes with essential biochemical processes. For example, desferrioxamine, which neutralises toxic doses of iron compounds does not remove essential iron atoms from haemoglobin or the cytochromes.

2 The maximum detoxicating clinical response will be seen in the early stages of therapy, when the body concentration of the poison is highest: so, *decrease the dose of chelating agent as the treatment progresses*. This ensures that an excess of the chelating agent will not be present to interfere with normal body function, e.g. dimercaprol in excess can inactivate enzymes requiring thiol (SH) groups, such as Na$^+$, K$^+$-activated ATPase.

3 In addition, allergic reactions or side- or toxic- effects can occur with these antidotes. Examples

• allergy to penicillamine, desferrioxamine (17.1) or N-acetylcysteine
• nephrotic syndrome or pyridoxine deficiency due to penicillamine (Table 5.13)
• renal damage with sodium calciumedetate.

21 Drug Development and Use

21.1 Drug discovery

This may be *accidental*—a chance observation by the doctor, patient or in the laboratory has often been productive. The best known examples are Withering's realisation that foxglove *(Digitalis purpurea,* which contains cardiac glycosides similar to digoxin) was the vital ingredient in a herbal remedy for 'the dropsy' (oedema), and Fleming's observation that staphylococcal colonies in culture were lysed by a contaminant mould *Penicillium,* which later resulted in penicillin. While such an event is still possible, the usual course nowadays is *intentional.* This process is initiated by the chemist producing

- botanical or zoological extracts. A valuable source, especially in developing countries where folk remedies can still yield effective constituents
- modifications of known body constituents (hormones, transmitters, autacoids) or drugs (e.g. morphine analogues)
- new chemical compounds.

Within all these categories, synthetic manipulation can produce changes in activity, pharmacokinetics and/or toxicity which are procured on the basis of structure–activity relationships (SAR, *see* 2.3 and 3.3). Hansch analysis (or one of its derivative techniques) is a more refined method whereby the effects of chemical modification are calculated for a number of parameters (e.g. molecular dimensions, electron distribution, lipid solubility) simultaneously. This is relatively naive, insofar as most drug molecules approaching their specific receptors are in various states of dynamic equilibrium (4.1), and has been replaced by *dynamic* structure–activity analyses (e.g. using computer-assisted graphics.) which take account of both

- conformational equilibria, which are the most favoured molecular configurations for activity under *in vivo* conditions, and
- ionised equilibria, the most effective charge distribution within the molecule which will affect not only its activity but also its pharmacokinetics.

21.2 Drug development: experimental

Pharmacological

As the chemist can synthesise new compounds much more rapidly than the pharmacologist can subject them to extensive tests, an initial broad evaluation is necessary to narrow the field. If the new compounds are variants of known drugs, appropriate experiments are carried out: otherwise, an observational test is performed (usually on mice) in which the drug effects on several easily measurable variables (e.g. motor activity, respiration, temperature) are noted and compared with the profiles of standard agents. Such tests, along with determinations of acute toxicity, result in the rejection of over 90% of new compounds—the rest pass on to a more detailed analysis. They are tested on a wide variety of isolated and whole animal preparations to discover their range of actions which are then compared quantitatively with those of appropriate familiar drugs. Any side-effects are noted, and toxicity specifically determined (following administration of the new agent in a range of doses, both acutely and chronically) by both macroscopic and microscopic examination of the major organs and tissues of common laboratory species of both sexes (including those at various stages of pregnancy). The therapeutic ratio, defined as:

$$\frac{LD_{50}}{ED_{50}} = \frac{\text{Dose which kills 50\% of animals}}{\text{Dose which produces an effective response in 50\% of animals}}$$

—a pharmacological shibboleth of the earlier part of this century—is not very useful by itself. For example, the therapeutic ratio of a general anaesthetic can be as low as two while that of thalidomide (20.7) is approximately 1000, i.e. other factors are involved: accuracy of dosage for general anaesthetics, teratogenicity for thalidomide.

Even with extensive testing, difficulties arise; a few examples follow. Most laboratory animals—unlike patients—come from inbred (genetically similar) strains. If a drug such as thalidomide produces its abnormality in (say) one human fetus of 10 000 exposed to the drug, how could this be detected using a few hundred pregnant animals? Further, any of the pharmacokinetic or pharmacodynamic criteria observed can differ significantly in a particular species compared with man; for example, an active metabolite may not be produced nor a toxic derivative formed. The objection that the experimental animal is not in a pathological condition similar to that of the human patient is often insuperable in our present state of knowledge (e.g. anti-migraine drug testing, 10.6); and, even if apparently the same situation is present (e.g. hypertension in rats given deoxycorticosterone acetate), the experimental and clinical circumstances may not be strictly comparable. Nevertheless, although preliminary animal experiments are gradually being phased out, they are still an unfortunate necessity for the development of most drugs and are essential evidence (along with clinical trial data, 21.3) which must be submitted to the Committee on Safety of Medicines.

Human volunteers

The use of human volunteers is an important ethical concern at the moment. It might be considered legitimate for relatively innocuous drugs (but how can this be determined?) particularly to test for minor side-effects or for pharmacokinetic experiments. But there are further pitfalls, for instance it must be appreciated that the subject is often in an artificial situation. For example, testing new analgesics by their ability to prevent the pain associated with the application of heat to the blackened forehead (a standard method which enables accurate quantitative control of the stimulus) is not analogous to the treatment of coronary pain—as the human volunteer can request that the painful stimulus be terminated, so that the psychological overlay (present in clinical cases) is absent.

21.3   Drug development: clinical trials

The moment of truth in a potential drug's life is the stage of clinical testing. Increased potency of an agent is not a justification for a clinical trial unless it is confidently expected that it is also significantly less toxic (including side-effects) than its currently used predecessor(s).

A full-scale clinical trial (which requires permission via the Committee on Safety of Medicines) is usually performed as follows. Patients with a particular condition entering a group of hospitals undergo the following procedures:

1   Screening for eligibility; for example, ailment definitely diagnosed, patient not treated with a similar drug previously, patient within age limits—not the very young or the very old, patient not pregnant. But do maintain a sense of proportion as too rigorous conditions may eliminate almost all the patients.

2   They are required to give consent after being fully informed of the possible benefits and likely dangers involved, and are randomly assigned to one of three groups:

- new drug regime
- currently best available treatment
- placebo (L: I will please), i.e. an inert substance such as a lactose tablet or a saline solution dispensed in an identical pharmaceutical preparation to that of the active agents in the other two groups.

It is not always ethical to include all these categories in a particular trial. If the disease is life-threatening, the placebo series must be omitted and, if the new drug appears capable of curing a hitherto fatal condition, there is no justification for including the current, best-available therapy either (such a situation arose in the treatment of tuberculous meningitis when streptomycin was introduced).

3   The appropriate medication is given using the 'double-blind' technique, i.e. neither the patient nor the medical attendant who is to monitor progress is aware of the group allocation.

4 Patients are assessed with regard to progress by *objective* criteria (e.g. sputum conversion and chest X-ray in the case of pulmonary tuberculosis). These are preferable as being more scientific but are not always definitive or possible, so that they usually have to be complemented or supplemented by *subjective* criteria, which are less reliable but the only means available at the moment for assessing, for example, psychotropic agents (Chapter 7).

A further consideration is that *relevant* criteria be used (*see* Table 21.1). At a time (or times) decided *before* the inception of the trial (to avoid bias), the results are collated statistically. If they are in favour of the new treatment, any side- or toxic effects assume significance: these should be carefully noted in questionnaire form during the trial.

Clinical trials are quite difficult to organise and are time-consuming but, when properly conducted, they yield a wealth of essential information for critical consideration by the Committee on Safety of Medicines. Experience suggests a number of possible pitfalls, including the following:

1 *Placebo usage.* This may be inadequate in at least two respects. First, there are 'placebo reactors' who either improve (positive), or deteriorate or show side-effects (negative) when given inert substances. Secondly, the side-effects of the drug under test may be so obvious that patients are very soon aware who is receiving the active agent. Such a situation arose in a trial of L-dopa for parkinsonism when those who were given the drug developed characteristic choreoathetoid movements, especially of the face (*see* Table 7.2)

2 *Tolerance.* If this develops slowly, it may be missed altogether in a clinical trial; if more rapid in onset, it can result in the sporadic occurrence of variations in drug effectiveness

3 *Compliance.* Therapeutic regimens in hospitalised patients can be closely supervised (and compliance tested, e.g. by measuring plasma concentrations of the drug) but outpatient administration introduces difficulties. For example, some tuberculous patients when they feel

Table 21.1 Which criterion would you take as establishing a beneficial effect of drug therapy in the treatment of angina pectoris?

Criterion	Relieved by	
	Glyceryl trinitrate	Ethanol
Symptomatic relief—less worried by the pain	+	+
Improvement of exercising electrocardiogram	+	−

+, Effective; −, not effective.

better, after a few weeks of triple therapy, may then stop taking the tablets. In this situation a spot-check can be made as rifampicin colours the urine red (p. 414); a more refined method involves measurement of isoniazid metabolites in the urine, having first determined whether the patient is a 'slow' or 'fast' acetylator (p. 400).

A variant of the above type of clinical trial, namely a *cross-over test*, is feasible when the disease is not curable, is chronic and progresses relatively slowly, e.g. essential hypertension. Here, two groups of patients are given (say, 3 months' trials) of two different treatments (A and B) successively applied in opposite order (A followed by B or vice versa). Thus, individuals act as their own controls. But sometimes 'carry-over' effects from the first treatment may complicate the interpretation of the second drug's actions.

The primary objective of a clinical trial is to determine whether the new drug possesses significant advantages over already existing therapy. It also gives information about the optimal route of administration, dosage schedule(s) and duration of treatment. If the point at issue is *solely* whether one of two treatments is more effective and there are ethical reasons for deciding this at once when it becomes statistically significant (so that all patients can be switched to the better therapy), a *sequential trial* is performed. In this, participants are paired and randomly assigned to groups receiving either drug A or drug B: the relative efficacy of the responses are assessed daily and plotted as shown in Fig. 21.1. One treatment is proved to be more effective when one of the lateral edges of the outline is crossed. It must be stressed that the sequential method takes no account of side-effects or other toxic actions and that it results in much less general information than the more

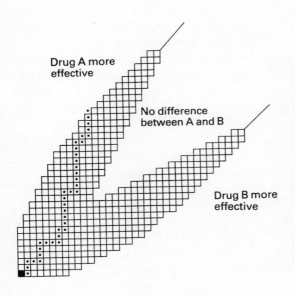

Drug A more effective

No difference between A and B

Drug B more effective

Fig. 21.1 Plotting of results in a sequential trial. Start at the filled square in the lower left-hand corner. For each pair of patients each day mark (dots in figure) one square upwards if drug A produces a better response than drug B or one square to the right if B is superior. When one of the *lateral* edge-lines is crossed one of the treatments is significantly more effective (e.g. A in the test plotted above). The outline illustrated is for 95% significance level, i.e. this result could only occur by chance 5 times in every 100 tests ($P = 0.05$).

elaborate clinical trial previously described; accordingly, its indications are *very limited*.

Finally, *orphan drugs* are possible treatments for conditions which are very uncommon and, so, not commercially viable. Under such special circumstances an individual physician may be given clinical responsibility to 'develop' the drug.

21.4   Committee on Safety of Medicines

This committee, an independent group of experts, is charged with the duty of obtaining optimal therapeutic benefit from drugs. It achieves this aim by the following means:

1   Initial study of pharmacological reports which, if satisfactory, allows the drug to proceed to clinical tests.

2   Assessment of clinical trial data which can then lead to marketing approval.

3   Adverse reaction monitoring (post-marketing surveillance). This system—reported by individual practitioners on 'yellow cards'—applies to *all* drugs in current use. Doctors must signify all side- or toxic effects of newly introduced agents (identified by an inverted black triangle, ▼, in the *British National Formulary*) and any unusual responses to established therapeutic substances. The latter is necessary not only to uncover rare or unexpected reactions but also to monitor any differences produced by changes in pharmaceutical formulation (a cogent example was an alteration in digoxin presentation in the early 1970s which accidentally roughly doubled the effective concentration of the drug). Difficulties for the busy doctor arise when patients are on multiple or frequently changing therapy, or when toxic effects develop slowly or in a disguised fashion.

21.5   Drug usage

The writer firmly believes in the Hippocratic tradition, namely that drugs should only be used therapeutically to aid the recuperative forces of nature. Ideally, the correct diagnosis should be followed, if necessary, by the exhibition of the most suitable, currently available drug by the route and in the dosage necessary to achieve an optimal effect at the required site. This treatment should be repeated at appropriate intervals for a length of time requisite to regain physiological equilibrium or, alternatively, to produce and maintain maximum correction of the underlying pathological condition.

Examples of the use and abuse of drugs in relation to the prescriber are summarised in Table 21.2. Ideal criteria for usage are indicated but, as in any other art, they may not always be wholly achievable due to the exigencies of any particular situation. Sources of information regarding the most appropriate drugs for specific conditions are contained in current editions of the *British National Formulary* and the *Prescribers' Journal*.

Table 21.2 Criteria for the use of drugs by practitioners contrasted with therapeutic misuse

	Use	Misuse
Diagnosis	Certain	Uncertain
Disease	Drug necessary	Drug unnecessary
Drug	Correctly indicated	Incorrectly indicated
Dosage	Adequate and at right intervals to maintain therapeutic concentrations	Under- or overdosage; wrong intervals
Distribution difficulties	Nil	Does not achieve a therapeutic concentration at the site of action due to, e.g. lack of activation, e.g. too rapid breakdown, redistribution or excretion
Duration of treatment	Satisfactory: correct supply of drug prescribed	Too short or too long; under- or overprescription
Dangers	Low toxicity (including side-effects)	High toxicity and/or prohibitive side-effects: iatrogenic effects*
Dependence	Nil	Present
Disadvantages	Nil	Any other problems in relation to usage, e.g. difficulty in administration, development of tolerance or bacterial resistance

* Iatrogenic effects are those produced by the physician (Gk: *iatros*, physician), almost always inadvertently. (For possibilities, *see* drug interactions, 20.5.)

21.6 Misuse of drugs

Some examples follows:

1 *Patient disobedience*—the opposite of compliance.

2 *Poisoning*. This can also include food ingredients or contaminants, and environmental hazards, including tobacco smoke, p. 444.

3 *Self-administration of dependence-producing substances* such as those shown in Table 7.9. Also abuse of certain volatile substances, for example.

4 *Non-dependent self-medication*. This, in our hypochondriacal society (bombarded with information which the laity find difficult to evaluate), is rather widespread but relatively trivial as far as drug abuse is concerned, e.g. many purgatives. The matter may become serious (if not divulged to the medical attendant), when it results in drug interactions or unexplained signs or symptoms, or interferes with diagnostic tests.

5 *Miscellaneous*. Further examples of drug misuse are the illegal employment of substances which either

a alter the psychological state of the individual

- acutely, e.g. 'truth' drugs, such as pethidine or hyoscine, which sedate and, reputedly, allow a more frank expression of 'secrets'
- chronically, e.g. psychotropic or antimitotic drugs which have been used to incapacitate (political) opponents over the long term *or*

b immobilise enemies (harassing agents)
- tear gas (CS gas) produces irritation of exposed surfaces including the eyes, skin and respiratory passages
- lethal chemical weaponry, e.g. nerve gases (pp. 53–4).

Strictly, the Misuse of Drugs Regulations apply to substances for which it is necessary to control possession, safe custody and/or prescription. In all cases, complete record keeping of supply and usage is mandatory. Further, known addicts must be notified to a central authority. In some countries ethanol can only be supplied to persons who are 'licensed addicts'.

Index

Note: Page numbers in **bold** refer to those pages on which figures appear; *italic* refer to pages on which tables appear.